The Essentials of NURSING AND HEALTHCARE RESEARCH

SAGE has been part of the global academic community since 1965, supporting high quality research and learning that transforms society and our understanding of individuals, groups and cultures. SAGE is the independent, innovative, natural home for authors, editors and societies who share our commitment and passion for the social sciences.

Find out more at: **www.sagepublications.com**

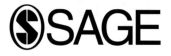

The Essentials of
NURSING AND HEALTHCARE RESEARCH

Edited by

Ruth Taylor

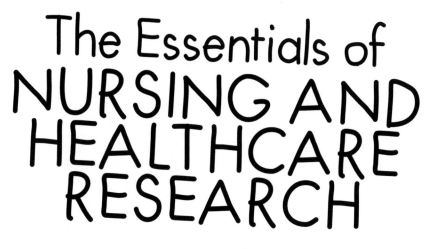

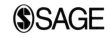

SAGE

Los Angeles | London | New Delhi
Singapore | Washington DC

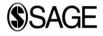

Los Angeles | London | New Delhi
Singapore | Washington DC

SAGE Publications Ltd
1 Oliver's Yard
55 City Road
London EC1Y 1SP

SAGE Publications Inc.
2455 Teller Road
Thousand Oaks, California 91320

SAGE Publications India Pvt Ltd
B 1/I 1 Mohan Cooperative Industrial Area
Mathura Road
New Delhi 110 044

SAGE Publications Asia-Pacific Pte Ltd
3 Church Street
#10-04 Samsung Hub
Singapore 049483

Editor: Alex Clabburn
Assistant editor: Emma Milman
Production editor: Katie Forsythe
Copyeditor: Audrey Scriven
Proofreader: Thea Watson
Indexer: Elske Janssen
Marketing manager: Tamara Navaratnam
Cover design: Wendy Scott
Typeset by: C&M Digitals (P) Ltd, Chennai, India
Printed in Great Britain by Henry Ling Limited, at
the Dorset Press, Dorchester, DT1 1HD

First published 2014

Library of Congress Control Number: 2013934731

British Library Cataloguing in Publication data

A catalogue record for this book is available from
the British Library

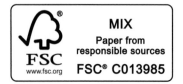

ISBN 978-1-4462-4946-8
ISBN 978-1-4462-4947-5 (pbk)

This book is dedicated to Dr Andrew McKie.
Andy was my friend, a true scholar, and is missed by all
who knew and worked with him.

CONTENTS

ABOUT THE EDITOR AND CONTRIBUTORS

Ruth Taylor is a Professor of Nursing and Deputy Dean at Anglia Ruskin University. She had previously worked at Robert Gordon University, Aberdeen for fifteen years. Her research and policy expertise relates to the student experience with a particular focus on the selection of student nurses and midwives. Her teaching expertise lies in clinical leadership, research (particularly in relation to qualitative research and case study research) and professional practice for compassionate care. In addition, she supervises students from undergraduate to doctoral levels. She has published and presented internationally. Ruth peer reviews and sits on editorial boards for a number of journals.

Dave Adams is a lecturer in the School of Nursing and Midwifery at Robert Gordon University, Aberdeen. He gained Mental Health and Adult Nursing qualifications in the 1970s, and held a number of clinical posts until moving to nurse education in 1989. His academic interests include health policy, health promotion and research methodology.

Dr Mary Addo is a lecturer in mental health nursing and a member of the Institute of Health and Welfare Research at Robert Gordon University, Aberdeen. She teaches and supervises undergraduate and postgraduate students up to PhD level. Her PhD (completed in 2006) was a hermeneutic phenomenological study of the experience of nurses working with sex offenders in maximum secure settings. She has academic publications on forensic and mental health nursing practice and related issues. Her research interests include bipolar disorder, clinical supervision, forensic and custody nursing practice, service users and informal carers.

Dr Winifred Eboh is the Course Leader for the Professional Doctorate at the Institute of Health and Welfare Research at Robert Gordon University, Aberdeen. She has led research and evidence-based practice modules in undergraduate nursing and midwifery curricula for over a decade and has combined this with supervision of doctoral students.

Neil Johnson is a senior lecturer in nursing in the School of Nursing and Midwifery at Robert Gordon University, Aberdeen. Teaching at both undergraduate and postgraduate levels, Neil's teaching interests include research and evidence-based practice. Neil has written a number of publications in relation to this theme including educational approaches to support knowledge and understanding in regard to research and evidence-based practice in undergraduate student nurses, discussion papers relating to tracing research impact in practice, evaluating the use and impact of practice procedure manuals in healthcare and the development of conceptual frameworks and models to assist in the implementation of research and evidence in practice.

Dr Colin Macduff is Reader in Nursing at Robert Gordon University, Aberdeen. After working in a number of clinical posts in mental health and general nursing, Colin worked as a researcher on several National Health Service evaluation projects. He has extensive experience of evaluation research, especially involving educational projects. He currently co-ordinates a research methods module undertaken by all PhD students in Robert Gordon University and supervises undergraduate nursing students in their dissertation work.

Colin MacLean is a librarian at Robert Gordon University, Aberdeen and provides library support for health related disciplines at the University, including Nursing and Midwifery. He has worked almost exclusively in academic libraries throughout a long career that has spanned a formative pre-digital and pre-internet era world of information. Outside of subject support he has interests in library technology, open access, e-learning and library service quality improvement methodologies and works with library colleagues to facilitate lean kaizen activities.

Dr Sheelagh Martindale is the Head of Professional Development, and is responsible for the post-registration/graduate portfolio within the School of Nursing and Midwifery at Robert Gordon University, Aberdeen. Current key research interests lie in asthma risk factors, COPD, quality of life and self-care. She leads the dissertation module for Master's level students and supports doctoral students.

Dr Andrew McKie was lecturer in the School of Nursing and Midwifery at Robert Gordon University, Aberdeen. He had teaching, scholarly and research interests in mental health nursing, ethics and in using the arts and humanities in professional healthcare education. His PhD (2011) centred upon a narrative exploration of the relationship between reading literature and poetry and ethical practice in student nurses. In addition to peer reviewing for three UK nursing journals, Andrew was a member of the scientific panel of Networking in Healthcare Education (NET), an annual conference for healthcare education.

ACKNOWLEDGEMENTS

I would like to thank the students who contributed their thoughts and views to this book. I am pleased to say that they are now all qualified nurses. They are: Jess Adam, Lisa Cameron, Jill Delday, Rachel Dempsey, Anne-Marie Johnstone, Karina McLean, Laura Minty, Nicola Reid, Lindsey Rhind, Mairi Thomson and Stuart Shand.

I would also like to thank all of the book chapter contributors who worked enthusiastically to complete the book alongside their busy professional lives.

Finally, thanks to Sophie, Jo and Chris for their support and encouragement.

PART 1

LET'S GET STARTED

PART 1

1

INTRODUCTION: THE BOOK ROADMAP

RUTH TAYLOR

Chapter learning outcomes

On completion of Chapter 1, you will be able to:

1 Appreciate the scope of the textbook and its relationship to your learning as a student.
2 Understand the format of the book and the kinds of activities you will be asked to undertake.
3 Begin to think about your own learning, and what you hope to gain from undertaking the activities within the textbook.
4 Formulate an early understanding of the meaning of some of the key concepts contained within the textbook (e.g. evidence-based practice, research).
5 Consider the importance of your learning to healthcare practice.

Key concepts

Evidence-based practice, research, application to healthcare practice.

INTRODUCTION

Welcome to our textbook on research for nursing and healthcare practice. As editor of the book, I am delighted to bring you a new approach to the development of your learning about evidence-based practice and research. As a nursing lecturer who has worked with students for a number of years now (I'm not saying how many!), I have found that students sometimes find research theory challenging. I have talked to my own students (some of whom have given their time and their insights to inform the focus of this book – thank you all!), and what I know is that the language of research can sometimes be intimidating. For some students learning about research can feel irrelevant, and for others it can feel like wading through treacle. Others, though, will engage with the theory and gain great satisfaction from thinking about how the theoretical insights relate to their own practice as they encounter different placement experiences.

In your reading of this book, I want to pass on to you my enthusiasm for research. I would urge you to use the book to engage with research as a topic worthy of your time and energy, to bring to you the excitement of knowing that you can make a difference to your practice through an understanding of the concepts described within the book, and to encourage you to see how engaging with this knowledge can lead to your own personal and professional development, and help towards the achievement of your potential. We have placed an emphasis on the use of knowledge as a way of improving practice and of feeling engaged with practice. On top of that, the book will provide you with the relevant knowledge base and pointers that will allow you to further explore particular areas of interest.

The book serves as a core textbook for student nurses undertaking degree courses. In addition, it will be useful as a 'revision' text for nurses undertaking 'top-up' degrees or embarking on research modules as part of research degrees (at a Master's or PhD levels).

The Standards for Pre-registration Nursing (NMC, 2010) emphasise the importance of research knowledge and expertise. The Standards have two major components:

- Standards for Competence.
- Standards for Education.

It is the former that we are most interested in here, although I would like to highlight one key area within the Standards for Education that relate to our reasons for developing this book: the required minimum outcome for a pre-registration nursing programme is now at degree level (you may know that previously the minimum outcome was at diploma level). While many nursing students have been graduating with degrees, it is the first time that this has become a requirement. Student nurses are therefore required to meet a graduate level, as the use of research in practice and the development of evidence-based practice are crucial to the development of this all-degree profession.

The Standards for Competence state that all new nurses will 'act to safeguard the public, and be responsible and accountable for safe, person-centred, evidence-based nursing practice' and 'use leadership skills to supervise and manage others and contribute to planning, designing, delivering and improving future services'. Along with the other key areas in which the NMC state that the public will have confidence in all new nurses, these two statements draw attention to the need for a strong grounding in research awareness and research literacy – these nurses will be in a strong position to provide excellent care and to lead service development for the future. The Standards for Competence are organised into four domains:

- Professional values.
- Communication and interpersonal skills.
- Nursing practice and decision making.
- Leadership, management and team working.

As a student nurse you will need to apply the competencies within each of the domains within your field of practice (adult nursing, mental health nursing, children's and young people's nursing, or learning disability nursing). In order to do so, you will also need to be able to appraise the evidence base across the four domains, and apply that evidence appropriately. These skills are at the forefront of what we hope to help you to achieve through your interaction with this book.

CHAPTER PURPOSE

The purpose of Chapter 1 is to help you to see how the learning activities have been planned so that you can use them as you work your way through your course of study. The authors of each of the chapters know that some readers will be undertaking a curriculum in which research and evidence-based practice are integrated into its modules and learning materials: some students will be working with distinct 'stand alone' research and evidence-based practice modules, and others will be using a combined approach. This book will suit your needs whichever approach your university uses. It has been designed to enable you to dip in and out of the chapters and learning activities and to go backwards and forwards between the chapters as you undertake the relevant learning on your course. You may even find that some of your lecturers will direct you towards relevant activities within this book in order to help you think about how your learning relates to practice. This latter point (how your learning relates to practice) is, for the authors of this book, the most important one: we want you to appreciate how the learning, the theories, and the concepts are relevant to your practice as a student (and later as a qualified practitioner). My students tell me that it is absolutely vital for their development as growing practitioners that learning activities help them to fully engage with what's required of them when they take up their practice placements. So whether you are an adult nurse, a mental health nurse, a learning disability nurse, a children's and young people's nurse, or even a different healthcare practitioner, you should find that we have provided examples which will facilitate your ability to think clearly about the theory and its application to practice.

Overview of the textbook's aims and objectives

The overall aim of the book is to enable you, as a student, to develop relevant knowledge and understanding for research and evidence-based practice. What we, the authors, want to do, is provide you with the appropriate theoretical knowledge, offer examples from practice so that you can begin to appreciate the relevance of the theory, and from there give you the opportunity to think about the theory in relation to your own practice as a student.

The book will enable you to achieve the following objectives:

1   To develop your enthusiasm for, and motivation to use, research knowledge in practice.
2   To appreciate the need for an understanding of research and the use of evidence in practice.
3   To apply research knowledge and an understanding of evidence in practice to the contexts that you work/learn in.
4   To value the ways in which that knowledge enhances relationships with, and the care of, patients, carers, and relatives, as well as relationships with colleagues.

So let's unpick these outcomes a little so that there is clarity about what you can expect from this book and how it will relate to your overall learning. Taking each objective in turn, I aim to uncover the relevant aspects of this textbook that will enable you to determine how you want to use the book as part of your overall learning experience. To begin with, however, Activity 1.1 will give you an early opportunity to consider your current knowledge base, your views on research, and the learning that you hope to gain from working your way through the activities that I, and the other authors, have prepared for you.

ACTIVITY 1.1

Take some time to think about the following thought-points:

1   What do you already know about 'research'?
2   What do you hope to learn through your engagement with the activities in this textbook?
3   How will you know if you have achieved what you set out to do?

You may have identified that you have very little knowledge about research – you might have heard some of the terms used in research but have little understanding of what these mean. On the other hand, you may have previously undertaken learning which has provided you with a strong understanding of the terminology, the processes, and the usefulness of research in practice. Whichever camp you sit in, you will benefit from using the activities to broaden your understanding and to really consider how research impacts on your practice as a student. In the next section in this chapter, I will describe the kinds of learning activities (*pedagogical approaches*) that each of the authors will use to facilitate your development.

In the meantime, let's go back to exploring how the textbook will enable you to achieve the relevant learning. Each of the chapters is described briefly below.

OVERVIEW OF THE BOOK CHAPTERS

Part 1: Let's get started

Chapter 2: Evidence-based practice and research

This chapter will provide a brief background and historical overview of research in nursing as well as evidence-based practice (and the differences) so that you can start to see where and how nursing research and evidence-based practice have evolved. It will describe the current situation so that you can clearly see the impact that taking the learning forward will have on practice and on your own personal and professional development.

Chapter 3: The importance of research for practice

Linking to the NMC Standards, case studies will be provided from some of the most significant contributors to nursing research which will demonstrate their personal impact both on the profession and on patient care – and from a UK and global perspective. The chapter aims to help you see how undertaking research advances knowledge for nursing practice and contributes to evidence-based practice and clinical effectiveness. The differences between research, audit and service evaluation will also be explored.

Part 2: Let's make this work: Skills for research and evidence-based practice

Chapter 4: Core skills for research and evidence-based practice

With a focus on the student nurse and your journey through your course (both in university and in practice), the purpose of the development of the core skills is explored. The kinds of skills that are relevant to you – both as a student and as you make the transition into professional practice – include literature and evidence searching, critical review and analysis of the evidence (we provide you with a step-by-step guide and the tools to facilitate critical analysis), and an introduction to statistics (particularly as they relate to your ability to impact positively on practice).

Chapter 5: Policy in research and evidence-based practice

As a student it is vital that you develop an appreciation for, and understanding of, policy and its importance in healthcare. This chapter gives you an opportunity to explore policy analysis, and how it relates to research and evidence-based practice. Examples of evidence-based national policy are provided from across the UK with vignettes that demonstrate how the policy directly impacts on practice. Inter-professional working (which is absolutely vital to integrated working practices) is explored in relation to the policy drivers for practice. In addition, the inclusion of stakeholders (patients, carers, and other service users) in the development of policy for evidence-based practice is explored.

Chapter 6: Practical approaches for understanding research and evidence-based practice

Keeping a research journal or a reflective journal can be a very helpful way for students (and experienced researchers) to reflect on their learning and development. A proposed approach is provided for you to consider or further develop to suit your own learning style. As well as this, the chapter gives you pointers to ways in which you can ensure that you keep reference sources so that they are easily accessible and make your life easier as you work your way through your studies (you will probably have realised by now that your learning will be evidence-based and this will there-fore require you to utilise reliable sources of evidence to support your work). The authors of this chapter will therefore offer you some tips to help you make the most of your university resources (complementary to the information that your university will have given you already).

Part 3: Let's get philosophical

Chapter 7: The philosophical background to nursing research

This chapter addresses some of the key issues that enable users of research to engage effectively with research findings and their implications for practice. The author of this chapter will explore theory, nursing knowledge, ways of seeing the world, enquiry perspectives and research approaches, as they relate to nursing and healthcare practices.

Chapter 8: Qualitative and quantitative research approaches

This chapter gives an outline of the key research approaches used in nursing and healthcare research with examples relating to the kinds of practice experiences that you will encounter. You will have the opportunity to get to grips with some of the words that can seem intimidating – phenomenology, quasi-experimental, ethnography, for example. Don't worry, you will soon be as enthusiastic as I am about the different approaches to research and how an understanding of them can really open your eyes to the wealth of evidence that exists for practice!

Chapter 9: Alternative and complementary research approaches

Drawing from a range of theoretical perspectives, Chapter 9 discusses action research, evaluation research and mixed methods within the contexts that these are utilised. There is a fantastic array of creativity in the research world, not least amongst researchers who push the boundaries to create new approaches so that the important research questions can be answered. *Creativity* is a key word for research – across both the qualitative and quantitative approaches.

Part 4: Let's do research

Chapter 10: The research process

The research process is described in detail using a tool that has been developed by one of the authors of Chapter 10 and other colleagues in the School of Nursing and Midwifery at Robert Gordon University. They are excited to be sharing this with you as they have found that students have benefited hugely from the interactive 'Research Pyramid'.

Chapter 11: Qualitative research and Chapter 12: Quantitative research

These two chapters mirror each other by providing an overview of the key aspects of the research process as they relate to each of the approaches to research – for

example, you will be able to see the differences between how you choose participants to take part in a qualitative research project and how you must do the same
for a quantitative research project. You will see that having knowledge of these
detailed aspects of the research process enables you to make judgments about the
usefulness of a piece of research. The chapters' authors have given examples from
practice so you can start to see the reality of the knowledge you are gaining as it
impacts on practice.

Chapter 13: Ethics in healthcare research

The ethical issues associated with nursing and healthcare research are immense, as
I am sure you can imagine. When you are working with patients, carers, staff and
others to inform your knowledge of healthcare practice, it is of primary importance
that ethical issues are addressed rigorously. An 'ethical journey' is taken so that you
can see the issues that arise and the processes that are undertaken to ensure ethical
practice. In addition, there are complex ethical issues associated with implementing
evidence-based practice, and Chapter 13 clearly addresses these in order to help you
work ethically in practice.

Chapter 14: Preparation for your dissertation

Some students will be undertaking a dissertation as part of their degree course (perhaps a research proposal, or a detailed literature review). This chapter provides some
tips around planning and focus as well as discussing how to make the most of supervisory relationships. The aim is to help you to really see the potential of this piece of
work for your future practice. You may be lucky enough to undertake your learning
in an environment where your practice colleagues are engaging with the focus of
your dissertation (either by identifying topic areas, or by discussing the pertinent
issues for practice). One of the exciting aspects of undertaking an extended piece of
work, such as a dissertation, is that you can contribute personally to the evidence
base for practice by producing a piece of work that draws together the relevant evidence for practice. Obviously you can then publish from your dissertation so that
your hard work is shared more widely!

Part 5: Let's implement research and evidence in practice

Chapter 15: Using research and evidence in practice

This chapter provides you with an opportunity to focus on how students use evidence in practice. The types of evidence that you already use – or will use – include

systematic literature reviews and evidence-based guidelines (for example, the Scottish Intercollegiate Guidelines Network develops evidence-based clinical practice guidelines for use within NHS Scotland), individual research studies in the journals that you will already be accessing, and other evidence which impacts on practice. As part of your development the chapter will help you to further develop your skills in critical analysis so that you are better able to critique the evidence and, from there, use appropriate skills to implement the evidence in practice (for example: leadership, change management and decision making). Getting the message 'out there' about evidence-based practice is important if you are to contribute to the growing knowledge base for nursing and healthcare practice. Don't think that this doesn't apply to you! I encourage my own students to start thinking about publishing or presenting at conferences as early as possible – I have one personal student who has published as part of a team on wound care management (Fumarola et al., 2010) and I have recently published with another student nurse (Carter and Taylor, 2012).

Part 6: Achieving your potential

Chapter 16: Achieving your potential

Why use the same title for a section and a chapter? I believe that the achievement of your potential as a student nurse, and then as a registered nurse, is *the* most important aspect to your development through your education. In this chapter I focus on your potential as a student nurse as you work your way through the course, and how a solid understanding of the theory in this book will help you to stand out as a student. I believe that if you work towards the achievement of your potential you will build satisfaction in your skills as a nurse and you will have a personal impact on healthcare practice. So, linking to the focus of this book, I will build on the previous chapter and ask you to consider how you can move forward as a developing professional.

Glossary

A glossary of key terms is provided for ease of reference, and the suggested reflective journal template in the Appendix is also included for your use. We hope that these practical items will assist you in your ongoing development as you work your way through the course.

I would also hope that the overview of each of the chapters has given you a feel for what to expect within the book. You should be able either to work your way through each of the chapters as they come, or to dip into particular chapters as you need to. As I've already said, this book's authors are well aware that each university uses a slightly different approach to the development of the required knowledge and skills for research and evidence-based practice. Therefore they would expect that each student will use this book slightly differently to help them achieve their learning in the way that most suits them.

PEDAGOGICAL APPROACH: 'HOW TO USE THE BOOK'

People have different learning styles i.e. various ways of interacting with the educational materials to enable them to come to an understanding of what is required. Have a think about how you learn best: for example, you may gain most from being in a lecture theatre listening to an inspiring lecture while taking notes, or you might prefer to look through the theoretical concepts yourself (using online lecture notes and books or articles) and then follow this up by taking the opportunity to discuss and debate the important issues for your learning. My own research on the first-year experiences of student nurses demonstrated that most of them got something from the big lectures, but that it was the interactive tutorial-based group working that most helped their learning (Taylor, 2009). My own view is that the majority of people will work best where there are a number of different kinds of learning activities for them to engage in as these provide variety and serve different purposes. To this end, the authors of this book have used a number of pedagogical approaches (learning approaches) to assist you with the development of the theoretical learning. I have listed some of the main approaches in Table 1.1 so you can see what we have in store for you, and to help you with planning your learning. The overarching aim of the activities is to *focus on real-life issues with tangible relationships to practice*. After all, you have been successful in achieving a place on a course that aims to provide you with the skills to deliver healthcare – the authors of this book therefore want to keep that focus in what we discuss in order that you can go into your practice placements and think about how your learning is relevant to your everyday working practices. You will find these different activities in 'call out' boxes within the chapters.

Table 1.1   Pedagogical approaches

Pedagogical approach	Potential benefits
Chapter learning outcomes: a bullet-pointed list of the learning outcomes in the chapter.	You will find these at the start of each chapter. They are provided so that you are clear, from the beginning, about what the author aims to cover theoretically, and what you should be able to do at the end of the activities.
Key concepts: a list of key words that are relevant to the chapter.	Again, the list of key words aims to provide a focus for your learning from the beginning, and also allows you to dip into the different chapters as your learning requires.

Pedagogical approach	Potential benefits
Student voices: these are questions, comments and ideas that our own students have offered us as part of the overall process of student engagement with the development of the book.	The student voices aim to talk to you, the learner, in a way that will help you relate to the learning expectations within some of the chapters. Our student group has enthusiastically engaged with all aspects of the book's development and their voices are crucial to your learning.
Directed activities: these will take different formats and link with the learning in the chapter.	The activities aim to enable you to consider the theory in relation to real-life situations (for example, the identification of a relevant area of practice and a related research article through to its critique and potential impact on practice).
Case studies: these are examples of research or situations where evidence has been implemented in practice and are based on real-life situations.	Case studies provide illustrations of concepts and theories that are explained and discussed in the main body of the chapter by the author. Case studies allow you to consider some reflective questions or critical thinking points so that you can continue to expand your learning.
Reflective exercises: these are critical questions or thinking points.	You are encouraged to engage with these tasks as they will enable you either to apply the theoretical concepts to a practice situation, or to think how the reflective points relate to the topic under discussion.
Group exercises: these are reflective exercises that will provide an opportunity to work together in small groups.	Collaborative working is an essential skill for learning and for healthcare practice. These activities will give you the chance to work with other students, to learn from and with each other.
Definitions.	Any complex or conceptual terms or expressions are defined within each of the chapters. Many of these definitions will find their way into the Glossary for you to reference quickly.
Practice vignettes: examples of practice situations where the theory is applicable.	The practice vignettes provide tangible examples of the application of theory to practice. Some of these specifically relate to the student nurse's role in healthcare practice.
Vignettes from nurses who have undertaken research and implemented research/evidence in practice.	The aim is to emphasise the impact that research/evidence has on healthcare practice, and help you to see that you personally have the potential to make a positive difference to practice.

(Continued)

Table 1.1　(Continued)

Pedagogical approach	Potential benefits
Further reading.	At the end of each chapter, the authors have identified some suggested further reading (books, chapters, journal articles, policy documents, websites) and annotated this to show why they might be useful. You are also encouraged to look more widely to the relevant evidence for other sources that will support your ongoing learning and development.
Text navigation.	These 'signposts' will guide you to other chapters that contain related or specific information on a particular theoretical concept that you are studying at the time.
Templates.	Examples of templates for your own personal use (which you are very welcome to modify) are provided in the appendices. We aim to offer you practical solutions to some of the approaches to implementing evidence in practice.

Each chapter's author(s) will ask you to use a number of these activities as part of the overall approach to learning. Remember, however, that they don't aim to provide you with every single piece of information you could possibly need for research and evidence-based practice – that would be impossible. What they do aim to do is assist you with developing the skills you will need in order to take forward research and evidence-based practice in an evolving healthcare context. The challenges in healthcare practice are immense – and they will provide you as a student nurse with incredible learning experiences. Alongside your lecturers and mentors in practice, this book is offering you a learning experience that aims to prepare you to take on these challenges. Box 1.1, for example, provides a brief overview of reflection – you will need to utilise reflective processes, so the information in this box may be of use. It is very likely that you are already familiar with reflection, so do feel free to move on to the next part of the chapter if you have covered this already.

Box 1.1　Reflection

You will be asked to undertake reflective exercises within this textbook. The aim of these exercises will vary, but overall the authors hope that the act of reflection will facilitate a deeper understanding of the key concepts and ideas that are being explored.

In the context of the learning that you will undertake as you engage with the activities in the book, I would define reflection as a process that involves six stages based on Gibbs' reflective cycle (Gibbs, 1988):

1 Review the theories and concepts addressed within the activity.
2 Describe the learning gained from the activity.
3 Evaluate the learning by relating it to a real-life situation (for example, a practice situation; a learning situation in the university; the findings from a research article).
4 Analyse the learning in order to make sense of the issues you are exploring.
5 Come to a conclusion relating to the learning/real-life situation.
6 Action plan for your future learning needs.

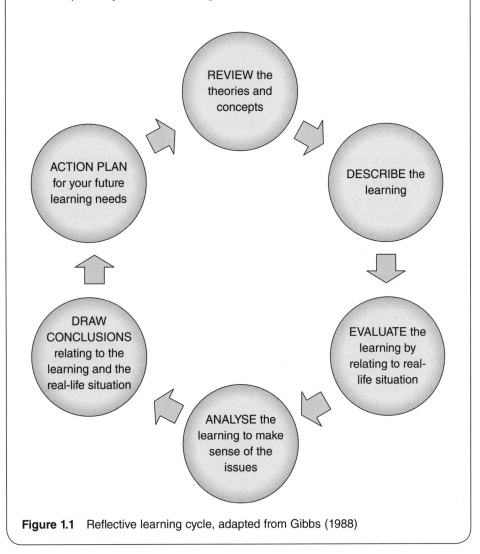

Figure 1.1   Reflective learning cycle, adapted from Gibbs (1988)

HOW WILL THE BOOK BENEFIT YOU?

This is an ambitious book. We aim to introduce you to research and evidence-based practice initially, and to work through the activities with you so that you will gain a good understanding of the relevant knowledge and skills for practice. We have used what we hope is an accessible approach that will engage you in such a way that you will feel enthusiastic about the topic area. We also hope that the learning you experience is just the starting point, and that the tools we have provided will give you the opportunity to continue to develop both personally and professionally as you move forwards from being a student nurse to becoming a registered nurse.

The book's objectives are reiterated below with an overview of how the achievement of these objectives will help you as a student nurse:

1 *To develop your enthusiasm for, and motivation to use, research knowledge in practice.*

   As we have already seen, you will have to be able to use research knowledge in practice. Whether you are dressing a surgical wound, communicating with a distressed child, undertaking observation of a person with mental health issues, or liaising with other services as part of an inter-professional team to improve care for a person with a learning disability, you will be using research and evidence.

2 *To appreciate the need for an understanding of research and the use of evidence in practice.*

   As I have already said, you will need to gain research awareness and research literacy. You will need to be able to appraise research papers to determine their appropriateness for your own practice. To do this, you will need to have an understanding of research concepts so that you can determine the usefulness of particular research and whether the findings are helpful as regards the development of healthcare practice in your context. In addition, you will have to be able to take forward the implementation of evidence in practice where you have established that this is appropriate.

3 *To apply research knowledge and an understanding of evidence in practice to the contexts that you work/learn in.*

   There would be little point in providing you with knowledge about research and evidence-based practice without finding ways to ensure that the relevance of that knowledge to real-life practice situations was also emphasised. This book keeps that aspect centre stage – by using examples from practice so that you can get a strong feeling for the ways in which the topic area impacts positively on healthcare practice.

4 *To value the ways in which that knowledge enhances relationships with, and the care of, patients, carers and relatives, as well as relationships with colleagues.*

   Person-centred care is a key policy driver, one that remains at the heart of nursing practice across all fields. As a student nurse we would recognise that you chose the academic course and profession because you wanted to impact positively on people's lives. As you work your way through the book, you will see that the authors have strived to ensure that the individual (whether a patient, carer, relative or colleague) is always at the centre of our thinking. It is vital you know how the theory in this book relates to the relationships you have in practice as these relationships are *the* fundamental aspect in delivering healthcare.

A short note here on our use of terminology – the word 'patient' is used within the book to reflect the various terms used across settings and fields of practice, as well as the work that nurses do with carers, relatives, and significant others. To do otherwise and incorporate all the relevant words each time would have been clumsy, so please read into the word 'patient' whatever is relevant to your setting and field of practice.

You have now had a chance to see how the book has been put together, what it aims to achieve, how we want to work with you, and what you could hope to gain by engaging with the learning. The next part of this chapter introduces you to the terminology (i.e. evidence-based practice and research). It then goes on to provide a rationale for the use of nursing research and other disciplines' research in healthcare practice – with an emphasis on the importance of inter-professional working. Before we get to that though, the next activity should help you to build on Activity 1.1.

Now that you have looked at what the book has to offer, revisit your thoughts in Activity 1.1 and complete the following questions:

1   What are your own personal learning objectives for this book?
2   How will you know if you have achieved what you set out to do?
3   How are you going to plan your time to use the book as you work your way through your course?

ACTIVITY 1.2

WHAT IS EVIDENCE-BASED PRACTICE?

In an article for *Primary Health Care* (Taylor, 2012), I wrote about evidence-based practice and noted that it is defined widely and with variation. One definition of evidence-based practice is:

> The process of integrating evidence into healthcare delivery. (Titler, 2011: 291)

The challenge for practice is to find effective ways of ensuring that evidence is appropriately utilised in practice, especially as there is a growing evidence base for nursing and healthcare practice. If you have had a chance to look at some of the nursing journals that are available (and remembering that our evidence base comes from a variety of disciplines), you will have had a taste of the vast array of information and evidence that is available to us for our practice. Some of this evidence will take the form of research (whether qualitative or quantitative – don't worry, we will be looking at these and other terms in depth later on so that they roll off your tongue!). However there are other approaches to the development of a good evidence base which can work in tandem with the use of research findings, for example clinical guidelines, objective information about a case (e.g. a patient's case notes), and subjective information about the patient experience (e.g. the views and opinions of the patient about their own experience) (Taylor, 2012). When you come to look at Chapter 2 and Chapter 3, you will have the opportunity to explore these as well as various other issues in some depth. As a starter, take a few minutes to complete Activity 1.3.

ACTIVITY 1.3

In a small group with some of the students in your class or on your placement, take some time to make a list of what you count as 'evidence'.

This is a starting-point for you. As you work your way through some of the other chapters you may wish to come back and add to your list as you learn more.

WHAT IS RESEARCH?

Thus far you will have briefly explored evidence and evidence-based practice. You will have noted that 'research' is a key aspect to the development of an evidence base. Remember however that the aim of this book is not to prepare you as a researcher, it is to help you become research aware and research literate, as I've already suggested (in other words, you need to develop your skills to access relevant sources of evidence, appraise the evidence, make decisions about its usefulness for practice, and implement it appropriately in practice – see Moule and Goodman, 2009). In order to develop these skills, you will need to have a good understanding of research (the approaches used to investigate a particular area of practice, and the processes undertaken within any investigation – again, more of these in later chapters!). As an opening, a definition of 'research' may be helpful to you in setting the context for subsequent chapters. Here is a fundamental definition:

> [Research is] A systematic approach to gathering information for the purposes of answering questions and solving problems in the pursuit of creating new knowledge about nursing practice, education and policy. (Hek and Moule, 2006: 10)

Keep this definition in mind as you progress through the book and in your learning. You may wish to add to it, or change it slightly, as your understanding develops.

RATIONALE FOR NURSING RESEARCH AND THE USE OF OTHER DISCIPLINES' RESEARCH IN PRACTICE

As I have said earlier on in this introduction, some student nurses can feel unsure as to the value of developing an understanding of research within their courses. What

I aim to do here is convince you that you *do* need to develop this knowledge, and that you will benefit immensely – both personally and professionally – if you take on this aspect of your learning with motivation and enthusiasm!

Having read the introduction to this textbook, can you relate to Sophie when she says:

> *Sophie*:   I don't really see why I need to learn about all these complicated ideas. When I go into practice I know what I have to do because the other nurses tell me. Why do I have to learn about research?

Does this reflect a little of what you are feeling? That's not a problem, but let's reflect on what Sophie says for a moment. Is she right to feel that she can go onto her practice placement and simply be 'told' what to do? What would you say to Sophie to help her understand why developing research awareness and becoming research literate would be helpful to her practice? What would you say to her about her responsibilities for the use of evidence in practice?

ACTIVITY 1.4

Remember that you are at the beginning of your own 'research journey'. As you progress through your learning, I am sure that you will be able to provide ever-more convincing arguments for the development of these particular aspects of your knowledge base for your nursing degree. You may however have suggested some of the following reasons for Sophie to engage with the learning:

- If Sophie does what she has been told to do without questioning or analysing the reasons for doing something in a certain way, she may not be using the best evidence for practice. You will, of course, learn so much from your mentors and other practitioners when you are on placement, but you will need to be aware that sometimes things are done on a place-ment because 'that's how they've always been done and it seems to work'.
- The implementation of good evidence can transform practice and improve the care of patients (Wood, 2006). Sophie will need to be able to interpret and use the evidence that is available in her area of practice if she is to be able to do this. She therefore needs to have an awareness and understanding of key research concepts so that she can interpret and use the evidence.
- Sophie has an ethical obligation to ensure that the care she is delivering is the most appropriate care for the context (ethical issues are covered in Chapter 13: Ethics in Healthcare Research). For Sophie, as a student nurse, this may mean that she engages in critical conversations with her mentors so that she gains an appreciation of the source of the evidence for her practice.
- As a student, Sophie has a responsibility to find out about the evidence for care within the particular context. She should access relevant sources of evidence (with help from practition-ers on her placement possibly), and ask questions when something does not make sense.
- You may also have noted that it can sometimes be challenging to implement the 'right' evi-dence in practice for reasons such as a lack of access to the relevant resources, a shortage

of time to access the resources, or not possessing the relevant skills to deal with the evidence (Upton and Upton, 2005). What this book aims to do is provide you with the relevant learning, skills and tools to make it easier for you to be research aware and research literate, as well as sufficiently confident in your skills to utilise the evidence base in practice.

- You may also have suggested to Sophie that she will gain great satisfaction in knowing that she is delivering care using the best available evidence.

I have already mentioned the need for professionals to work together 'inter-professionally'. What this means is that care is integrated rather than fragmented, and that the relationships between professionals and with the patient are collaborative. There are, unfortunately, numerous examples of where care falls down (e.g. the Francis Report, 2013) and inquiries into these failings will often reveal that a lack of collaborative working was partly to blame. There needs to be a coming-together of working practices, and by implication, the implementation of evidence-based working practices across the professions. If you are interested in having a look at an inquiry, you could access the Victoria Climbié Inquiry Report (www.publications.parliament.uk/pa/cm200203/cmselect/cmhealth/570/570.pdf) (House of Commons Health Committee, 2003). It makes distressing reading at times, but clearly and succinctly paints a picture of services that had gone wrong and provides clear pointers for future evidence-based working practices.

SUMMARY

This chapter has provided you with some early pointers towards the key areas that are addressed throughout the book. The critical points for your learning so far are:

- Your enthusiasm and motivation for research and evidence-based practice can grow from this starting-point and these will enable you to deliver safe, effective, and person-centred care.
- The terminology can be challenging – we will support you in understanding the meaning of terms and appreciating their relevance to your practice as a student nurse.
- Remember that the book is designed to allow you to dip into chapters appropriately as you work your way through your university course.

FURTHER READING

The websites listed below may prove useful to you in gaining an appreciation of the resources that are available to healthcare practitioners to support evidence-based practice. You might wish to refer to them on an ongoing basis to support your learning through the activities in this book, and as a useful resource for when you are on placement or undertaking an academic assignment.

National Institute for Health and Clinical Excellence: www.nice.org.uk/
NICE provides guidance to practitioners on conditions and diseases, public health and treatments, procedures and devices.
Scottish Intercollegiate Guidelines Network: www.sign.ac.uk/index.html
Evidence-based guidelines are available (with categories as wide-ranging as cancer, child health and mental health) for healthcare professionals.

REFERENCES

Carter, G. and Taylor, R. (2012) The influence of a personal patient experience on student nurse development, *Nursing Times*, 108 (20): 21–23.

Francis, R. (2013) *Report of the Mid Staffordshire NHS Foundation Trust Public Inquiry Executive Summary*. London: The Stationery Office.

Fumarola, S., Butcher, M., Cooper, P., Gray, D., Russell, F., Springfellow, S., Betram, M., Duiguid, K., Pirie, G., and Shand, S. (2010) A clinical audit of Suprasorb® X+PHMB, *Wounds UK*, 6 (3): 78–87.

Gibbs, G. (1988) *Learning by doing: A guide to teaching and learning methods*. London: Further Education Unit.

Hek, G. and Moule, P. (2006) *Making sense of research: An introduction for health and social care practitioners* (3rd edition). London: Sage.

House of Commons Health Committee (2003) *The Victoria Climbié Inquiry Report*. London: The Stationery Office.

Moule, P. and Goodman, M. (2009) *Nursing research: An introduction*. London: Sage.

Nursing and Midwifery Council (NMC) (2010) *Standards for pre-registration nursing education*. Available online: http://standards.nmc-uk.org/PreRegNursing/Pages/Introduction.aspx

Taylor, R. (2009) Creating connections: An investigation into the first year experience of undergraduate nursing students. Available online at: https://openair.rgu.ac.uk/bitstream/10059/373/1/Ruth%20Taylor%20thesis.pdf

Taylor, R. (2012) Using and developing the evidence base in primary health care, *Primary Health Care*, 22 (1): 31–36.

Titler, M.G. (2011) Nursing science and evidence-based practice, *Western Journal of Nursing Research*, 33: 291–295.

Upton, D. and Upton, P. (2005) Nurses' attitudes to evidence-based practice: Impact of a national policy, *British Journal of Nursing*, 14 (5): 284–288.

Wood, M.J. (2006) Nursing practice research and evidence-based practice, *Clinical Nursing Research*, 15: 83–85.

2

EVIDENCE-BASED PRACTICE AND RESEARCH

NEIL JOHNSON

Chapter learning outcomes

On completion of Chapter 2, you will be able to:

1 Appreciate the historical development of research in the nursing profession.
2 Outline key influences in the evolution of evidence-based practice in healthcare.
3 Discuss the ways in which research informs evidence-based practice.
4 Consider contemporary drivers in research and evidence-based practice.
5 Reflect upon the impact of research and evidence-based practice on personal and professional development.

Key concepts

Research in nursing, evidence-based practice, development of research and evidence-based practice in nursing, professional development, research impact.

INTRODUCTION

Research is for researchers, nursing is for nurses. From my experience as a lecturer in nursing, this is a relatively common perspective taken by students as they begin to learn about research and evidence-based practice. Indeed this viewpoint is borne out by literature exploring student nurses' attitudes and perceptions toward research (Ax and Kincaid, 2001; Johnson et al., 2010). Apprehension about research as a subject has been reported amongst nurses, both qualified practitioners and new students of nurse education. You may yourself be concerned about such aspects as understanding research methodology, and engaging in nursing practices in placements where the translation of research to practice can be evidenced. What this book aims to do is assist you in the process of reducing your apprehension by providing the tools to understand and appreciate research and evidence for practice.

Common questions that are asked of lecturers who teach research, and that you may also have about research for nursing and healthcare practice, may include *why* the topic is included in nursing curricula. My reflections have led me to firmly believe that I cannot expect learners to understand a topic (and its relevance to nursing) if I cannot articulate its importance to practice. I think back to the numerous research studies that I have read, that had a personal and professional impact in terms of my practice, my self-awareness, personal beliefs and attitudes, the ability to see things from the perspective of others (e.g. patients/families/carers), and in some instances humbled me by my lack of insight into how individuals cope and deal with crisis events in their lives. Without a knowledge of research in healthcare and the ability to be research 'literate' (i.e. to be able to read and understand original research studies as published in professional journals), I would still hold those initial expectations and images that I had accumulated as I embarked on a career in nursing.

The quote 'Research is to see what everybody has seen and to think what nobody has thought' (Szent-Gyorgy, 1957, cited by Field and Morse, 1995: 1) conveys to me the answer to the questions posed by my students. The ability either to undertake or to read and appraise research evidence opens up a whole new world for us as healthcare providers. It has the ability to provide new perspectives, to help us make sense of our experiences in practice, to advance our knowledge and understanding, to make us more effective practitioners/teachers, to influence our careers/roles, and to shape and change our beliefs and attitudes about the world in which we work and live. Crucially, it enables the delivery of safe, effective, and person-centred care. We have a duty to provide the best care possible for our patients and clients, using the best available evidence. This ability either to engage in real-world research or to become research literate provides us with the key skills that will underpin how we develop as individual professionals, enhance the care that we provide to patients, solve problems, make decisions, and build knowledge and understanding.

This initial introduction has served to acknowledge some of the concerns that you may have regarding your learning. The rest of the chapter seeks to provide you with an understanding of the development of research in nursing, the evolution of evidence-based practice in healthcare, the ways in which research informs evidence-based practice and the contemporary drivers that shape the ways in which research and evidence are applied in healthcare provision today. In doing so, the aim is to facilitate your understanding of the need for research and evidence-based practice in healthcare to inform your personal and professional development.

PERSONAL IMAGES OF NURSING AND THE ROLE OF THE PROFESSIONAL NURSE

Thinking back to the statement made earlier in this chapter regarding personal expectations and images of nursing roles, and to assist you in clarifying and reflecting upon your own personal images of the role of the nurse, as well as the notion of research in nursing, take some time to consider Activity 2.1:

ACTIVITY 2.1

Take some time to consider your current attitudes, beliefs and images of nursing.

1 What has shaped and formed these?
2 What types of knowledge underpin what nurses do in caring for their patients – where does this knowledge originate?
3 What are your current attitudes and beliefs toward research as a subject in nurse education?

The purpose of having this activity at the start of this chapter is three-fold. Firstly, it will facilitate your own personal understanding of the role of the professional nurse. Secondly, it challenges you to consider what types of knowledge underpin the practices of the professional nurse – this should generate a broad spectrum of responses. Finally, the activity challenges you to think about why research is included in nursing and healthcare education and when considering this question to ask yourself this: how is the knowledge underpinning what nurses do in practice created? You may find, following discussions with your peers and/or tutors, that learners hold a variety of attitudes, beliefs, and images of nursing: some may suggest that a key role of the nurse is to be a kind and caring professional with good communication skills; others may see the nurse as a professional who needs to have an excellent knowledge base in relation to human anatomy and physiology, or a professional who requires technical mastery in procedures such as wound care, injections, or taking a patient's vital signs. It is also important to identify both the positive and less well-informed responses to these questions in order to identify where further learning, self-awareness and reflection are required. This is crucial in your developmental journey, recognising the impact of where your learning about research and evidence-based practice will take you, both in terms of practice and your ongoing continuous personal and professional development.

Other discussion points from this activity may include asking such questions as where do our attitudes, beliefs and images of professional roles come from, what influences these, and what types of knowledge do nurses draw upon in caring for patients and clients? The responses to the second question in this activity may take a little more time to clarify as the issue of knowledge in nursing is a complex and well-debated one. Later chapters in this book will help you understand this concept in terms of how differing approaches to research can help expand certain types of nursing knowledge, and how specific questions that we have about our practice can be answered with the most appropriate types of evidence. However, a useful starting-point here is the seminal paper by Barbara Carper (1978) 'Fundamental patterns of knowing in nursing'. It would be helpful in respect of the notion of identifying differing types of knowledge utilised in nursing to read Carper's paper. This should be accessible either via your library or online search databases.

RESEARCH AND EVIDENCE-BASED PRACTICE: AN EXPLANATION OF TERMS

Although the terms 'research' and 'evidence-based practice' have been introduced to you in Chapter 1, it is worthwhile spending a little more time exploring their definitions. These terms are frequently used interchangeably and it can be easy to become confused! Thus, before exploring the development of research and evidence-based practice in nursing, it is vital to define these two terms and highlight how they *differ*.

What do we mean by 'research' in nursing and healthcare?

Within Chapter 1 of this book, research is defined as, 'A systematic approach to gathering information for the purposes of answering questions and solving problems in the pursuit of creating new knowledge about nursing practice, education and policy' (Hek and Moule, 2006: 10). Parahoo (1997: 7) defines nursing research as 'the systematic review and collection of data on the organization, delivery, uses and outcomes of nursing care for the purpose of enhancing a client's healthcare. It is not only about what nurses do but also about clients' behavior, knowledge, beliefs, attitudes, perceptions and other factors influencing how they make use of, and experience, care and treatment'. Parahoo's definition is significant here as it emphasises and recognises that the knowledge required for professional practice is not solely based on one domain of knowledge, but that instead – as nurses – we must integrate knowledge from the health and social sciences, knowledge of patient experiences, circumstances and perspectives, knowledge from the arts and humanities, as well as knowledge of the attitudes and experiences of healthcare providers, in order to provide holistic care for our patients and clients.

One key theme can be identified across definitions – the fact that research is a *systematic* and *planned* process which seeks to investigate given issues or questions in order to enhance our knowledge and understanding. At this juncture, it is worth pausing and thinking about how the outcomes of research impact upon us professionally. Nutley et al. (2007) usefully considered this question in presenting a continuum of research impact. Research does not always translate into practice directly (e.g. by altering the way we *do* things for our patients or undertake particular procedures), but it can alter the way we think about things, change our attitudes, influence our values, and enhance our self-awareness. The utilisation of research outputs can be considered, according to Nutley et al. (2007), on an instrumental and conceptual impact continuum (see Figure 2.1).

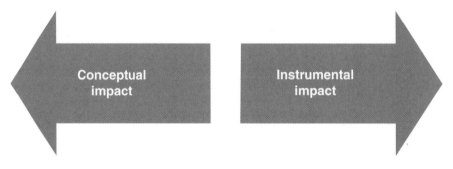

Figure 2.1   Research impact continuum

Source: Nutley, Sandra (2007) *Using evidence: How research can inform the public services.* ©Republished with kind permission of The Policy Press.

Instrumental impact relates to the ways in which research outputs directly lead to demonstrable changes in practice – for example, the practice of intramuscular injection technique is well documented. Publications by Workman in the late 1990s highlighted the practice of the Z tracking technique when administering medication via intramuscular injection in order to provide enhanced patient outcomes, in terms of patients receiving the full therapeutic dose of the medication as well as the prevention of tissue or skin damage during the procedure: a demonstrable outcome which one could witness nurses applying when performing an intramuscular injection (Workman, 1999). Further instrumental impacts can be seen by the way in which research translates into local policies and procedures – for example, local hospitals providing clinical procedure guidelines for practices such as indwelling urinary catheterisation by basing these on the best available research.

Conceptual impact relates to the ways in which the outcomes from research shape our attitudes, help us understand the experiences of others, and develop insight into the lived experiences of healthcare providers and users. For example, Dunniece and Slevin (2000) published research which explored the lived experiences of nurses being present when a patient was given the diagnosis of cancer. This work presented a number of useful findings and made one think about how one would feel, act and react while being present with a patient when they were receiving such a diagnosis: this should encourage us to reflect upon our interpersonal skills as well as to seek out further knowledge and understandings about conceptual impact.

What do we mean by 'evidence-based practice' in nursing and healthcare?

All of us use 'evidence' in the regular decisions we must make throughout life (e.g. when deciding upon where to rent or buy a property we would review the evidence in relation to location, services and amenities, transport or costs). As a learner you will constantly be faced with decisions and challenges which you will need to resolve by using an evidence-based approach.

As with the definitions provided for the term 'research', a number of researchers in this field have provided their position on what is implied by the term 'evidence-based practice'. Sackett et al. (1996: 71) define this as the 'conscientious, explicit and judicious use of current best evidence in making decisions about the care of individual patients'. In Chapter 1, evidence-based practice was defined as 'The process of integrating evidence into healthcare delivery' (Titler, 2011: 291), while Moule and Goodman (2009) refer to this as the process of making choices about what are the most appropriate/effective approaches to care for individual patients. Considering all these definitions, evidence-based practice is a *process* of making decisions about the care of patients and clients based on not only the best available valid research but also a consideration of:

- Professional expertise.
- The needs, abilities, preferences, circumstances, attitudes and beliefs of the individual patient or client.

Evidence-based practice is therefore a *process* about making the right decisions for individuals and does not imply the translation of research outcomes and recommendations in a prescriptive manner. Even when the best available current evidence is translated into a practice guideline or standard, consideration must be given toward patient preferences, circumstances and beliefs.

The main *differences* between the aims and purpose of research and evidence-based practice are helpfully outlined by Carnwell (2000), and these can be reviewed in Table 2.1 below.

Table 2.1   The three essential differences between research and evidence-based practice (adapted from Carnwell, 2000)

	Research	Evidence-based practice
1	The research process is applied to investigations or enquiry with the primary aim of providing new knowledge/insights.	Evidence-based practice is the process by which all the relevant evidence available (of which original research forms part) is appraised and reviewed, thereby generating recommendations about the best approaches to practice/care.
2	The outcomes of research relate to the initial aims of the study which may provide findings relating to the effectiveness of particular interventions or improved insights into specific phenomena.	The outcomes of evidence-based practice are decisions about the best course for clinical actions which may lead to changes in approaches to practice.
3	The research process uses existing evidence to justify new study/enquiry/investigations.	Evidence-based practice draws on existing research and evidence (including patient needs and preferences) on which decisions about approaches to care are based.

How does research inform evidence-based practice?

In applying an evidence-based approach to care, one has to consider what counts as evidence. Research evidence in the form of original, credible research studies is generally considered to be more reliable than sources of evidence that are not derived from original research studies (e.g. non-research based literature, evidence from the opinions of clinicians). The general consensus around the ranking of sources of evidence in terms of value/strength is outlined in Figure 2.2. (Don't worry if some of these terms are alien to you at present as they will be explained in more depth in later chapters of this text.) Although this hierarchy exists, outlining the relationship between research and evidence, differing sources of research evidence will be reviewed for differing types of questions that we may have about our practice. Qualitative research – an approach which seeks to understand human experiences – would be reviewed if our questions about practice were related to understanding the experience of nurses or service users as regards specific phenomena. So whilst not acknowledged as being the strongest type of research evidence, the point that is made here is that in answering questions about practice we must source the most appropriate types of evidence. In doing so, we will need to utilise the best research evidence currently available to us with our expertise and experience as healthcare providers, whilst also considering the preferences and circumstances of the individual

Research-Based Evidence

- *Systematic reviews and meta-analysis*
- *Randomised controlled trials*
- *Non experimental studies, surveys*
- *Qualitative research studies*
- *Published, evidence-based practice guidelines*

Non-Research-Based Evidence

- *Opinions and the consensus of experts*
- *Case studies*
- *Evaluations and audits of practice*

Figure 2.2 Hierarchy of sources of evidence

patient, to provide evidence-based practice. Note however that there may be instances in practice where no research evidence is available and therefore the consensus opinion of experts or data from local evaluations of care may influence our decisions.

Research and evidence-based practice in nursing: A historical perspective

Contemporary healthcare provision has an established approach to care that is firmly based upon the best evidence available (for which research makes a significant contribution). For many years, however, healthcare was delivered in what could be described as a ritualistic manner, one that was based upon the ways things were done rather than considering what was best for the patient. In reviewing nursing practice based upon rituals, Walsh and Ford (1989) discovered that much of what nurses did for their patients was based upon exactly that – ritual with no evidence to justify the practices. Some examples here include the use of unorthodox methods for moving and handling patients which had the potential for harm just because it was the done thing in a ward, insisting that pre-operative patients fasted for a length of time that was more excessive than required, recommending bed rest for patients with back pain when it had been shown to make that pain worse, and using the application of egg white in the management of wounds without any credible evidence that it was effective. As Muir Gray (2001) states, healthcare has shifted away from practices that were based solely on personal opinion and preferences as to how patients were treated and cared for, towards an era where decisions are firmly underpinned by justification and rationale via the use of evidence.

Megan is a second year student studying to become an adult nurse. She is on placement in a busy minor surgery unit. She has studied pain and the management of pain in a university module prior to this placement and is aware of the differing analgesic groups of medicines (medicines prescribed to manage patient pain) and she also understands the different ways in which a patient's pain can be assessed. She has observed that all patients are prescribed the same analgesic medication post-operatively even though different patients have had differing procedures, and as her tutor at university emphasised, pain is a subjective phenomenon and therefore the management of pain must be based on individualised assessments. She asks her mentor why all patients are prescribed the same analgesic medication following surgery. Her mentor replies 'because that is the preferred medication within the ward that we have been prescribing for years ... it seems to work'.

In this scenario what are the risks of basing care on ritual and routines to the:

- Nurse?
- Patient?

Your responses to this activity may vary depending upon your level of experience, however it is important to consider the consequences of such approaches both from the perspective of the consequences for patients (e.g. the prevention of harm and promotion of safety) and the implications that ritualistic approaches could have in terms of a nurse's ability to account for, and justify, all that he or she does for the patient. What would you do if faced with Megan's experience in practice placement?

By basing our practice on evidence of interventions that have a proven value, we aim to eliminate ritualistic care and provide positive patient outcomes. Even with good intentions at heart, compassionate but ill-informed care can be dangerous if based on interventions that could potentially harm patients.

The historical development of research in nursing has had an interesting journey and it is worth taking some time to examine the pathways to research and evidence-based practice in contemporary healthcare which in many ways also reflect the development of nursing as a profession.

Pre-1970s: Much of the activities of early nursing pioneers were aimed toward enhancing the recognition of nursing as a profession, enhancing the educational preparation of nurses, and raising the standards of care for the sick. The work of Florence Nightingale during the Crimean War, in which she recognised the need to review the way in which sick and injured soldiers were cared for, can be seen as the first evidence of research in nursing. Nightingale, and her empirical observations and collections of data, gave rise to changes in practice for the sick and wounded as regards nutrition, cleanliness, and water, as well as the importance of considering the environment in which care was provided. Other notable pioneers in nursing research in this pre-1970s period included:

- Jeanne Quint Benoliel: a researcher devoted to the study of death and dying who worked with the sociologists Strauss and Glaser examining communication between healthcare providers and dying patients (Quint, 1967).

- Lisbeth Hockey: an internationally renowned researcher in the field of community nursing research who was responsible for the initiation of the Queen's Nursing Institute in Scotland, she recognised and emphasised the need for continuous quality improvement in care and the importance of nurses questioning and challenging ritualistic approaches to care.
- Marjorie Simpson: acknowledged as being instrumental in the development of nursing research in the UK in the 1950s, as Smith (1992: 893) states: she was 'totally dedicated to fostering "research mindedness" among nurses, midwives and health visitors worldwide'.

Although nursing academics had begun to write theories and models of nursing, notably in the USA, within this pre-1970s period, and in spite of the aforementioned devoted pioneers, the ethos of altruism, vocation and service before professional development in nursing was not truly challenged until the late 1960s (Bradshaw, 2010).

1970s: In reviewing as its remit the professional role of the nurse, educational preparation of nurses and the use of nursing as a resource in healthcare, the Briggs Report (Department of Health and Social Security, 1972) encouraged the nursing profession to become more mindful of the need for a nursing research base in practice, and to develop its own professional knowledge base grounded in empirical research – much of the knowledge utilised by nurses up until this point had been derived from other disciplines such as medicine, psychology, and sociology. Partly as a result of the report's recommendations, over the following decade nursing research output increased, and in the 1970s itself prominent nurse researchers (including some of the pioneers of the pre-1970s period) started to publish more seminal work which provided nursing with research on which to guide and base practice: for example, Stockwell's (1972) *The unpopular patient*, Franklin's (1974) *Patient anxiety on admission to hospital*, Hawthorn's (1974) *Nurse – I want my mummy!*, and Hayward's (1975) *Information – A prescription against pain*, are all good examples of studies administered by the Royal College of Nursing (RCN) and sponsored by the then Department of Health and Social Security in the UK government. Around the same time a British epidemiologist, Archie Cochrane, questioned the effectiveness of healthcare interventions and emphasised that they needed to have evidence that they promoted desirable patient outcomes. Cochrane's work would eventually lead to the establishment of the Cochrane Collaboration in 1993, a non-profit making organisation that publishes systematic reviews of studies of clinical effectiveness, providing practitioners with evidence of which clinical interventions promoted positive patient outcomes.

It would be useful to look at Hayward's 1975 study and read the introduction to this paper (pp. 8–9). This provides an interesting insight into the context of research in nursing in the 1970s and the underpinning social and historical factors influencing it. It also provides insights into the developing rationale for nurses to move away from ritualistic practice and towards an approach to care that could be challenged with the use of research evidence. This can be accessed by typing the search term, the title of the study *Information – A prescription against pain*, into your internet browser.

ACTIVITY 2.3

The Briggs Report also made recommendations for changes in nurse education and training, as well as recommending the establishment of a new statutory body for nursing (which eventually led to the creation of the United Kingdom Central Council for Nursing, Midwifery and Health Visiting in 1983, later to be renamed the Nursing and Midwifery Council (NMC) in 2002). These recommendations would ultimately impact upon the nature and use of research in nurse education and practice in that these bodies provided and, in the case of the NMC, continue to provide, guidance for registered nurses on the standards of conduct, performance and ethics for nurses and midwives (NMC, 2008), as well as guidance as to the standards for pre-registration nurse education (NMC, 2010). In both practice and educational preparation, the NMC continues to emphasise the ethos of basing care on best evidence and nurses developing research literacy skills as core values.

1980s: Throughout the 1980s, nursing research activity continued to grow steadily and the notion of individualised care was becoming more apparent in the field of health and social care, coupled with the need to recognise the rights of individuals and patients that was embedded in government reports around this time. This being the case, some commentators implied that nursing had not realised the recommendations made by Briggs (i.e. that nurses did not understand research, were unable to apply research findings to their practice, or did not accept the need to utilise research in that practice). The Report of the Taskforce on the Strategy for Research in Nursing, Midwifery and Health Visiting (Department of Health, 1993) sought to address some of these perceived deficiencies and acknowledged that not all nurses would be expected to be researchers. However, there was a need for nurses to be research literate.

In 1983, a new UK statutory body for nursing, midwifery and health visiting (the UKCC) informed a radical reform of nurse education in the UK, with a new philosophy for the education and preparation of student nurses with an emphasis upon learning in the classroom. National Boards for each of the four countries within the UK were also set up with a brief to monitor the quality and standards of nursing programmes. Concurrent with this was an increase in research capacity within educational institutions delivering nurse education. The introduction of the Research Assessment Exercise (RAE) (now known as the Research Excellence Framework (REF)) by the then Conservative government in 1986 resulted in educational institutions devising strategies to increase the level and quality of nursing research. The REF is undertaken approximately every five years and academic departments of nursing strive to improve their rating (in terms of the quality of research output) to obtain funding from one of the four funding councils in the UK. Indeed the need for research and scholarly output has now become imperative within academic department strategies, thus enhancing not only the level and quality of research produced but also the numbers of nurses undertaking Master's and Doctoral level study. This latter trend is also reflective of the modernisation of nursing careers and the new roles that nurses have developed and undertaken in healthcare provision, resulting in nursing career frameworks which expect individuals to undertake these higher degrees.

At the end of the 1980s, government policy shifted toward the notion of assuring quality and standards of care, rather than what had been a focus upon finance and ensuring budgets were achieved. Concurrent with this policy shift, toward the later part of this decade, work undertaken by researchers at McMaster University in Ontario, Canada, would become pivotal in the creation of the evidence-based practice movement in healthcare. The work of the researchers was focused upon decision making and problem solving in medicine and involved students as well as professionals searching and reviewing evidence for specific medical practice interventions/ treatments. The positive results generated by this project in terms of evidence of clinical and cost effectiveness gave rise to other healthcare professional disciplines drawing from this work and developing the process of evidence-based practice.

1990s: Since the beginning of the 1990s there has been a global drive toward basing practice on the best evidence available. Initially this notion was known as evidence-based medicine. The work of the researchers at McMaster University sought to change the culture of decisions made by medical professionals from one based upon individual opinion and preferences to one based upon evidence of effectiveness and improved patient outcomes. There were also a number of key drivers during the 1990s which served to enhance the notion of healthcare systems being based on an awareness and use of research and evidence of what works in terms of improving the quality of care provided to patients. Initially centring on ensuring the best value for money within the health service, the term 'quality' toward the end of this decade became synonymous with the delivery of care of a consistently high standard with minimisation in variations in the way in which care was provided (i.e. a patient with a similar condition or healthcare need could expect to receive the same care and treatment irrespective of where the care was provided in a geographical sense). Around this time national review bodies were implemented within the UK (e.g. the National Institute for Health and Clinical Excellence (NICE) in England and Wales and the Scottish Intercollegiate Guidelines Network (SIGN) in Scotland). Such bodies continue to develop evidence-based clinical practice guidelines which are published following a rigorous and methodological appraisal of the research evidence (mainly from randomised controlled trials and experimental studies) involving specialists from all the healthcare professions as well as service users. Governmental drivers were therefore centred on addressing the perceived fall in standards of care.

By 1997 pre-registration nurse education provision had moved from what were termed Colleges of Nursing and Midwifery to Higher Education Institutions (HEIs). Additionally commissioned reports such as the Peach Report in 1999 (UKCC, 1999), in reviewing nursing and midwifery education, placed an emphasis upon the future direction of healthcare provision and the roles that these professional groups would play in a changing healthcare system which, according to Peach, would impact upon nursing and midwifery by placing 'greater demands upon nurses and midwives for technical competence and scientific rationality' (UKCC, 1999: 3).

2000–present: As we entered the twenty-first century the focus of governmental policy was clearly centred on the notion of clinical effectiveness and enhancing the quality of care for patients and clients. This has continued to the present day with publications such as the *Healthcare quality strategy* (Scottish Government, 2010) focusing upon safe, effective, person-centred care. Coupled with this is a range of other factors which have shaped and altered the ways in which care is provided, the places where care is provided, the roles of healthcare professionals, and the nature of the needs of the public. There is now a multitude of standards, guidelines, and research-based studies published annually. Electronic databases and methods of communication have improved to enable ease of access to such resources.

IMPLICATIONS FOR HEALTHCARE PROVIDERS

All professional groups that provide health and social care must articulate and develop their practice by utilising best available evidence. There is a wide range of

Table 2.2   Contemporary drivers influencing the provision of health and social care

Patient/service user expectations	Demographics
• Access to services. • Consultation in the planning, evaluation and reviewing of healthcare provision. • Increased access to health related information resulting in users having higher levels of understanding regarding their illness, disease or health. • Quality of care. • Safety and risk of harm.	• Populations are living longer. • Increase in complexity of care needs. • Increase in populations living longer with a long-term condition. • Increased dependency upon health services.
Advances in knowledge	**Changes in the provision of services**
• Epidemiology. • Advances in health science knowledge. • Advances in Arts and Humanities knowledge. • Advances in technology. • Advances in medicines. • Increase in research outputs. • Improvements in the management of healthcare.	• Shift in location of care delivery e.g. care in the community. • Changes in duration of care delivery. • Changes in the roles of professionals in the delivery of healthcare. • Shifts in emphasis toward focus of care delivery e.g. public health and promotion of health in populations. • Telemedicine.
Professional expectations of practice	**Media and societal influences**
• Expectations of professional regulatory bodies e.g. standards and professional codes. • Expectations around service provision. • Personal professional accountability. • Changes in the educational preparation of student nurses in the UK.	• Increased scrutiny of health services. • Increase in issues of public confidence. • Increased threat of litigation.

drivers underpinning the continued advancement of evidence-based practice in all areas of healthcare provision (see Table 2.2). As you will see, the impact of these drivers is huge in relation to the direction and delivery of nursing and healthcare provision.

In responding to changes in healthcare provision with changing priorities and environments, the NMC *Standards for pre-registration nurse education* (NMC, 2010) aim to prepare nurses of the future with the knowledge, skills and behaviours that will meet future challenge, thereby enabling nurses to base decisions upon best available evidence. The learning that you are undertaking in research and evidence-based practice will also impact upon your future career pathways – roles such as clinical nurse researcher and advanced and specialist practitioner, as well as leadership and management roles, education roles, and practice development. The fundamental skills of research literacy and the ability to understand and engage in the process of evidence-based practice are a core requisite for the advancement of knowledge beyond pre-registration education (e.g. Master's and Doctoral research degrees). As regards public expectations, the NMC has stated that there are a number of values that mean the public or service users can have confidence in these nurses of the future. Of particular relevance to the context of this text is the public's confidence in nurses being able to:

Act to safeguard the public, and be responsible and accountable for safe, person-centred, evidence-based nursing practice. (NMC, 2010: 5)

You will already be familiar with the NMC's competencies and, as you will be aware, there are *generic* competencies (i.e. competencies that must be achieved irrespective of your chosen field of practice) and competencies that are *specific* to each field of nursing, organised into four domains. These are:

- Professional values.
- Communication and interpersonal skills.
- Nursing practice and decision making.
- Leadership, management and team working.

Table 2.3 offers some examples of where there is a reference to evidence-based competencies – emphasising the need for all student nurses to engage in evidence-based learning and practice.

Irrespective of your chosen field of practice, it is clear that research and evidence-based practice are fundamental areas of learning that will equip you with the knowledge and skills to ensure that the care you provide for your patients and clients is of a high standard, as well as contributing to your own personal professional development and the multifaceted array of career pathways open to nurses following registration. Activity 2.4 aims to bring together your learning from this chapter and help prepare you better as you go on to subsequent chapters.

Table 2.3　Examples of competencies for evidence-based practice for entry onto the register

- **All nurses** must act first and foremost to care for and safeguard the public. They must practise autonomously and be responsible and accountable for safe, compassionate, person-centred, evidence-based nursing that respects and maintains dignity and human rights.

- **All practice** should be informed by the best evidence and comply with local and national guidelines. Decision making must be shared with service users, carers and families and informed by critical analysis of a full range of possible interventions, including the use of up-to-date technology.

- **All nurses** must use up-to-date knowledge and evidence to assess, plan, deliver and evaluate care, communicate findings, influence change, and promote health and best practice. They must make person-centred, evidence-based judgments and decisions, in partnership with others involved in the care process, to ensure high quality care. They must be able to recognise when the complexity of clinical decisions requires specialist knowledge and expertise, and consult or refer accordingly.

- **All nurses** must appreciate the value of evidence in practice, be able to understand and appraise research, apply relevant theory and research findings to their work, and identify areas for further investigation.

- **Adult nurses** must recognise and respond to the changing needs of adults, families and carers during terminal illness. They must be aware of how treatment goals and service users' choices may change at different stages of a progressive illness, loss and bereavement.

- **Mental health nurses** must be able to apply their knowledge and skills in a range of evidence-based individual and group psychological and psychosocial interventions, to carry out systematic needs assessments, develop case formulations and negotiate goals.

- **Mental health nurses** must be able to apply their knowledge and skills in a range of evidence-based psychological and psychosocial individual and group interventions to develop and implement care plans and evaluate outcomes, in partnership with service users and others.

- **Mental health nurses** must work positively and proactively with people who are at risk of suicide or self-harm, and use evidence-based models of suicide prevention, intervention and harm reduction to minimise risk.

- **Learning disabilities nurses** must use data and research findings on the health of people with learning disabilities to help improve people's experiences and care outcomes, and the shape of future services.

- **Children's nurses** must use recognised, evidence-based, child-centred frameworks to assess, plan, implement, evaluate and record care, and to underpin clinical judgments and decision making. Care planning and delivery must be informed by a knowledge of pharmacology, anatomy and physiology, pathology, psychology and sociology, from infancy to young adulthood.

What strategies, goals and actions could you adopt during your practice placement experiences which would enhance your knowledge and awareness of evidence-based practice in action?

SUMMARY

The key points for your learning in this chapter include:

- Understanding that research and the process of evidence-based decision making are core fundamental attributes of the registered nurse.
- Recognising that healthcare provision is changing: there a number of factors presenting new challenges to nursing and healthcare in terms of the roles that must be undertaken as regards the changing healthcare needs, priorities and developments that exist in health-care. Even for nurses who do not pursue a career in research, research literacy skills are crucial in engaging with evidence-based decision making.
- Recognising also that career pathways in nursing are changing: information and research literacy skills are core requisites for Master's and Doctoral-level degrees.

FURTHER READING

International Council of Nurses (2012) *Closing the gap: From evidence to action*. Geneva: International Council of Nurses.
http://nursingworld.org/MainMenuCategories/ThePracticeofProfessionalNursing/Improving-Your-Practice/Research-Toolkit/ICN-Evidence-Based-Practice-Resource/Closing-the-Gap-from-Evidence-to-Action.pdf
From a global perspective this 2009 publication by the International Council of Nurses is helpful in clarifying further the notion of evidence in practice, where evidence comes from, how evidence can change practice, and how the outcomes of evidence-based practice can be evaluated.

National Institute for Health and Clinical Excellence: www.nice.org.uk/
The National Institute for Health and Clinical Excellence provides clinical guidelines for healthcare professionals, guiding best practice that is based upon an appraisal of the evidence currently available.

Rycroft-Malone, J., Seers, K., Titchen, A. et al. (2004) What counts as evidence in evidence based practice, *Journal of Advanced Nursing*, 47 (1): 81–90.
This paper by Rycroft-Malone et al. provides some interesting discussion around what is seen as 'evidence' in relation to evidence-based practice. It also covers the debate around the notion of four differing types of evidence: research, clinical experience, patient experience and local context, and how these are melded together to inform decisions about patient care.

Veermah, V. (2004) Utilization of research findings by graduate nurses and midwives, *Journal of Advanced Nursing*, 47 (2): 183–191.
This work by Veermah presents an original research study which evaluated the impact of research education on the attitudes toward, and utilisation of, research by nurses and midwives. It is especially interesting as there may be some similarities between the study's findings and your own personal current perspectives upon research as a topic.

REFERENCES

Ax, S. and Kincaid, E. (2001) Nursing students perceptions of research: usefulness, implementation and training, *Journal of Advanced Nursing*, 35: 161–170.
Bradshaw, A. (2010) An historical perspective on the treatment of vocation in the Briggs Report (1972), *Journal of Clinical Nursing*, 19: 3459–3467.
Carnwell, R. (2000) Essential differences between research and evidence-based practice, *Nurse Researcher*, 8 (2): 55–68.
Carper, B.A. (1978) Fundamental patterns of knowing in nursing, *Advances in Nursing Science*, 1 (1): 13–24.
Department of Health and Social Security (1972) *Report of the committee on nursing (the Briggs Report)*. London: HMSO.
Department of Health (1993) *Report of the taskforce on the strategy for research in nursing, midwifery and health visiting*. London: HMSO.
Dunniece, U. and Slevin, E. (2000) Nurses' experience of being present with a patient receiving a diagnosis of cancer, *Journal of Advanced Nursing*, (32) 3: 611–618.
Field, A.P. and Morse, J.M. (1995) *Nursing research: The application of qualitative approaches*. London: Croome Helm.
Franklin, B.L. (1974) *Patient anxiety on admission to hospital*. London: RCN.
Hawthorn, P.J. (1974) *Nurse – I want my mummy!* London: RCN.
Hayward, J. (1975) *Information – A prescription against pain*. London: RCN.
Hek, G. and Moule, P. (2006) *Making sense of research: An introduction for health and social care practitioners* (3rd edition). London: Sage.
Johnson, N., List-Ivancovic, J., Eboh, W.E., Ireland, J., Adams, D., Mowatt, E. and Martindale, S. (2010) Research and evidence-based practice: Using a blended approach in teaching and learning in nurse education, *Nurse Education in Practice*, 10: 43–47.
Moule, P. and Goodman, M. (2009) *Nursing research: An introduction*. London: Sage.
Muir Gray, J.A. (2001) *Evidence-based healthcare: How to make policy and management decisions* (2nd edition). Edinburgh: Churchill Livingstone.
Nursing and Midwifery Council (NMC) (2008) *The code: Standards of conduct, performance and ethics for nurses and midwives*. London: NMC.
Nursing and Midwifery Council (NMC) (2010) *Standards for pre-registration nursing education*. London: NMC.
Nutley, S.M., Walter, I. and Davies, H.T.O. (2007) *Using evidence: How research can inform the public services*. Bristol: Policy Press.
Parahoo, K. (1997) *Nursing research: Principles, processes and issues*. Basingstoke: Palgrave.
Quint, J. (1967) *The nurse and the dying patient*. New York: McMillan.
Sackett, D.L., Rosenborg, M.C., Muir Gray, J.A. et al. (1996) Evidence based medicine: what it is and what it isn't, *BMJ*, 312: 71–72.

Scottish Government (2010) *The healthcare quality strategy for NHS Scotland*. Edinburgh: Scottish Government.

Smith, J.P. (1992) Majorie Simpson: pioneering nurse researcher, *Journal of Advanced Nursing*, 17: 893.

Stockwell, F. (1972) *The unpopular patient*. London: RCN.

Titler, M.G. (2011) Nursing science and evidence-based practice, *Western Journal of Nursing Research*, 33: 291–295.

United Kingdom Central Council for Nursing, Midwifery and Health Visiting (UKCC) (1999) *Fitness for practice*. London: UKCC.

Walsh, M. and Ford, P. (eds) (1989) *Nursing rituals: Research and rational actions*. Oxford: Butterworth Heinmann.

Workman, B. (1999) Safe injection techniques, *Nursing Standard;* 13: 47–53.

3

THE IMPORTANCE OF RESEARCH FOR PRACTICE

NEIL JOHNSON

Chapter learning outcomes

On completion of Chapter 3, you will be able to:

1 Understand how research relates to your learning and development.
2 Identify the ways in which nurse researchers can and have influenced nursing practice.
3 Discuss the ways in which research advances knowledge for nursing practice.
4 Define the term 'clinical effectiveness'.
5 Understand global perspectives on research and evidence-based practice.
6 Discuss the differences between the terms 'research', 'audit', and 'service evaluation'.

Key concepts

Research, research impact, clinical effectiveness, global perspectives, research, audit and service evaluation.

INTRODUCTION

In Chapter 2 evidence-based practice and research were explored from the perspective of their relevance to learning as well as to practice. It is clear that evidence-based practice and research will continue to have a significant role in the development of nursing as a profession, nursing as an academic discipline, and in shaping the future direction of services and the evolution of new nursing roles and career pathways in a modern healthcare system. Evidence-based practice and research are now synonymous with one another and form part and parcel of all pre-registration nursing programmes, as well as courses offered at the post-registration level. As you will have already seen, the NMC *Standards for pre-registration nurse education* (NMC, 2010) have a philosophy of developing nurses to meet future healthcare challenges, in order that they can apply an analytical and evidence-based problem-solving approach, challenge practice, and develop ways in which the standards and quality of care can be enhanced. Whilst Chapter 2 provided a general overview of the development of research and evidence-based practice, I start here by focusing on research and in particular researchers who have provided examples of significant contributions to nursing research, nursing as a profession, and nursing practice. Examples for all four fields of practice are provided (i.e. adult, children and young people, mental health, and learning disability nursing). Following on from this I explore the ways in which research advances knowledge for nursing practice before turning my attention to what could be described as practice development activities (i.e. activities that are designed to assist in the evaluation of practices and patient outcomes as well as in informing decisions around service provision development). I then finish the chapter by exploring global perspectives on research and evidence-based practice.

THE WAYS IN WHICH RESEARCHERS HAVE INFLUENCED PRACTICE AND THINKING IN THE FOUR FIELDS OF NURSING

When considering researchers who have influenced practice and provided a major contribution to nursing in terms of changing our ways of thinking and knowing and acting as a catalyst for further research and literary outputs, our first question must be 'where to start?' Whilst the scope of this chapter cannot possibly make reference to *all* significant contributories to nursing research (this would require a sizeable text in itself), it is important to capture some examples of individuals who have had impact in terms of both instrumental and conceptual forms (see Nutley et al., 2007, Chapter 2). A wealth and multitude of nursing research, nursing researchers and publications now exist, and as a learner entering the field of research and evidence-based practice for the first time, accessing this can be a daunting prospect − where to start, how to work out if you have found something of relevance and quality, how to manage this considerable body of evidence? Glasziou (2005: 6) uses the phrase 'practice famine amidst the evidence glut' to describe the fact that (circa 2005) Medline (an online database) had indexed more than 560,000 articles and the Cochrane Collaboration had added around 20,000 new trials to its database (this totalled 1500 new articles and 55 new trials per day!). There are a number of relevant points here: you must develop the appropriate skills for searching for research evidence; you must be able to read, understand and review the research evidence; and you must also be aware of sources of evidence where this process has already been undertaken for you (e.g. SIGN and NICE guidelines: later chapters will assist you in these respects).

There have been (and indeed still are) a number of eminent nurse researchers in specific fields of practice or undertaking research in key areas of nursing. As you learn and explore specific themes or topics in your educational development certain names may appear repeatedly, and you will therefore become more familiar with those researchers who are at the cutting edge of knowledge and practice development.

ACTIVITY 3.1

Whether you are just starting a nursing programme, or are just about to complete one, what topics of interest do you have in relation to your chosen field of practice?

Try and find some examples of the research that has been published, and the researchers' names, in relation to this topic. Please note that you will be doing some detailed work in relation to searching for evidence in later chapters, so all I want you to do here is get a 'feel' for some of the research that is relevant to your field of practice.

You may find this activity relatively straightforward, particularly if the topic you chose has a good body of research behind it. In others, you may discover that little or no research has been undertaken – remember, however, that this should not surprise you as evidence will not exist for every single question we may have about healthcare. You may also notice that some of the researchers were not nurses. Indeed a number of studies which have had an impact upon nursing over the years have been undertaken within other professional disciplines such as psychology, sociology, and medicine. Given that contemporary healthcare is interprofessional, nurse researchers are more likely to find themselves working collaboratively with other professional groups on research questions that will have transferability across disciplines (e.g. bereavement care). Working collaboratively with other professional groups will advance nursing in the practical sense and in the creation of new knowledge.

Significant contributors to nursing research are presented below. Note that they come from differing backgrounds, differing fields of practice, and indeed differing eras. They are:

- Doreen Norton for her work on the prevention of pressure ulcers.
- Phil Barker and Poppy Buchanan-Barker for the Tidal Model for mental health nursing.

- Alison Twycross for her research in the field of children's nursing.
- Ruth Northway for her work in the field of learning disabilities and in particular the adult protection agenda.

I am sure you can or will, as your knowledge, understanding and experience grow, be able to identify others. So why have I chosen these individuals? Because all of them have influenced practice directly and this can be seen in the manner in which their research has translated into differing ways of thinking as well as different ways of practising. Their work has also translated into motivating others to undertake research and to develop and evaluate new ways of caring for patients and clients across age spans and in differing fields of practice.

Doreen Norton: The Norton Scale (1962)

Nowadays we will often take the practice of ensuring that pressure is not a contributory factor in the formation of pressure ulcers for granted. We work in practice with tools to assist us in assessing risk and grading pressure ulcers and we receive specialist support from tissue viability nurses. We realise that there are groups of patients who are at a higher risk of developing pressure sores (e.g. the elderly, immobile or incontinent), but we forget that it took one nurse and her research in the 1950s to provide the scientific evidence that would change practice not only in the short term but also in the years and decades to follow. Doreen Norton, an English nurse working with the elderly, used research to provide evidence that the most effective way of preventing pressure ulcers was by eliminating pressure by turning patients at regular intervals. Her work was instrumental in changing practice as well as contributing to a fall in pressure ulcers – and pressure ulcers were a factor that had previously led to many patients dying.

Until Norton's research, nurses were following ritualistic, opinion-based practices (of which there were many!) that had little or no proof of clinical effectiveness (we will explore this term later in this chapter). As one of the first risk assessment tools used by nurses, Norton developed her assessment scale to help nurses assess a patient's risk of developing a pressure ulcer. The Norton Scale, based on research conducted within elderly care, was finally devised and provided a method by which nurses could assess risk. The tool was presented as five risk factors and within each of these verbal descriptors provided nurses with an ability to assess and score a patient's level of risk of developing a pressure ulcer. Each risk factor was assessed individually and a score apportioned to each. The scores for each risk category were then added to give a total: the lower the score the higher the risk, and a cut-off value of 14 was identified to show patients at risk. Table 3.1 presents the Norton Scale.

Norton's work changed practice considerably, and although her tool was effective in improving patient outcomes (e.g. a reduction in pressure ulcers) in elderly settings, its validity (i.e. the tool's ability to do what it was intended to do, namely reduce the incidence of pressure ulcers) in others was less convincing. The tool has since been superseded (although it still forms the basis for assessment in many areas globally) in

Table 3.1　The Norton Scale

Physical condition	Mental condition	Activity	Mobility	Incontinent	Score
Good	Alert	Ambulant	Full	Not	4
Fair	Apathetic	Walk-help	Slightly limited	Occasional	3
Poor	Confused	Chair bound	Very limited	Usually urine	2
Very bad	Stupor	Stupor	Immobile	Doubly	1

assessing a patient's risk of developing a pressure ulcer. As you can probably see, this research represents a good example of how one nurse's questions about her patients and their risk of developing a pressure ulcer led to the development and implementation of an assessment tool, globally, at a time where nursing practice was based on ritual and routine. Norton's work, although criticised by some, provided impacts at a number of levels: it made nursing more aware of the risk factors associated with pressure ulcer formation; it made nurses think about how they viewed the risks associated with the factors identified in the tool; and crucially, it provided the basis for others to expand knowledge through research and the development of new tools. Contemporary risk assessment tools, based on best available evidence, enable learners and nurses to realise standards of competence for entry onto the register as well as maintaining the Standards of Performance made explicit within the Code (NMC, 2008). Such tools enable adult nurses to 'use up-to-date knowledge and evidence to assess, plan, deliver and evaluate care ...' (NMC, 2010: 17). It is a great example of an initial clinical question that gave rise to a nurse researcher transforming thinking, knowledge and practice, and sustaining new enquiry.

Phil Barker and Poppy Buchanan-Barker: The Tidal Model

Phil Barker was the UK's first Professor of Psychiatric Nursing and has a forty year history of working in the field of mental health nursing. Along with Poppy Buchanan-Barker he co-authored the Tidal Model of Mental Health Recovery. In the field of mental health nursing, the Tidal Model is a humanistic representation of nursing which has now been utilised globally in mental health settings and has influenced government policy on mental healthcare. The model's origins can be traced back to research undertaken by Professor Barker and Dr Chris Stevenson (Barker et al., 1999b). Described as a recovery model, this approach to the care of individuals with a mental health problem aims to help individuals realise their own health, a process that had traditionally been led by professionals (Barker and Buchanan-Barker, 2005). Barker saw recovery in mental health as a process of reclaiming one's identity and therefore requiring therapeutic conditions for personal recovery within institutional mental health settings. To prevent what can be described as institutionalisation, the Tidal Model emphasises that recovery begins when an individual is admitted to hospital (i.e. at their lowest point) and not at any point later in their care when institutionalisation can occur.

The Tidal Model was the first research-based model of recovery in mental health that was developed by nurses with the assistance and support of past and current service users. It was based upon two empirical research studies: firstly, a study that developed theory around the perceptions of professionals, patients and carers in regard to the need for psychiatric nursing (Barker et al., 1999a); and secondly, a study exploring mental health nurses' empowerment of patients with long-term mental health problems (Barker et al., 1999b). Recognised internationally and used interprofessionally, the model focuses upon the person's, not the 'patient's', capacity to recover their health from its lowest point: 'by using their own language, metaphors and personal stories people begin to express something of the meaning of their lives. This is the first step towards helping *recover* control over their lives' (Barker and Buchanan-Barker, 2005). For more information on the Tidal Model you should visit: www.tidal-model.com.

Again, this provides an excellent example of nurse-led developments in practice based on research. The Tidal Model is now recognised internationally and is shaping and changing traditional approaches to mental health nursing. Unlike the previous example of Doreen Norton, the model is currently implemented extensively in the field of mental health nursing and its philosophy resonates with the new NMC Standards. For example, it enables nurses in the field of mental health to:

> work with people in a way that values, respects and explores the meaning of their individual lived experiences of mental health problems, to provide person-centred and recovery-focused practice. (NMC, 2010: 23)

Since its implementation, evidence from evaluative studies has demonstrated the positive impacts of the Tidal Model with reported satisfaction from service users and nurses, a reduction in violent events and patients requiring to be sectioned under the Mental Health Act, shortened stays in hospital, a shortened gap between admission and assessment, less use of restraint, and improvements in the delivery of primary care in substance misuse (Fletcher and Stevenson, 2001; Young, 2010).

Alison Twycross: Children's Nursing Research and Practice Development – Pain Management in Children

Dr Alison Twycross has a background in children's nursing and has focused research outputs on acute pain and post-operative pain management in children. She is recognised as a significant researcher in the field of children's nursing. Her studies have reviewed pain management practices, methods of improving pain management, and the education of healthcare professionals regarding paediatric pain management. It is this area that is used here as an example of research impact.

Raising the profile of pain management in the field of children's nursing has ensured that both educational and healthcare providers are focused upon ensuring that current and future children's and young people's nurses improve upon practice. Twycross's work identified significant shortcomings in the management of pain in children and also provided recommendations as to how this could be improved. Factors identified as contributing towards poor practice in this area included knowledge deficits, inaccurate and out-dated beliefs about paediatric pain management, decision making strategies, and the culture of the organisations where care was provided – even when national clinical guidelines on paediatric pain management were available (Twycross, 2010). In recognising these shortcomings, Twycross has provided evidence-based recommendations for the improvement of pain management practices in paediatric settings (e.g. pain management policy and guideline utilisation in all organisations, the regular monitoring of standards, ongoing education for all levels of clinical staff, and the implementation of a pain management service including pain link nurses). Twycross also undertook research to explore the perceived importance that paediatric nurses attached to the task of pain management, again illuminating the fact that regardless of the perceptions held, a number of factors continued to contribute toward sub-optimal post-operative pain management in children (e.g. nurses' beliefs and attitudes toward pain, the effect of role models, the lack of knowledge, and the organisational culture: see Twycross, 2008). In another example from an earlier study, Twycross (2002a) demonstrated that in surgical paediatric nursing settings the general care relating to pain assessment and pain management was poor and the approaches adopted by nurses were unsystematic. She has also provided guidance to educational providers in terms of how to assist learners to gain an awareness, knowledge and understanding of pain management via innovative learning approaches (Twycross, 2002b). The work of Alison Twycross has therefore raised the profile and importance of the management of pain in children, which in turn has translated into greater emphasis on this topic area both in practice and educational settings.

Professor Ruth Northway: Learning Disability Nursing Research – Advocacy

Professor Ruth Northway is a significant contributor to research in the field of learning disability nursing. Having a considerable public output record, Professor Northway has published on a number of topics relating to learning disability nursing, including advocacy and the role of the learning disability nurse, adult protection, and the health and quality of life of people living with an intellectual disability. In regard to the role of the learning disability nurse as an advocate, Professor Northway and her colleagues have provided research outputs which have helped to inform knowledge and understanding, and as such have assisted individuals, service providers, policy makers and decision makers in enhancing advocacy for individuals with a learning disability. For example, Northway has explored the notion of advocacy in learning disability nursing and has identified some of the key challenges faced by advocates in the role, as well as providing expert guidance on the role of learning disability nurses as advocates for people with a learning disability (Jenkins and Northway, 2002). Northway's work has identified the perceived barriers to advocacy (as perceived by learning disability nurses); the educational needs of learning disability nurses (by engaging in research in the real world with learning disability nurses); and the use of independent advocacy services, clarifying definitions and the role of the advocate as well as the specific requirements for advocacy training (Lllewellyn and Northway, 2007). This body of work has – like that of Twycross in the field of children's nursing – been instrumental in bringing the notion of advocacy to the forefront of learning disability nursing, both in respect of the instrumental impact on practice and the conceptual impact in terms of shaping and influencing belief and attitudes. This is of particular relevance to learning disability nurses and those training to become registered learning disability nurses. The NMC Standards (2010) are explicit in stating that for entry to the register, the learning disability nurse must:

- Always promote the autonomy, rights and choices of people with learning disabilities and support and involve their families and carers, ensuring that each person's rights are upheld according to policy and the law.
- Use their knowledge and skills to exercise professional advocacy, and recognise when it is appropriate to refer to independent advocacy services to safeguard dignity and human rights. (NMC, 2010: 31)

Without the scholarly work of researchers such as Northway, learning disability nursing would be the weaker for lack of guidance around the role of the learning disability nurse as an advocate.

ADVANCING NURSING KNOWLEDGE FOR PRACTICE THROUGH RESEARCH

Nursing research influences nursing practice in that its primary purpose is to generate new knowledge that helps to inform and enhance approaches to care. Thinking back to Chapter 2, and the reference made to the differing bodies of knowledge that nursing draws upon (e.g. science, aesthetics, ethics and personal experience: see Carper, 1978), there is a broad scope of research activities that are undertaken to expand knowledge in each of these four domains. There is therefore a range of research questions that assist in the development of nursing as a profession, as a discipline, and in practice. These include questions related to the *effectiveness* of interventions (e.g. are silver-coated urinary catheters more effective than non-silver-coated urinary catheters in preventing catheter associated urinary tract infections?). These types of question seek to establish therapeutic interventions that will promote health and reduce the consequences of ill health. Other research questions may relate to questions of *meaningfulness*, focusing on the investigation of human experience (e.g. human responses to health and illness). An example of this type of investigation may be the exploration of an individual's experience of living with a long-term condition such as diabetes. A plethora of research interests exists:

- Research with patient and service users.
- Research with care providers.
- Research with learners in education.
- Research which evaluates the impact of new approaches to care or initiatives to improve health.
- Research on attitudes and behaviours (and so the list goes on ...).

This is not an exhaustative list, rather it has been designed to provide you with some examples of the scope of nursing research. The outcomes from such research can help improve the quality of care, contribute to nursing knowledge, and enhance the educational preparation of nurses of the future. A key message here is this: nursing research should always aim to promote excellence in practice.

Research therefore not only enables us scientifically to measure, compare or test the effectiveness of a clinical intervention (e.g. the example of silver-coated *vs* non-silver-coated urinary catheters and incidence of infection), but also to expand knowledge in the personal, ethical and aesthetic domains of nursing. This is vital as the philosophy of the NMC Standards is safe, effective, *and* person-centred care. The journey from novice learner to expert in nursing is not one that is solely dependent upon building knowledge and expertise about the things we *do* for our patients (e.g. giving an injection, dressing a wound, taking a patient's vital signs). That journey is also one of personal discovery, understanding one's self as a developing professional, understanding how humans respond to a variety of phenomena (e.g. reacting to illness, recovering health). In realising such understanding you will gain knowledge through engaging with research that seeks to explore these questions. At this point in the discussion there are two key issues to consider. Firstly, that knowledge in nursing can never be considered fixed. As Gerrish and Lacey (2010) imply, as the world evolves and changes in society occur, so new knowledge is gained, and past research outputs can become outmoded by new findings and recommendations. Secondly, that it is important to remind you that knowledge can take differing forms, as you saw in Chapter 2. You will gain knowledge through understanding and the use of research, and you will also gain knowledge through your growing competence and experience taken alongside your theoretical learning.

For example, Nicol (2011: 35) defines the term 'empathy' as 'your capacity to understand another's situation, to identify with their emotions and to use this to respond in an appropriate manner'. Empathy is therefore an ability to see the world as if through the eyes of someone else – an essential skill for any nurse regardless of the field of practice. The NMC Standards (2010: 114) state that by the second progression point in a pre-registration nursing education programme, the graduate nurse will 'contribute to care based on an understanding of how different stages of an illness or disability can impact on people and carers'. To help you become more aware of how research can help in your own personal development, consider the following practice scenario and the questions that follow.

Betty is a 75 year old lady who lives with her husband Stan in a small terraced house. She is an active lady and has no health complaints: she remains independent and has a good network of friends and family. Stan is 82 and has suffered from dementia for the last five years: his condition has gradually worsened, making him more dependent upon Betty for his needs. In addition, Stan has recently been diagnosed with prostate cancer and receives treatment for this at his local hospital outpatient department. You visit Betty and Stan on a daily basis during a placement with your community nurse. Over the course of this placement, Betty appears to be becoming more and more upset about her and Stan's circumstances. She confides in you when you visit that she cannot cope anymore.

What are your feelings and responses to this scenario? How would you react if faced with a similar situation in practice? Could you truly empathise with Betty? How could you enhance your understanding of Betty's experience as a carer?

ACTIVITY 3.2

RESEARCH AND DEVELOPMENT: CLINICAL EFFECTIVENESS, RESEARCH, AUDIT, SERVICE EVALUATION – CLARIFYING THE TERMINOLOGY

The terms research and development, or 'R and D', are ones that you may read about or hear being mentioned either in university-based classes or on a clinical practice placement. As has been discussed in the earlier parts of this book, research aims to provide us with new knowledge to utilise in order to enhance our professional development and practice. Much of the research in nursing can be considered 'applied research' (i.e. the outputs from research aim to be utilised in practice/applied to practice). As research activities are constant within nursing, development (the D in 'R and D') refers to the process by which organisations, policy makers, practitioners and decision makers will *utilise* research outputs to address the need for improved services to patients – or what has now become known in policy terms as quality improvement.

Central to governmental policy drivers relating to *continuous* quality improvement, research and evidence-based practice is now embedded in healthcare education, policy and practice. Research contributes to new knowledge that can be utilised in the evidence-based practice decision making process.

Clayton (2003: 4) defines continuous quality improvement as 'the never ending pursuit to raise standards in health and social care'. As a key stakeholder in healthcare provision, nurses must not only be aware of such a concept, they must also become active participants in its realisation. After all, as part of the inter-professional team, nurses will spend more time with patients on a continued basis than any other professional discipline. Indeed the NMC (2010) states explicitly that the public can be confident that all new nurses will:

- Deliver high quality essential care to all.
- Act to safeguard the public, and be responsible and accountable for safe, person-centred, evidence-based practice.

- Act with professionalism and integrity, and work within agreed professional, ethical and legal frameworks and processes to maintain and improve standards.
- Use leadership skills to supervise and manage others and contribute to planning, designing, and improving future services. (NMC, 2010: 5)

We therefore do not have a choice as to whether we participate in quality improvement initiatives, be it at a ward, hospital, national or international level: it is implicit within professional standards. So what does quality mean to you?

ACTIVITY 3.3

What does the term 'quality' mean to you? How can quality care be evidenced in nursing and how would you observe or measure this? What might the term 'quality' mean to:

- Patients and service users?
- Nurses?

You may wish to discuss these questions with your peers, tutors and/or mentors. You may also wish to ask this question of your patients during a practice placement. Are there differences between what the term 'quality' means to patients and service users as opposed to nurses?

Equally important in quality improvement are the mechanisms by which approaches to healthcare, treatment and interventions are measured and monitored (i.e. the development activities – those that seek to evaluate the implementation of evidence-based approaches to care). To this end it is important to discuss the methods by which this occurs. Definitions of four key terms related to this development activity are provided in Table 3.2.

It is beyond the scope of this chapter to provide a lengthy and detailed discussion as regards the intricacies of all activities related to quality improvement. However, it is vital that you have an awareness of what these activities seek to achieve and why they are of importance. The term 'clinical effectiveness' is considered as an overarching term to describe the activities, tools and skills used in the pursuit of quality improvement (e.g. research, clinical audit, service evaluation, education and professional development, risk management). In regard to the three terms (research, audit, and service evaluation), it is important that you understand not only the basic principles behind each but also what makes them distinct.

Research is a systematic process whereby relevant steps in the research process are followed with the aim of generating new information data and knowledge that will benefit education, practice and policy. A research study is designed in such a way that others can replicate it. It can be used to investigate and explore phenomena, test relationships between differing variables, and evaluate new or existing approaches to care, and it is undertaken by researchers with appropriate skills in the research

Table 3.2 Key definitions – research, clinical effectiveness, audit, and service evaluation

Key term	Definition
Research	'A systematic approach to gathering information for the purposes of answering questions and solving problems in the pursuit of creating new knowledge about nursing practice, education and policy' (Hek and Moule, 2006: 10).
Clinical effectiveness	'The effectiveness of an intervention, from single treatments through to services including the professionals within them, is the degree to which the desired health outcomes are achieved in clinical practice' (Muir Gray, 2001: 185).
Audit	'Clinical audit is a professionally-led initiative which seeks to improve the quality and outcome of patient care through clinicians examining their practices and results and modifying practice where indicated' (NHSE, 1996: 16).
Service evaluation	'Service evaluation seeks to measure the standards that a particular service achieves. It aims to answer the question – "what standard does this service achieve?"' (NHS Direct, 2012).

process. Research in nursing also requires ethical permission from a research ethics committee prior to the actual research being undertaken.

An audit – or clinical audit as it has been described by some – is a continual process of evaluating particular practices in terms of how close these match best practice or recommended standards of practice. A clinical audit can be likened to a cycle whereby practice is evaluated against agreed best practice standards, evaluations are reviewed, and changes and amendments are made to practice as a result. Figure 3.1 provides a diagrammatic representation of the audit cycle.

An audit has at its core the aim of improving services for patients and clients. It does not seek to generate new knowledge and it is undertaken in one specific location or client group, meaning the outcomes of the audit are applicable only to that group or location and therefore cannot be generalised to encompass other comparable areas: it is used purely as an evaluative tool and does not require ethical permission.

Service evaluation is a method by which the current service provision is evaluated without any mapping or comparing it against the agreed standards. It therefore utilises a range of methods (e.g. questionnaires, interviews) to establish the current standard of care. The process may involve care providers or service users. It can utilise data from a range of other sources but does not require ethical permission.

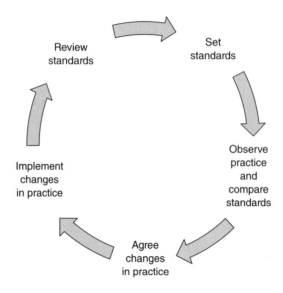

Figure 3.1   The audit cycle (adapted from Sasaru et al. 2005)

ACTIVITY 3.4

During your next placement, ask your mentor about any audit activities that are taking place locally. What is being audited and what standards of practice is it being audited against? Which professionals are involved in the audit?

GLOBAL PERSPECTIVES ON RESEARCH AND EVIDENCE-BASED PRACTICE

Research and evidence-based practice in nursing (and indeed in all healthcare professions) is a well and truly established global phenomena. Most western society healthcare systems have philosophies of continuous service improvement at their core, though perhaps for differing reasons (e.g. clinical effectiveness, accountability, the threat of litigation). These philosophies are apparent in the nature of nursing research globally, with technological advances meaning that access to international research can be sought at the click of a mouse. Just as important as the generation of new knowledge through research is the need to find more effective ways in which research can translate into knowledge use (i.e. closing the gap between what we know (evidence) and what we do (practice): see Chapter 15). This challenge is particularly important in nations where real issues surrounding health inequalities, the lack of a health service infrastructure and poorly performing health services are found (ICN, 2012). In respect to this challenge it would be advisable to read the

International Council of Nurses (ICN) publication *Closing the gap: From evidence to action* (2012) as a precursor to Chapter 15 where the notion of implementation is discussed further. The ICN also supports evidence-based practice through additional publications and the ICN Research Network: this can be accessed at www.icn.ch/networks/research-network/

There are also a number of international organisations that provide support for healthcare providers in implementing care that is based upon a systematic review of available best evidence. In the UK, the Scottish Intercollegiate Guidelines Network (SIGN) and the National Institute for Health and Clinical Excellence (NICE) can supply busy healthcare professionals with advice regarding best practice in relation to a range of health areas. The Cochrane Collaboration is a non-profit making international body which comprises over 28,000 people from over 100 countries, helping professional care providers, patients and policy makers with informed decision making regarding healthcare. Another good example of an organisation which on an international level has made a significant contribution to evidence-based practice is the Joanna Briggs Institute (JBI). This institute is an international non-profit making organisation which is based in Adelaide, Australia. With many centres located across the world, JBI assists healthcare professionals in a number of ways by providing the education and skills required for evidence-based practice:

- Critical appraisal skills.
- Systematic reviews for practice in a range of areas and translating these into practical tools to assist individuals.
- Organisations to embed evidence into policy and practice.
- Best practice guidelines and procedure manuals.

The ultimate aim of this as well as that of other international organisations is the global pursuit of knowledge transfers, the sharing of best practice, and realising the aims of evidence-based practice.

CONCLUSION

Research and the generation of new knowledge that then translates into practice (e.g. in the form of clinical guidelines or local policies) is central to the development of nursing as a profession and a discipline as well as for practice. Key researchers in each of the four fields of nursing continue to engage in research which expands nursing knowledge in each of the four domains cited in this chapter, with the aim of not only enhancing patient care but also enabling learners to develop self-awareness and insights into the ways in which individuals react to illness or recover their health. Not only this, but also the work of key researchers (and in the scope of this chapter, only four have been cited as examples) should inspire future generations of nurses to engage in careers where practice and research are conducted as concurrent activities or where practice and quality improvement strategies take place synonymously. Research and evidence-based practice in nursing are truly international activities.

SUMMARY

The key points for your learning in this chapter include:

- Continuous quality improvement is central to governmental policies on health and health-care provision.
- Nurse researchers have played, and continue to play, a key role in the development of nursing as a profession and a discipline as well as for practice.
- Graduate nurses of the future will be at the forefront of continuous quality improvement and service redesign: leadership skills, research literacy and an understanding of the tools required to achieve clinical effectiveness will be required.

FURTHER READING

Access the Cochrane Collaboration at: www.cochrane.org/about-us
Access JBI at: www.joannabriggs.edu.au/
Access NICE at: www.nice.org.uk/
Access SIGN at: www.sign.ac.uk/

REFERENCES

Barker, P., Jackson, S. and Stevenson, C. (1999a) The need for psychiatric nursing: Towards a multidimensional theory of caring, *Nursing Inquiry*, 6: 103–111.

Barker, P., Leamy, M. and Stevenson, C. (1999b) *Nurses' empowerment of people with enduring forms of mental illness*. Newcastle: Report to the Northern and Yorkshire Regional Research Committee.

Barker, P. and Buchanan-Barker, P. (2005) *The Tidal Model: A guide for mental health professionals*. Hove: Brunner-Routledge.

Carper, B.A. (1978) Fundamental patterns of knowing in nursing, *Advances in Nursing Science*, 1 (1): 13–24.

Clayton, J. (2003) Clinical governance and best value: a toolkit for quality. In S. Pickering and J. Thompson (eds), *Clinical governance and best value: Meeting the modernisation agenda*. Edinburgh: Churchill Livingstone.

Fletcher, E. and Stevenson C. (2001) Launching the Tidal Model in an adult mental health programme, *Nursing Standard*, 15 (49): 33–36.

Gerrish, K. and Lacey, A. (eds) (2010) *The research process in nursing* (6th edition). Oxford: Wiley-Blackwell.

Glasziou, P. (2005) The paths from research to improved health outcomes, *Evidence-based Nursing*, 8: 36–38.

Hek, G. and Moule, P. (2006) *Making sense of research: An introduction for health and social care practitioners* (3rd edition). London: Sage.

International Council of Nurses (ICN) (2012) *Closing the gap: From evidence to action*. Geneva: International Council of Nurses.

Jenkins, R. and Northway, R. (2002) Advocacy and the learning disability nurse, *British Journal of Learning Disabilities*, 30 (1): 8–12.

Llewellyn, P. and Northway, R. (2007) An investigation into the advocacy role of the learning disability nurse, *Journal of Research in Nursing*, 12 (2): 147–161.

Muir Gray, J.A. (2001) *Evidence-based healthcare: How to make policy and managment decisions* (2nd edition). Edinburgh: Churchill Livingstone.

NHS Direct (2012) About research, service evaluation and clinical audit. Available at www.nhsdirect.nhs.uk/Commissioners/WhatWeOffer/ResearchServiceEvaluationClinicalAudit/AboutResearchServiceEvaluationAndClinicalAudit [last accessed 1 June 2012].

NHS Executive (NHSE) (1996) *Promoting clinical effectiveness: A framework for action*. London: NHSE.

Nicol, J. (2011) *Nursing adults with long term conditions*. Exeter: Learning Matters.

Nursing and Midwifery Council (NMC) (2008) *The code: Standards of conduct, performance and ethics for nurses and midwives*. London: NMC.

Nursing and Midwifery Council (NMC) (2010) *Standards for pre-registration nursing education*. London: NMC.

Nutley, S.M., Walter, I. and Davies, H.T.O. (2007) *Using evidence: How research can inform the public services*. Bristol: Policy Press.

Sasaru, R., Sheward, Y. and Sasaru, S. (2005) Audit in allied health professional practice. In T.J. Clouston and L. Westcott (eds), *Working in health and social care*. Edinburgh: Elsevier.

Twycross, A. (2002a) Managing pain in children: an observational study, *Journal of Research in Nursing*, 7 (3): 164–178.

Twycross, A. (2002b) Educating nurses about pain management: the way forward, *Journal of Clinical Nursing*, 11 (6): 705–714.

Twycross, A. (2008) Does the perceived importance of a pain management task affect the quality of children's post-operative pain management practices? *Journal of Clinical Nursing*, 19: 3205–3216.

Twycross, A. (2010) Managing pain in children: where to from here?, *Journal of Clinical Nursing*, 19: 2090–2099.

Young, B.B. (2010) Using the Tidal Model of mental health recovery to plan primary health care for women in residential substance abuse recovery, *Issues in Mental Health Nursing*, 31 (9): 569–575.

PART 2

LET'S MAKE THIS WORK: SKILLS FOR RESEARCH AND EVIDENCE-BASED PRACTICE

PART 3

4

CORE SKILLS FOR RESEARCH AND EVIDENCE-BASED PRACTICE

COLIN MACLEAN AND WINIFRED EBOH

Chapter learning outcomes

On completion of Chapter 4, you will be able to:

1 Relate your experience of the internet to the application of online resources to research.

2 Distinguish the characteristics of sources of information that make them appropriate for use in learning and research.

3 Apply the search functionality offered by Google, Google Advanced Search and Google Scholar to locating internet resources.

4 Recognise some important library information resources and be clear about the identity management systems in place to access them.

5 Appreciate sources of statistical information about the health and wellbeing of populations and their role in understanding and preventing disease.

Key concepts

Internet, worldwide web, social media, search engines, academic publishing, journals, articles, records, databases, open access, authentication, identity management, epidemiology, health statistics.

INTRODUCTION

Surveys consistently show that an overwhelming majority of students will begin their search for academic information using a search engine (Griffiths and Brophy, 2005). This chapter will explore issues about using information resources from the internet, search engines and library databases.

Social networking and micro blogging, synonymous with Facebook and Twitter, occupy 20% of the time that internet users spend online (Comscore, 2011). But what does that statistic tell us? It confirms that Facebook and Twitter are immensely popular. Indeed, you probably use them. They possibly don't seem too relevant in a textbook like this yet they give us access to valid sources of information. If you use Facebook or Twitter there is no need to discount them. What we are suggesting in this chapter is that you think about how to incorporate the academic and scholarly information discussed in this chapter into your 'likes'.

Besides helping you find ways to incorporate the skills that you already have into your academic routine, this chapter will explore additional resources that are available through your university and more widely. The aim here is to enhance your ability to identify useful sources of information and to streamline approaches to searching so that you can more easily tap into the wealth of information that is readily available. Related to this important area of skill development, we will provide an early introduction to statistics and their use within nursing and healthcare research. You will then go on to explore statistics and epidemiology in more detail as you progress through the textbook, but our experience tells us that an incremental approach to the development of statistical knowledge is helpful to many students.

We shall start by analysing resources that you may already be familiar with before going on to discuss additional resources.

INTERNET SOURCES FOR LEARNING

Wikipedia

For most people it is a need for information that leads them to the internet. The web has replaced the role of encyclopaedias and other sources of reference information. *Encyclopaedia Britannica* used to be a set of volumes that households aspired to own (Jack, 2012) as an authoritative source of knowledge, but today it is no longer available to buy in printed form. It is still authoritative, but with Wikipedia omnipresent and free online it is hard to see a need for anything else for fact checking. Some research published in the journal *Nature* suggests Wikipedia is just as reliable as the *Encylopaedia Britannica* (Giles, 2005). Note however that the wiki content creation process is an interesting one, so it is you who must decide whether or not it is flawed.

The eleventh edition of *Britannica*, published between 1910–11, was highly regarded because it contained contributions from eminent scholars of the time and was the first edition to have contributions from women writers. It is no longer a wholly reliable source of information but it still offers a fascinating insight into the state of knowledge in the early part of the twentieth century. Florence Nightingale died in 1910 and the article on 'Nursing' is interesting to read 101 years on (Lovetoknow, 2006a) as are other articles on health and disease. We will return to *Britannica* later in this chapter.

Wikipedia could not have existed in an equivalent printed format. It is wholly a creation of the web. It is a 'wiki' which means anyone can contribute to it, placing its authoritativeness in question. People worry about Wikipedia. At university you might be advised not to refer to or use it for projects and essays at all. Bear in mind that your tutor is looking for you to use information from lots of different sources wisely, critically and creatively in order to support your own written ideas. Wikipedia might help you get started, and will probably give you some helpful links, but you will need to go beyond it. Below are two activities for you to undertake: the first one could be a group exercise, and the second is one that you will come back to as you work your way through this chapter.

One advantage that Wikipedia has over printed encyclopaedias is to provide direct links to hundreds of other articles and references that, were you to follow them, would give you enough information to help validate the Wikipedia article. Create a discussion around the statement, 'Wikipedia – love it or hate it'. Have someone facilitate and gather statements from the group (for example, five things for and against), and try and arrive at a balanced conclusion.

If you can't do this in a group, brainstorm the discussion points and come up with your own conclusion.

ACTIVITY 4.1

Now think of an area of practice that you are particularly interested in. As you work your way through the activities in this chapter, make a note of the resources that come up as you use each of the search approaches. For example, you might want to find out more about breast cancer or adolescent mental health issues. Whatever terms you use, analyse the types of information/evidence that are made available to you through your searching (more on the analysis of evidence later):

ACTIVITY 4.2

(Continued)

(Continued)

- Wikipedia:
- Google:
- Google Advanced Search:
- Google Scholar:

Google

The internet didn't arrive on our screens fully developed. The usefulness of the web relies first of all on people creating content: text, images, video and file attachments. Search engines allow us to search that content. You might be familiar with Yahoo Search or Bing, but for most people the number one search engine is Google (Alexa, 2012). Google is an innovative company, founded as recently as 1998 by Larry Page and Sergey Brin (Google, 2012a). Google is a search-friendly place and among its company values you will find this:

> Even if you don't know exactly what you're looking for, finding an answer on the web is our problem, not yours. (Google, 2012b)

Google carries out hundreds of thousands of searches every minute (Crowd Science, 2011) so let's try one now. You are probably familiar with a UK healthcare body called NICE (the National Institute for Health and Clinical Excellence). NICE exists to 'help those working in the NHS, local authorities and the wider community deliver high-quality healthcare' and 'develop evidence-based guidelines on the most effective ways to diagnose, treat and prevent disease and ill health' (NICE, 2012). If you try a search on Google for 'nice' (no double quotes necessary), the National Institute for Health and Clinical Excellence comes out top of the list. Similarly 'nice organisation' does the same. While 'organisation' and 'body' in this context are synonymous ('nice body' as a search phrase produces quite different results!), Box 4.1 provides an overview of the way in which search strategies are developed through the use of keywords and phrases.

Box 4.1   Practice vignette

Search Strategies 1: Keywords and phrases

Sometimes 'organisation' is spelled 'organization' or is known as 'a body'. In the English language it is quite common for a word to have a different spelling in US English and British English. It is also quite common for different words to mean much the same thing. These are called *synonyms*. Computers can help you spot them but really it is a task for you to think about in your searches. Search engines generally don't recognise the differences between **cases** either, so that search-wise there is no difference between 'nice' and 'NICE'. *Abbreviations* are also common in all walks of life and are prevalent in medicine, health and social care, although the Nursing and Midwifery Council specifically recommend that they should not be used in patient documentation (Wood, 2003).

Singular, plural, past and present / future forms of words may occur and be relevant to a search. In English we can use a method called 'stemming' to pick up many of these forms at once: for example, 'nurse', 'nurses', 'nursed', 'nursing' could all be retrieved by using the stem 'nurs'. You will notice this when typing if search engines enable 'type ahead' or with predictive text on your phone. In search engines you can achieve it by cutting the characters of the word back to the common stem. You do this with an asterisk, *, – like this: 'nurs*'. Google and Google Scholar will automatically apply stemming.

As you search, other words will emerge during the process and these words may end up being even more important than the ones you started with.

You may wish at this point to go back to the area of practice that you identified in Activity 4.2 and consider ways in which you could use some of the techniques described here to enhance your search.

Google Advanced Search

Often when we use Google we will be trying to find a specific website. Google is built in such a way that it uses information gathered from trillions of searches to make predictions about what you are searching for. You can take Google into a different arena however by making use of its advanced features. Google 'Advanced Search' is available from a link in the gear wheel at the top right of the Google home page and offers to find pages with the following criteria:

All of these words	The exact word or phrase	Any of these words	None of these words	Numbers in a range

The number of results may be further refined:

- By language.
- Sourced from a geographical region.
- By when it was last updated.
- From a particular website or domain.
- By where the text appears on the page.

Finally, filters permit the exclusion of website content that wouldn't be suitable for people under 18, reading level, file type and so on. It's not necessary to apply these search tools together at one time. Just consider their effects and think of them as approaches or strategies you might adopt when searching the web.

Google Scholar

Depending on your previous experiences, you may or may not be familiar with academic journals. An academic journal article is a text – the length can vary from very short pieces of one A4 page or less through to extended articles of 20 to 30 pages. Estimates suggest there are around 50 million published scholarly articles in existence (Jinha, 2010). Academics employed by universities and health services are the wellspring of this material. When people talk about 'literature searching', it is this collection of articles and the body of scholarly publishing in the fields of science, technology and medicine that they mean.

Google Scholar is a great place to start to become familiar with journal articles. You can use Google itself to lead you to Google Scholar through the scholarly article links that it suggests, or go directly to the Google Scholar website which features an Advanced Search, matching:

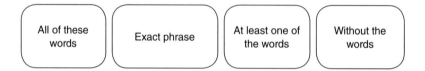

Google Scholar works with websites developed by academic and scholarly publishers to bring resources straight to your desktop. The names of some publishers will crop up again and again as you search – SAGE, the publisher of this book, is one. Wiley, Elsevier, Taylor and Francis, Springer, and the Oxford and Cambridge University Presses are others. Their published output is immensely important and is the essence of what is truly known about the world. Google Scholar reaches deep into this body of knowledge and it is impossible to overstate its significance. Box 4.2 takes you into a further stage of searching – the use of Boolean operators.

Box 4.2   Practice vignette

Search Strategies 2: Boolean operators

Google Advanced Search and Google Scholar Advanced Search options for 'all of the words', 'at least one of the words' and 'without the words' are techniques that can be applied in most search engines and library databases. Most books that refer to literature searching and searching for evidence (e.g. Roberts and Priest, 2010: 65) call these techniques 'Boolean operators'. 'Boolean operators' are simply the words 'AND', 'OR' and 'NOT'. They have a direct equivalent to three of the options offered by either Google or Google Scholar, so:

1 'all of the words' = AND
2 'at least one of the words' = OR
3 'without the words' = NOT

To put it crudely, AND narrows a search and makes the results more relevant to the question; OR broadens a search and makes some of the results less relevant but includes some results you might otherwise miss; NOT also narrows a search by excluding a word/phrase that you are not likely to need and which could otherwise lead to you finding results that are not relevant. From a practical point of view AND is by far the most useful of these, OR has occasional applications, and it is unlikely you would ever need NOT.

The academic publishing business

The commercial publishers mentioned above dominate the market for academic journals. You may see copies of their publications on the shelves of some of the high street bookshops in their specialist sections, but university, health service and research libraries also buy them to support the work of their academics, clinicians and students. It is a kind of symbiotic arrangement that has stood the test of time. Nowadays the medium is largely a web-based electronic one and it has become less common for the print equivalent to be found on library shelves, at least for the current content. You will be strongly encouraged to read and use information from journal sources in your work at university. In fact access to them is one of the privileges of being a student and will be encouraged, as using resources wisely is a strategy that will more or less guarantee success.

The greatest proportion of spending by universities in the UK on their libraries is on electronic journals (Economist, 2011). To put a figure on it, in 2010 JISC (Joint Information Systems Committee – JISC champions the use of digital technologies in UK education and research) reported that university libraries in the UK were spending up to £121,000,000 on these resources (Look and Spark, 2010). The need for more open and free access has exerted a pressure on the publishing industry that is bringing about quite rapid changes. New approaches to scholarly publishing, such as Open Access (JISC, 2010), offer alternatives to the commercial approach (Wellcome Trust, 2011). Open Access cannot yet rival the commercial relationship that exists among publishers, scholars and libraries, but there are notable successes where the quality of freely available published output is considered to be just as good academically. Biomed Central and the Public Library of Science are two examples of bodies leading the way in promoting open access to research.

e-Journals from publisher databases, e-journal content and inter-library loans

Each publisher owns its own content and many have developed websites where that content can be accessed. Some also licence their content to other information providers. These kinds of websites are known as bibliographic databases and many are accessible to Google Scholar searches. Generally you are able to read only a restricted amount of information, namely the bibliographic details of the article (the information you would use to create a reference) and possibly an abstract or summary of its contents. Accessing the entire article, known as the full text, often requires the payment of a fee. Box 4.3 explains the use of bibliographic databases. Once you feel comfortable with this information, complete Activity 4.3.

Box 4.3   Case study: Bibliographic databases

Databases that consist of structured information about books, journals, journal articles and other equivalent types of publication are called bibliographic databases. A bibliography is a list of works (i.e. books and so on). A library catalogue and Google Scholar are examples of bibliographic databases.

Books and journal article data consist of fields (author, title, edition, year of publication, place of publication, publisher – in the case of books: author, article title, journal title, year of publication, volume, part and page numbers – for journal articles).

Bibliographic databases may contain other information. Often included are lists or tables of content and short summaries about the content of a book (i.e. what it is about). The summaries are referred to as abstracts. Sometimes keywords used in the book are also offered, again to briefly represent what the content of the work is about. Other descriptions may be added, so that bookshops, libraries and online retailers can categorise the book in question, so that other books about the same or similar topics can be found together by a person browsing on the bookshop or library shelves.

For 'books' read 'works' because what we are talking about may just as well be physical objects such as DVDs or videos, or electronic documents such as a file from a website, a journal article, an image jpg file, or a guideline published in a pdf format. A word often used in the context of education to describe these is 'resources'.

ACTIVITY 4.3

It is important for you, as a learner, to be aware of the varied resources that are available to assist with your learning. List the types of resources and file formats you encounter in your learning environment:

The internet has raised expectations about what is available online. Your university library won't be able to give you direct access to everything, but it will offer a service called 'inter-library loans' where you can request that a book or copy of an article be obtained for you from another library in the network. Check locally with library staff to find out how the service works.

University, college and NHS authentication for library resources

Because most university journal subscriptions are now online, university libraries are able to provide access to these only to students and staff of their own institution. NHS services also provide access to journals but again the access is for NHS staff, students and partners only. Once enrolled on a university course you will be given a user ID and password and shown how to use these to login to the network, email, student portal, the Virtual Learning Environment and the library. One user ID and password will often serve to give you access to everything. The actual systems in place will vary but the facilities offered will be more or less consistent with those discussed here.

The range of internet addresses (IP addresses) used by campus computers and wireless networks will have been registered with publishers and others providing online journals and databases, so anyone logged in on campus can have direct access to online journal articles. An easy way to access the journals that the library has paid subscriptions for is to try Google Scholar on campus. Check if 'library links' has been enabled on Google Scholar. If it has you will also be able to set this up for when you are not on campus so that you can tell which articles are directly accessible without having to go on campus to do it or double check the library catalogue. This means you can do journal article research work at home or on placement.

A valid campus IP address is proof for the provider of electronic resources that the person accessing it is genuinely permitted to do so. However, because of the internet and new ways of delivering courses online students are studying off campus just as much as on. For this reason there are methods of identity management that vouch for the authenticity of students' affiliation when they are away from campus altogether. So long as the internet is available, access to learning materials and the library online is assured using identity management systems such as Athens. The Athens administration system is available to universities and other organisations to enable access to subscribed electronic resources for their students and staff. Usually administered by library staff, users are required to register and are then given an Athens user ID and password. When presented with a link to a full text journal article the user clicks on 'Athens login', supplies their Athens credentials in the boxes provided and gets access, provided the affiliated organisation has a paid-up subscription.

The Athens system is relatively simple to use and because it authenticates to networked library resources which have no association to patient records or confidential data online, it is the identity management solution favoured by the NHS in the UK. In universities, systems were developed that used Athens for authentication but built on the fact that students already had a university user ID and password that provided proof of their affiliation. More recently, universities have begun to adopt a different identity management system called Shibboleth. Shibboleth is often paired with Athens and labelled 'Athens/Institutional login' on publisher websites. It is important to be clear about the authentication systems your university library uses and practise following the links to access the resources available. At this point you need to complete Activity 4.4.

ACTIVITY 4.4

Go back to your findings from Activity 4.2 and update your search using your university and/or NHS library resources. Once you have done this, you could draw together all your findings into a bibliographic list that will enable you to easily access the resources in future if you wish to do so. You can, at this point, also determine which of the search approaches has provided you with access to resources that are of the standard required for academic work and evidence-based practice.

Internet and library research databases

Twenty years ago, to undertake any kind of literature search you would have needed to use a library that had within its collection publications called 'abstracts and indexes', which are a type of publication that contained detailed lists of journal articles, arranged by different indexed lists, usually for author, title and subject. These had names like 'Index Medicus', 'Cumulative Index of Nursing and Allied Health Literature', 'Applied Social Science Index and Abstracts' and 'Excerpta Medica', and occupied hundreds of metres of library shelves. This type of publication could be readily adapted for computer searching. Computer disks took up a fraction of the space, and with search software designed with the end-user in mind, bibliographic records could be readily retrieved, saved, and results printed. Improved computer networks later resulted in networked equivalents, where files were hosted online and licensed as services to which organisations could subscribe. The abstracting and indexing sources listed above are now known as the databases Medline, CINAHL, Assia, and Embase. They are fully online files, hosted by companies such as Ovid, Ebsco and Thomson Reuters, who in turn have developed sophisticated software tools that make comprehensive literature searching a realistic prospect for anyone at university.

Paralleling the growth in accessibility of academic and scholarly information to the professional community has been the availability of consumer health information. From the United States the National Library of Medicine (NLM) published the Medline database to the world free and online, under the name PubMed, in 1997 (National Library of Medicine, 1997). The NLM also enabled a gateway to other information databases owned by the National Center for Biotechnology Information and the US National Institutes of Health. There are links to all three organisations from the PubMed home page. There are also links to full text where this is freely available, from open access journals or where the publisher has allowed free access.

The NLM also lease the database contents of PubMed by the name of Medline. It is as Medline that the database will be made available from your university library. NLM leases Medline to Ebsco, Ovid and Proquest among others, who in turn combine the database with leased online journal packages from other academic publishers to make the combined product available as 'Medline with Full Text', where full text is attached to the bibliographic information as pdf or html files. Your university library may also offer this resource.

The contents of an individual database represent a slice of the published literature, not the whole. How much of the published literature the slice represents is hard to picture but some facts may help:

- Medline indexes the contents of more than 4,000 journal titles from 1966.
- CINAHL has over 1,200 journal titles indexed since 1982.
- Web of Knowledge has over 5,500 journals since 1945.

Some journals are uniquely indexed for each database, others are not, so that records for the same articles may be retrieved from different databases. Therefore to obtain results about a topic, and be confident of having retrieved most of what is relevant, you will need to search more than one database. This is standard practice for a literature review. Box 4.4 below deals with a further step in searching for evidence.

Box 4.4   Practice vignette

Search Strategies 3: An approach to clinical questions

Jo is a 35 year old woman with a BMI of 19. She suffers chronic low back pain for which she takes the maximum permissible daily dose of painkillers. These can be effective but she worries about the amount of medication and is genuinely interested in other strategies to manage the pain.

We can try to help Jo. Begin by formulating a clinical question based on the scenario, *Does the use of alternative therapies in the treatment of patients with non-specific lower back pain lead to improved pain control?*

You need to search for answers here so you will require keywords/phrases. The keywords in this question are: *alternative therapies, treatment, patients, non-specific lower back pain, improved pain control.* The key phrases are: 'alternative therapies'; 'non-specific lower back pain'; 'pain control'.

Google Scholar can easily handle all of the keywords in a single search, or a combined keyword phrase search, each of which is a valid approach, but you can also think about others:

(Continued)

(Continued)

1 'All of the words': alternative therapies treatment patients non-specific lower back pain improved control.

2 'All of the words': treatment patients non-specific lower back pain improved control AND 'Exact phrase' alternative therapies.

The components can often be deconstructed using the mnemonic PICO. Various definitions exist about what the letters stand for – something you can research yourself – but these are adaptable. This is how it works and the search strategies it leads to:

Table 4.1   PICO

P	I	C	O
Patient	Intervention	Control	Outcome
Patient with lower back pain	Alternative therapies	None	Improved pain control
Search for: 'low back pain'	Search for: 'alternative therapies'	No search terms	Search for: 'pain control'
Synonyms?	Synonyms?	Synonyms?	Synonyms?

'Control' could be a comparison with, say, painkillers. CINAHL and Medline don't work as well as Google Scholar for long strings of keywords. The phrases in this scenario would be good, but the danger of combining all three with AND would perhaps be to find no results. Searching for 'alternative therapies' in the context of (i.e. AND) 'low back pain' would be sufficiently precise. The search software will help work out synonyms. Have a plan, but keep track of what you are doing and modify that plan according to what you find.

Stating the method by which you set about a task is itself academic, scientific, and systematic. Fully realised, the process and its writing up are known as a 'systematic literature review'. For such a review, the choice of databases demonstrates the scope of the coverage of the literature undertaken. The selection of keywords and phrases and their combinations demonstrate the thought process about the question being researched. Simple record-keeping techniques, such as noting the number of records returned by the searches and the duplication of results from the different databases, help build the methodology. Analysis of the abstracts and appraisal of the published papers themselves enable a judgment to be made about the quality of what is known about the question being asked. Not every question requires a literature review, but having this understanding of the process will allow you to adopt as much or as little of it as you need to address a research question with confidence.

There are some organisations whose publications or resources you can turn to where this process has already been undertaken, as discussed previously in Chapter 3. NICE, Scottish Intercollegiate Guidelines Network (SIGN), the Cochrane Collaboration and the Joanna Briggs Institute (JBI) provide excellent authoritative resources where evidence has been assessed and turned into forms of advice that you can rely on. JBI Connect may be available as a subscription through your library but the others are free on the internet.

JBI and online information providers Ebsco, Ovid and Proquest are leading information providers whose database and full text journal packages libraries subscribe to. Ebsco publishes the CINAHL database (the letter 'C' at the beginning is pronounced 'S'). Like Medline, CINAHL is published as a database in its own right but also in conjunction with full text from Ebsco in two 'flavours' (as CINAHL with Full Text or CINAHL Plus with Full Text). Your university library or the health service that supports your practice placement will offer CINAHL in one of these forms. CINAHL is the most important source of research knowledge in the field of nursing and one of the most important health-related databases of all, alongside Medline.

If your library or health service doesn't offer either CINAHL or Medline with full text, it is very likely that they will provide a linking facility (the same linking facility that is used for library links in Google Scholar, often labelled as 'Find it @ my University' or 'Full Text @ my University').

We are now going to introduce you to statistics and epidemiology in a way that fits together with the skills you have developed so far through your reading and the activities in this chapter. We aim to help you to see their significance within the context of your practice so that when you come on to more in-depth learning later in this book, you will feel confident with some of the terminology and its application to practice.

STATISTICS AND EPIDEMIOLOGY

The 1911 *Encyclopaedia Britannica* (Lovetoknow, 2006b) has a section that lists diseases, describing the state of contemporary knowledge. The article on diabetes described the prevalence of the disease by believing it to be hereditary, more likely to occur in towns and cities than in the country, and most common among Jewish people. Excessive consumption of sugar was considered a cause although observers believed that obesity itself was culpable. According to the *Encyclopaedia* it occurred in people of all ages, although most commonly in adult white males aged 50 years and older.

It was possible to make these assertions because of the systematic collection of data about patients and the diseases, and the creation of what we would know nowadays as databases. Information about the population of a community, such as that collected by registers of deaths or a national census, allowed agencies to form questions and help establish patterns from which the variables exerting influence over public health could be extrapolated. There are striking health differences among populations: factors such as age, gender, ethnicity, geography, income and education have a part to play, before even adding on behavioural ones like smoking, diet, exercise and alcohol. Knowledge about how these factors influence health is obtained through applying statistical analysis techniques to data collected by health service authorities, and national and international health agencies. Box 4.5 links the use of databases with epidemiology.

Box 4.5   Databases and epidemiology

The rows and columns in a spreadsheet offer powerful possibilities in terms of sorting data. These rows and columns become fields and records in databases. The structured form of databases support query language, allowing the records to be browsed or searched. A database could be used to list women who live in Aberdeen, are aged between 20 and 30, are unemployed, and have one or more children. Spelled out for a computer to understand, the question would look something like this:

- Gender equals female.
- Address contains 'Aberdeen'.
- Age equal to or greater than 20 and less than or equal to 30.
- Employment equals no.
- Children greater than or equal to 1.

In healthcare research, statistical information can reveal a great deal about the social structure of a city, for example. Mapping other layers of data about ethnicity, household income, attendance at healthcare centres, education and so on enables complex pictures of the population and the drivers influencing health outcomes to be understood. The study of the health of populations is called epidemiology and is fundamental to the concept of public health.

Statistical analysis in healthcare is used to differentiate real risk factors from those that would happen by chance. Using statistics to explain the incidence and prevalence of disease and predict its spread in populations is part of the role of epidemiologists. It also has an important part to play for public health practitioners, including nurses. Epidemiology makes sense of health data, calculates 'risk', and provides a sound scientific background to how we contain and manage diseases in populations.

Epidemiology originally focused on the spread of infectious diseases. The origins of the science stem from the work of the Ancient Greek physician Hippocrates (c470–360 B.C.), who suggested that the occurrence of disease was due to the environment and behaviours, a scientific opinion that was held in stark contrast to the contemporary view that supernatural influences were the cause. Last century, epidemiologists moved beyond the study of infectious diseases to diseases of behaviour, ones that could be influenced by knowledge and attitudes: for example, the 1911 *Encyclopaedia Britannica* recognised obesity as a factor in the prevalence of diabetes. A significant landmark here was a study by Doll and Hill (1950) that linked smoking with lung cancer. Today, lifestyle factors dominate the health agenda due to their impact on cardiovascular disease and the global surge of type 2 diabetes.

Media reports of research studies regularly emerge suggesting that, for example, certain foods contain nutrients that can reduce the risk of heart disease, or that regular reasonably energetic exercise helps prevent heart disease. Nurses talk to patients about health issues so it is important to ensure that advice is based on information that is as reliable as it can be. Throughout this chapter we emphasise the importance of finding and using information from authoritative sources to validate your knowledge. When you read articles and consider statistical data it is important to be critically aware of bias, chance, and confounding factors.

Lanoë (2002) defines bias as a tendency to present results that do not reflect a true picture. Bias comes from the researcher, from the sample or the statistical method. You can probably assume that all research will contain some degree of bias. However, it is important that the researcher has put measures in place to minimise its effects. For example, it is recognised that the random selection of participants in a clinical trial is crucial to exclude the partiality of the research team. Organisations like the BBC have a reputation for fairness and accuracy, a reputation that applies to its health and lifestyle reporting as much as it does to political news. A BBC Online report, from December 2011, stated that:

> Nearly half of cancers diagnosed in the UK each year – over 130,000 in total – are caused by avoidable life choices including smoking, drinking and eating the wrong things, a review reveals. (Roberts, 2011)

That the BBC chose to highlight research that itself stemmed from a journal article published in an authoritative source (the *British Journal of Cancer*) lends credibility to the story. In fact there seems little doubt that eating a balanced diet, taking regular exercise and achieving a work/life balance will help improve health. Nevertheless it is vital to look beyond the media story to find out more about the methods employed by the researchers. Questions that may be asked are: what measures were used, were measurement errors accounted for, or could the results have arisen by chance alone? Doubt about the methods employed could mean reliable conclusions cannot be drawn and applied to the wider population. Presumably the BBC ran the story because the reporter believed that the editors of the *British Journal of Cancer* wouldn't have published the article if the methods that the researchers employed hadn't been sound. The important thing is to apply critical awareness to this chain of events and the validity of the factors on which the assumption is based.

Statisticians make predictions based on samples of the population (we will discuss samples and some of the other terminology used in this chapter in greater depth as you progress through the textbook). Even the most carefully selected sample may be subject to potential bias. In articles you will see the sample size described using a capital letter or lower case 'N', for example $N = 1503$ or $n = 64$. Because of sampling there will always be some uncertainty in the results of scientific predictions (Simon, updated by Forland, 2008). Probability is the science used to determine whether or not something is likely to happen. The probability, or p value, gives an indication of whether an occurrence in a sample being studied is likely to have happened by chance or is evidence of an effect. A p value at or below 0.05 is said to demonstrate evidence that the effect occurred as a result of a cause and said to be statistically significant. Epidemiologists express the probability of occurrences in terms of confidence intervals. These are a range of values that attempts to give a more realistic appraisal of the probability of an occurrence being more than just chance. The narrower the confidence intervals, the greater the likelihood that the effect being measured is supported by evidence. However, wider intervals mean the evidence becomes less reliable and any inferences based on it are more likely to be flawed.

Other statistical considerations worth noting at this point include *confounding* variables which are factors that are more difficult to eliminate from a study. For example, while we may say with certainty that smoking causes lung cancer (Peto et al., 2000) we can also observe that lung cancer does not occur among the entire population of smokers and does occur among non-smokers too. Other factors which cannot always be controlled, including genetics and the environment, may also contribute to the incidence of the disease. Statistics give a fascinating insight and are also fundamental to an understanding of nursing. We will consider statistical test methods in more depth in Chapter 8 and Chapter 12, but their influence on the data sourced to inform practice needs to be understood by practitioners in order to make informed decisions.

EPIDEMIOLOGICAL DATA AND HEALTH POLICY

Statistical data inform policy (NICE, 2009) and are reflected in best practice documents such as those published by bodies like NICE and SIGN. Policy is also driven by evidence obtained from clinical trials and the economic realities of affordable and effective interventions. The absence of epidemiology data can pose problems for health service planning. For example, cancer registries do not record the incidence of Basal Cell Carcinoma (BCC) in England and Wales. The absence of data means that the prevalence of this condition is unknown (NICE, 2010). Without such data, the patterns for this form of cancer cannot be determined. Examples of this include the increase in the prevalence of skin cancer amongst young girls: this information provides an insight into the desire among teenagers for cosmetically tanned skin. Consequently, with the lack of data about the cancerous effect of exposure to ultraviolet radiation and evidence-based public health messages, young people were unknowingly putting themselves at exceptional risk of disease (Cokkinides et al., 2002).

In contrast, monitoring the prevalence of type 1 and 2 diabetes is heavily reliant on epidemiological data. These data provide useful insights into the pattern of disease, the age groups that experience the highest incidence, the factors that contribute to this and how targeted health education can help reduce it. The existence of epidemiological data for the incidence and prevalence of disease across a population gives governments the necessary information to plan and budget for healthcare services and allocate more resources to areas with the greatest risks. The final activity below offers you the opportunity to explore an area of practice that is of particular interest to you.

Think about a disease that is relevant to your field of practice and find out some information relating to the epidemiology of the disease and the impact that this knowledge has on current practice.

ACTIVITY 4.5

SUMMARY

Critical points for your learning from this chapter are:

- Sources of information vary in terms of their reliability and it is always good practice to validate one source against others.
- Even authoritative sources have a threshold of accuracy that diminishes over time. Good healthcare demands practice based on the best evidence available from the current state of knowledge.
- Sharing information through research publications and statistical data opens it to scrutiny. Learn to recognise the values that help you to evaluate and trust the sources you use.
- Statistics and epidemiology are sources of evidence that can lead to the development of health policy and also impact on nursing and healthcare practice.

FURTHER READING

Biomed Central: www.biomedcentral.com/
Cochrane Summaries (an approachable gateway to evidence of the effectiveness of healthcare interventions): http://summaries.cochrane.org/
Encyclopedia Britannica 1911 edition (Nursing topic): www.1911encyclopedia.org/Nursing
Google Scholar: http://scholar.google.co.uk/
NICE Guidance (a gateway to clinical guidelines): http://guidance.nice.org.uk
Public Library of Science (PLOS): www.plos.org/
PubMed: www.ncbi.nlm.nih.gov/pubmed
US National Library of Medicine (NLM): www.nlm.nih.gov/
World Health Organization: www.who.int/en/

REFERENCES

Alexa (2012) Google.com. [online] Oakland, CA. Alexa Internet Inc. Available from: www.alexa.com/siteinfo/google.com+yahoo.com+altavista.com (last accessed 1 June 2012).

Cokkinides, V.E., Weinstock, M.A., Connell, M.C. and Thun, M.J. (2002) Use of indoor tanning sunlamps by US youth, ages 11–18 years, and by their parent or guardian caregivers: prevalence and correlates, *Pediatrics*, 109 (6): 1124–1130.

Comscore (2011) It's a social world: Social networking leads as top online activity globally, accounting for 1 in every 5 online minutes. [online] Reston, VA: Comscore. Available from: www.comscore.com/Insights/Press_Releases/2011/12/Social_Networking_Leads_as_Top_Online_Activity_Globally (last accessed 1 June 2012).

Gizmodo (2011) What happens in 60 seconds on the Internet. [online] Available from: http://gizmodo.com/5813875/what-happens-in-60-seconds-on-the-internet (last accessed 19 August 2013).

Doll, R. and Hill, A. B. (1950) Smoking and carcinoma of the lung, *British Medical Journal*, 2 (4682): 739–748.

Economist (2011) Of goats and headaches: one of the best media businesses is also one of the most resented, *Economist*, May 26.

Forland, L. (2008) Category: Confidence intervals, Category: Statistical evidence. [online] Available from: www.childrensmercy.org/stats/journal/confidence.aspx (last accessed 1 June 2012).

Giles, J. (2005) Wikipedia rival calls in the experts, *Nature*, 443 (493), published online 4 October. http://news.bbc.co.uk/1/hi/technology/4530930.stm (last accessed 1 June 2012).

Google (2012a) Google's mission is to organise the world's information and make it universally accessible and useful. [online] Mountain View, CA: Google. Available from: www.google.co.uk/about/corporate/company/ (last accessed 1 June 2012).

Google (2012b) Our philosophy: Ten things we know to be true. [online] Mountain View, CA: Google. Available from: www.google.com/about/company/tenthings.html (last accessed 1 June 2012).

Griffiths, J.R. and Brophy, P. (2005) Student searching behavior and the web: Use of academic resources and Google, *Library Trends*, 53 (4): 539–554. [online] Available from: http://hdl.handle.net/2142/1749 (last accessed 1 June 2012).

Icerocket (2012) Latintos: When in doubt: look it up. [online] Reno, NV: Axel.

Jack, I. (2012) Printed encyclopedias were once a rare source of knowledge: but no more. [online] *The Guardian*, 16 March, p. 37. Available from: www.guardian.co.uk/commentisfree/2012/mar/16/encyclopedia-britannica-sum-of-human-knowledge (last accessed 1 June 2012).

Jinha, A. F. (2010) Article 50 million: An estimate of the number of scholarly articles in existence, *Learned Publishing*, 23(3): 258–263.

JISC (2010) Open access. [online] London: JISC. Available from: www.jisc.ac.uk/openaccess (last accessed 1 June 2012).

Lanoë, N. (2002) *Ogier's reading research: how to make research more approachable.* London: Ballière-Tindall.

Look, H. and Spark, S. (2010) The value of UK HEIs to the publishing process: Summary report. [online] London: JISC Collections. Available from: www.jisc-collections.ac.uk/Global/report%20on%20HEIs%20non-cash%20contribution%20to%20the%20journal%20publishing%20process%20final.pdf (last accessed 1 June 2012).

Lovetoknow (2006a) 1911 Classic Encyclopaedia: Nursing. [online] Available from: www.1911encyclopedia.org/Nursing (last accessed 1 March 2012).

Lovetoknow (2006b) 1911 Classic Encyclopaedia: Disease. [online] Available from: www.1911encyclopedia.org/Category:Disease (last accessed 1 June 2012).

National Library Of Medicine (NLM) (1997) Free web-based access to NLM databases. [online] NLM Technical Bulletin, May–June, 296. Washington, DC: NLM. Available from: www.nlm.nih.gov/pubs/techbull/mj97/mj97_web.html (last accessed 1 June 2012).

NICE (2009) Methods for the development of NICE public health guidance (2nd edition). [online] www.nice.org.uk/media/2FB/53/PHMethodsManual110509.pdf (last accessed 1 June 2012).

NICE (2010) Individual research recommendation details. [online] www.nice.org.uk/research/index.jsp?action=researchando=2176 (last accessed 1 June 2012).

NICE (2012) What we do. [online] Available from: www.nice.org.uk/aboutnice/whatwedo/what_we_do.jsp (last accessed 1 June 2012).

Oberdan, T. (2009) Google and Gödel, *Bulletin of Science, Technology and Society*, 29 (6): 464–469.

Peto, R., Darby, S., Deo, H., Silcocks P. et al. (2000) Smoking, smoking cessation, and lung cancer in the UK since 1950: Combination of national statistics with two case-control studies, *BMJ*, 321 (7257): 323–329.

Roberts, M. (2011) Over 40% of cancers due to lifestyle, says review. [online] Available from: www.bbc.co.uk/news/health-16031149 (last accessed 1 June 2012).

Roberts, P. and Priest, H. (2010) *Healthcare research: A textbook for students and practitioners*. Chichester: John Wiley.

SIGN (2010) Management of diabetes – A national clinical guideline. [online] Available from: www.sign.ac.uk/pdf/sign116.pdf (last accessed 1 June 2012).

Wellcome Trust (2011) *Position statement in support of open and unrestricted access to published research*. [online] London: Wellcome Trust. Available from: www.wellcome.ac.uk/About-us/Policy/Policy-and-position-statements/WTD002766.htm (last accessed 1 June 2012).

Wood, C. (2003) The importance of good record-keeping for nurses, *Nursing Times*, 99 (2): 26.

5

POLICY IN RESEARCH AND EVIDENCE-BASED PRACTICE

DAVE ADAMS

Chapter learning outcomes

On completion of Chapter 5, you will be able to:

1 Understand what is meant by the term 'policy'.
2 Appreciate the importance of policy in relation to health and healthcare.
3 Understand the relationship between policy analysis and evidence-based practice.
4 Outline the formats in which research evidence is used in health policy documents.
5 Discuss some of the ways in which research evidence is used in health policy documents.

Key concepts

Policy, policy drivers, policy analysis, policy process, context of policy, use of research evidence.

INTRODUCTION

I have found that using the words 'policy' and 'research' in the same sentence can be a risky business from a lecturer's perspective – students' eyes start to glaze over and you can sense the will to live slipping away at the thought of the lecture to follow. However, much to their surprise and my delight, many students go on to find that not only is the subject more interesting than they had expected, but also that the content has a practical application that continues to be of use to them in their future careers.

The intent of this chapter then, is to help you to gain an understanding of the links between policy and research and to appreciate their potential to impact on clinical practice. I will use relevant examples from current policy documents to illustrate the discussion and consider the real world implications of the sometimes tenuous relationship between policy and research.

The chapter is broken down into four sections with the first section providing an overview of what policy is – just so you are clear what it is I am talking about. The second section gives some insight into the importance of policy to the philosophy, organisation, and delivery of healthcare. After all, you can't be expected to appreciate the importance of research in this context if you are not convinced that there is a need for policy in the first place.

The third section considers the relationship between policy analysis and research and evidence-based practice. Here I look at how the ability to critique policy can help you identify where and how research has played a part in its development. The final section looks at the kind of research and evidence that policy makers use, bringing into play relevant policy from the four countries of the United Kingdom.

As you work through the material in this chapter keep in mind that, just like research, policy has its own jargon too. Remember, however, that no-one is expecting you to be fluent in two new languages at the end of this chapter – just to be familiar with a few key concepts that will make you feel more comfortable in working with this kind of material (the academic equivalent of being able to ask for directions, order drinks or a meal, or find out where the toilets are on a holiday abroad!). I am aiming to enable you to add to your understanding, increase your enjoyment, and prevent embarrassment!

WHAT IS MEANT BY 'POLICY'?

To appreciate the importance of policy to health and healthcare you first need to be clear about just what is meant by the term 'policy'. It does tend to be one of those concepts that mean different things to different people, so I have developed a working definition as a focus for this chapter. There are a number of different kinds of 'policy' and when you start looking at these it can be confusing to say the least. I hope to ease the confusion!

In its widest sense policy is a statement of intent: an actual or potential problem has been identified and the policy has been developed to give direction to how this problem is to be dealt with. In effect it is saying 'this is what I intend to do' – or sometimes 'this is what you need to do'. Scriven states that:

> A policy is a broad statement of the principals of how to proceed in relation to a specific issue and can be at a number of levels from international to national, regional and organizational level. (Scriven, 2010: 223)

Policy can take a number of forms. Public policy is developed by a public body and is intended to impact on a wide section of the general population. (By the way, this also means that there is a political element in the process of developing policy in relation to government policies – this is another point I will return to later in the chapter.)

In 1986 the World Health Organization (WHO) used the term 'Healthy Public Policy' in its Ottawa Charter (WHO, 1986), referring to the belief that any policy being developed (on any topic, not just those directly concerned with health) should take into account the impact on health.

Policy which is concerned with specific issues surrounding the welfare of the population and the role of the state in dealing with these issues is referred to as social policy. Health policy is social policy that is focused on health issues – such as (in the UK) the way in which the NHS is run and the approach to public health. Activity 5.1 below is a way of confirming your understanding of the term 'policy'.

ACTIVITY 5.1

Make short notes on the following thought points (you can do this as a group if you wish):

1 What does 'policy' mean to you?
2 Which area of policy do you feel affects you the most?

Try to put together an explanation of the concept of policy to deliver to someone with no prior knowledge of it as a subject.

SO WHY IS HEALTH POLICY SO IMPORTANT?

Now you have some idea of what it is I am talking about, let's consider the question which forms the heading for this section – why is health policy so important? Well in a nutshell it's important because nothing would get done without it. Without policy to use as a tool the social changes that have improved and increased the human lifespan over the past centuries may not have progressed as quickly as they have – improvements in housing, sewage, water supplies and working conditions, or advances in medicine. Policy is all around us in the sense that it affects everything we do – from where we are born, where we live, where and how we are educated, to how we are employed and looked after if we fall on hard times or become ill, and how we spend our twilight years (the latter is referring to old age by the way and nothing to do with vampirism!). But like the air we breathe, most of us pay no attention to policy – at least until it has a direct effect on us. Policy to many of us is something that other people create, and is no business of ours.

But let's stop a minute and consider just how much impact health policy has on us as healthcare professionals. It's no exaggeration to say that policy has an effect on every aspect of our professional lives as well as our personal ones (Cook, 2006). Policy dictates how the health service is organised and run, it dictates the kind of institutions we work in and how they are staffed and equipped, it dictates if healthcare is a state responsibility or a private sector one, or a mixture of both. 'But what does that have to do with me?' I hear you ask, 'Surely someone else is going to organise and get involved with that?' I hope to be able to persuade you to look again, so that you can see why a knowledge of health policy is an important tool for any health professional.

Nurses make up the biggest group of trained healthcare workers, with front-line responsibility for the direct delivery of care to patients both in the UK (Audit Scotland, 2007; Department of Health, 2012; Health and Social Care Information Centre, Workforce and Facilities Team, 2012) and abroad (Kunaviktikul et al., 2010). Given the nature of these crucial roles it would seem only right that their knowledge, experience and skills should be called upon to inform policy change which will have a direct impact on their working practice, and indeed the expectation that this group of workers should be key players (or actors, to use the jargon) has long been recognised (WHO, 2002). The reality is, however, that policy engagement amongst these professionals has not been evident in practice, with key policy changes affecting nurses sometimes being made by others. By not engaging with policy development, we lose our opportunity to influence the services we work in, and indeed, our own working practices. While in more recent times this trend has started to change, there is still a call for nurses to take a more active role in the process of policy development (Fyffe, 2009).

Almost as much of a problem as a lack of involvement in the policy process can be a lack of knowledge of the current policy imperatives, and this is something which can impact not just on you, but also on those you care for. In relation to this point, it is almost certain that at some point in your professional career you will either be on the receiving end of change, or will wish to make changes within your clinical area. Change is inevitable. Without it we would stagnate and advances in clinical practice would never be implemented. One advantage of keeping your finger on the pulse of current policies is that they will give you some insight into what their impact is likely to be on your area, either immediately or in the near future. Forewarned is forearmed, as they say. Even now, while you are undertaking your education for professional practice, a knowledge of policy content will give you some insight into how services will be structured and where their main focus will be by the time you are qualified and looking to obtain a post.

But what do you do if a change is proposed that you feel is not going to be of benefit to you or your staff and patients? Well, just saying you are unhappy is not likely to achieve much, but if you have a knowledge of current policy, then you can see if the proposed change is in keeping with it – if not, you will have a much surer footing for mounting your opposition.

Likewise, you may well find that you want to make changes within your area – introduce a new way of organising care or a new treatment regime for example. Again, if you can link your proposal for change to recommendations or intentions that are outlined in relevant policy then you will strengthen your case for change, and be more likely to be able to implement it.

Finally, consider that, for nurses in particular, we are called upon to act as patients' advocates – to be able to speak up on their behalf (Nursing and Midwifery Council, 2008). In order to do so we need to be aware of what our patients' rights are. And where do we find that out? Health policy documents can be a source for that kind of information as well.

So a knowledge of policy is an essential part of any health professional's toolkit, both for healthcare professionals' benefit and the benefit of patients. In Activity 5.2 you will have an opportunity to seek out some policy documents that are of particular interest to you. You can do a simple Google search, or you may wish to go onto your country's Health Department website as an easy way to access relevant health policy.

ACTIVITY 5.2

Identify health policy documents that have an impact on:

1 Your personal life.
2 Your professional life.

Try to give a brief outline of the manner in which they have an effect on both these areas.

POLICY ANALYSIS AND RESEARCH

In the early 1990s there was a movement towards evidence-based medicine which aimed to ensure that there was more use of research evidence to underpin clinical practice (Buse et al., 2005). Towards the end of the that decade this movement was extended to the area of policy making to encourage the adoption of research evidence to form the basis of evidence-based policy decisions (Sykes, 2011). It would therefore be logical to assume that by now all policy is supported by sound, research-based evidence – however, as I will discuss in this section, it's a bit more complicated than that.

It is not the intention of this section, you may be relieved to know, to go into great detail about the topic of policy analysis: this is an area which has entire books devoted to it, so it would be difficult to do it justice as part of a chapter. Rather, we will consider here – as the focus of this book is research – just what part research plays in the policy process, and how analysing policy can help us uncover how and why research has been used within the process of policy development.

What I will look at is how to go about finding where research has been used in a policy, and what kind of factors might have an effect on how it is used. The best way to do this is to undertake a bit of policy analysis. While there are a number of different frameworks you could use, some quite complex in nature, I will use one of the simpler formats, which will suffice for the purpose of your learning here: the Policy Analysis Triangle (Walt and Gilson, 1994) (see Figure 5.1), which is useful for guiding us through a systematic assessment of all the different factors which might have an effect on a policy and its content.

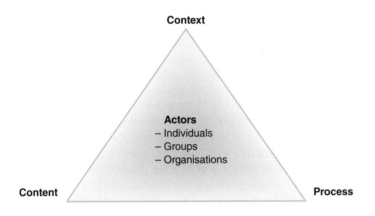

Figure 5.1   The Policy Analysis Triangle (source: Walt and Gilson, 1994)

As you can see from the diagram, there are four key areas which I will explain briefly:

- **Actors**: These are all the individuals, groups, organisations and governments that can exert influence on a policy. Not all actors will have the same degree of influence of course – some by virtue of their position will be able to exert more power than others.
- **Context**: This part of the framework refers to the range of different factors that can have an effect on the development of the policy. These factors are broken down into four sub domains (Sykes, 2011):

  - *Situational Factors* – are the unexpected and usually temporary incidents which require a policy response; the outbreak of a disease epidemic for example, or the realisation that health services need to change due to an ageing population.

- ○ **Structural Factors** – refer to the relatively stable features of a society, such as its political, financial and educational systems, its levels of employment and technology.
- ○ **Cultural Factors** – relate to religious viewpoints and the ideas, attitudes and perspectives of the various groups within a society, and how they interact with each other.
- ○ **International Factors** – recognise that there are issues outwith our own society which may have the potential to affect national policy, the impact of World Health Organization policy on our own, for example.

- **Process**: This refers to the stages of policy development – the four stages of getting issues on the policy agenda, developing, implementing, and then evaluating the policy.
- **Content**: This is, as the name suggests, what is in the policy – what it is trying to do and how it proposes to do it.

The idea of Walt and Gilson's framework is that when applied to a specific piece of policy it can help you to understand the policy better by breaking it down into the four key areas. It would be a mistake though to consider these areas in isolation from each other, as you will also need to think about how the different areas have affected each other (Buse et al., 2005).

Of particular interest is how you can use some of the key areas addressed by the framework to try and tease out not just where but also why research has been included within a policy. Starting with the actors in the policy, the first thing to do would be to try and identify all those who had some involvement in giving insight into the agenda for the policy. If the main players are governmental for example, then from their political ideology you might get some idea as to the kind of research evidence they are likely to use to support something they wish to introduce or to argue against an existing practice which they wish to change.

Looking at the context in which a policy has been developed can also give you some insight as to why certain evidence has been used. If the policy can be seen to have arisen as the result of some sudden crisis resulting in raised levels of public concern then it may be that there is a scarcity of supporting evidence available. Indeed one of the things the policy may recommend is that research should be undertaken to investigate the particular issue. If, on the other hand, the issue being dealt with is a long-standing one then you might expect there to be an abundance of objective evidence available – and to ask questions if there is not. Religious, cultural, international or political perspectives may influence the quality and range of the available evidence put forward to support the proposed change. For example, understanding the wider policy context in which political drivers are pushing efficiencies in healthcare will help you appreciate the reasons for particular policy proposals that will impact on the care you deliver.

As you will have already seen, the policy process can be understood in its simplest sense as a series of four stages that are framed in the questions below (Naidoo and Wills, 2008):

1 How are issues first raised?
2 How should these issues be addressed?

3 Who should be involved in policy development (usually involving some degree of consultation)?
4 How can we determine the effects of the policy on the issue it was designed to deal with (evaluation)?

Research may potentially find its way into any of these stages in the policy process. It may, for example, find its way into the first stage, acting as a policy driver. A policy driver can be thought of as something which gives direction to a policy, the kind of things which decide whether or not something is seen as an actual or potential problem requiring a policy response, and what degree of priority it should be given – it is how things first find their way onto the policy agenda (Sykes, 2011). A recent example of this in practice might be research that demonstrates that there continues to be an increase in obesity in the UK amongst both children and adults. Policies have been developed across the UK aiming to address the problem of obesity. Examples of this would be 'Healthy Eating, Active Living' (Scottish Government, 2008) or 'Food and Fitness' (Welsh Assembly Government, 2006).

Research may also be involved in the decisions about how an issue should be dealt with by providing evidence of the effectiveness of a specific approach or type of initiative. Research may also have a role to play in evaluating the impact of the implementation of the policy on the issue that it aims to address.

Of course, in reality it is not as straightforward as that, as a number of other matters must be factored in. Let's take the first example of research being used as a policy driver. It sounds logical – a piece of research identifies a problem and it becomes incorporated into a policy which aims to address the problem. The other factors (aside from the strength of the evidence) that need to be considered in this context include the political ideologies of those involved in making key decisions within the policy. To look at this rather simplistically, left of centre political parties (such as Labour in the UK) see state involvement and intervention as part and parcel of dealing with health problems, while right of centre parties (such as the Conservative Party) see health issues as more of an individual responsibility with choice as a key factor.

Perhaps one of the prime examples of this in the UK was that of the Black Report. This report ('Inequalities in Health: Report of a research working group', to give it its full title) which had been commissioned in 1977 by the then Labour government, was chaired by Douglas Black. But by the time they were ready to report in 1980, there had been a change following a general election and Labour had been replaced by a Conservative government.

The report incorporated research in the form of epidemiological data (epidemiology examines patterns of health and illness in a society: see Chapter 4) which seemed for the first time to show a clear relationship between an individual's social class and their health. It suggested, amongst other things, that the lower the social class of a person, the worse their health would be, and the earlier they would die. It seemed to be clearly demonstrated that inequality was the biggest determinant of the health of the country, and drastic action would need to be taken to deal with it (Townsend and Davidson, 1982). The report made a range of suggestions about how inequalities could be addressed involving massive social change and state intervention. This is not how a right of centre party (such as the Conservative government of the day) views health problems, or how it feels they should be dealt with, and consequently no policy was produced in response to this report until 1997 when a Labour government came back into power.

Public opinion – sometimes reflected in and sometimes apparently driven by the media – can also be a powerful driver of policy. Politicians are influenced by the media and potential voters in the decisions that are taken when they determine the focus and content of policy which may be at odds with research evidence. Governments also want to stay in power and so will not want to alienate those who can keep them there: if they get it wrong they may find themselves returned to the backbenches.

And let's not forget the extent to which financial considerations can have an effect on policy decisions. In the present economic climate there is international recognition that the need for countries to reduce their national debts means that governments are looking to cut costs in all areas, including health (Oberlander, 2011). Timescales too may be an issue. Policy makers may make use of research findings if they are readily available, but might not be able to wait for them to be produced if they are under pressure to develop a response to an important issue.

So the process by which research finds its way into policy is not as simple as it may first appear – a range of other factors has to be taken into account, along with the research evidence itself, before decisions are made about how much influence that research will have on policy content. It is your chance at this point to consider some of these issues: the aim of Activity 5.3 is to get you to use the ideas that I have presented so far so that you can critically review a policy that is relevant to your own area of practice (perhaps a specific policy that relates to your field of practice – adult, children and young people, mental health, learning disability).

ACTIVITY 5.3

Using the policy document you identified in Activity 5.2 which was relevant to your professional life:

1   Identify the key actors who may have influenced its development.
2   Describe, as much as you can, the context in which this policy was developed. Try to do this in relation to Situational, Structural, Cultural and International factors, as far as you are aware of them.

EXAMPLES OF RESEARCH IN POLICY

Having looked at the nature of policy and the policy process – and considered the part research evidence may play in all this – let's now find some examples of research within existing policy documents. To do this I will take one major health policy document from each of the four countries that make up the United Kingdom (England, Scotland, Wales and Northern Ireland), ones which have had a direct impact on the running of the National Health Service in each of these countries, and try to see how, if at all, research has influenced their content. Why look at examples from the four countries? Well, it is important to remember that though we speak of 'the NHS', in reality it is four separate institutions (Bain and Adams, 2011), and since devolution in the UK, the four different countries have been responsible for the development of their own health policies. So it will be interesting to see if each of the countries uses research evidence in the same way. Weiss (1991) suggested that there are three ways in which research evidence might influence policy:

- *Research as data and findings* – when facts and figures generated by quantitative research studies are used. These data may help to highlight areas which require attention and so will get things onto the policy agenda, or help with the prioritisation of targets or the resources.
- *Research as ideas and criticisms* – can be seen when research findings are communicated to policy makers, informing them and perhaps challenging some of their existing ideas. It is a long-term strategy based on the premise that such an approach may gradually wear down certain preconceptions and result in change.
- *Research as briefs and arguments* – involves researchers taking a dynamic approach to how the findings of their research would best be utilised. It may involve a degree of lobbying (actively trying to influence people in power to accept your point of view) in order to get the research findings utilised as the researchers think they should be.

In almost all cases the most visible type of evidence used will be objective evidence from quantitative studies – surveys, epidemiological studies, randomised controlled trials (all of which you will learn more of within the book) – and so will fit into the first of Weiss's categories. It is much more difficult to find clear evidence of qualitative evidence or Weiss's other two categories when critiquing health policy.

So let's look at these key policies and see what can be found in terms of the evidence used. The four key documents chosen are those which have probably had the most impact in shaping the delivery of healthcare, in its current form, in each of the four countries at the time of writing. It is important to remember that each of the policies is tied into other national policy documents, and I am only considering them in isolation as an aid to understanding how research evidence gets used in policy. The four documents are:

- England – *Equity and excellence: Liberating the NHS* (Department of Health, 2010).
- Scotland – *Better health, better care: Action plan* (Scottish Government, 2007).
- Wales – *Designed for life* (Welsh Assembly Government, 2005).
- Northern Ireland – *Investing in health* (Department of Health, Social Services and Public Safety, 2002).

I will start with a quick summary of each policy, and then look at commonalities in the type of evidence, and the way that evidence has been used. Finally, I will look at how evidence is often carefully selected to support a particular viewpoint or agenda.

England – *Equity and excellence: Liberating the NHS* (DH, 2010)

This is the most recent of the four documents, published in 2010 by the Conservative and Liberal Democrat (coalition) UK government. The politicians were the principal actors, and their politics provides some of the context for the policy development. We would expect a right-wing agenda from the Conservative members of the coalition, perhaps pulled a bit towards the centre by their Liberal Democrat partners.

The policy has a stated main focus on patient choice and control. Success in clinical areas is to be measured in terms of outcomes – principally in improvements in patient survival rates. Changes are also proposed which aim to result in 'liberating the NHS', with more control being given to 'frontline staff', such as doctors and nurses, and government backing off from 'micromanagement'. General Practitioners in particular were to become responsible for the direct commissioning of services for their patients, a major change in the existing service.

Scotland – *Better health, better care: Action plan* (Scottish Government, 2007)

This policy was published by the Scottish government formed by the Scottish National Party (SNP) quite soon after they took power in 2007. The SNP are left of centre and have a primary political objective of obtaining full independence for Scotland from the UK – both important points when looking at the context of the policy.

Much of the content of Scotland's policy is similar to that of the previous Labour/ Liberal Democrat Scottish Executive (whom the SNP replaced in power) 2005 policy 'Delivering for Health', with a focus on addressing the health problems presented by an ageing population, a change in the presentation of illness from acute to chronic conditions, and continued high levels of inequality within Scottish society. Some additional 'new' elements of policy content were put forward, including an aim to reduce the waiting time between initial GP consultation and hospital treatment, the abolishment of prescription charges, and direct elections to Health Boards.

Wales – *Designed for life* (Welsh Assembly Government, 2005)

This policy was introduced in May 2005 by a Labour-led Welsh Assembly, which had replaced the previous Labour/Liberal Democrat alliance in 2003.

A prominent feature of Welsh health policy in past years has been a focus on improving health by trying to reduce the underlying causes of ill health, with a more 'joined up' approach to health and social care, rather than treating these as separate concepts.

Designed for life continued the strong public health agenda of previous policies, and also announced the decision to radically change the planning system for health and social care in Wales. User involvement was to be paramount and access to services was to be improved. A main focus of the policy was to be the achievement of a sustainable level of health and wellbeing for the population, along with a reduction in levels of inequality.

Northern Ireland – *Investing in health* (Department of Health, Social Services and Public Safety, 2002)

Politics in Northern Ireland is perhaps more complex than in any other part of the UK. The need to maintain broad agreement between adversarial political parties, and the suspension of devolved government for periods of time in response to 'The Troubles', have led to a degree of political stasis that is not present elsewhere. Greer (2004) describes Northern Ireland as having a high degree of stability in its policy-making process. Another way of saying this would be that change, when it does occur, happens rather slowly, and thus a 2002 document is still at the heart of healthcare reform here. The context of the political situation in Northern Ireland is perhaps one of the greatest drivers of its policy.

Investing in health was published by a coalition government, formed by the left of centre Social Democratic and Labour party and the right of centre Ulster Unionist Party. The main focus of the policy is on trying to improve the life expectancy of the population, particularly in relation to healthy life expectancy, while also acknowledging the need to deal with health inequalities between different groups within Northern Irish society.

Analysis

- Commonalities in the use of evidence: facts and figures

All of the four countries make some use of research evidence in the form of descriptive statistics (statistics which describe some aspect of the sample group from which they are taken: see Delaney, 2009) within their policy documents, though the sources for some of the evidence given are not always made clear. The Northern Irish document makes the most use of statistics by far, with most of the four chapters in Part 1 of the policy (around 24% of this hefty 242-page document) using descriptive statistics to support the need for a change of approach. In part this extensive use of descriptive statistics may be a reflection of the time it was written – some older documents seem to have used more statistical evidence than newer ones. However, if we put it in the context of Northern Ireland's political process, an alternative explanation may be that it might also be a reflection of the difficulties of getting very different parties to compromise and come to an agreement on any political issue. Statistics may be the 'best' evidence to put forward in this kind of arena, and may be more readily accepted as the kind of 'proof' that all concerned can trust.

Statistical evidence is perhaps the most 'traditional' use made of research by policy makers, especially when the statistics given are related to mortality (death) and/or morbidity (illness). Numbers are attractive to use and are often accepted as the ultimate decider of what is true and what is not (Wales alone does not use statistics in this form within its 2005 document, but instead uses them to high-light achievements made between 2001 and 2005). However, as Taflinger (2011) suggests, statistical evidence may only paint a partial picture and we should not simply accept the data at face value but instead be more critical. We need to give some consideration to the source of the data and the purpose for their collection. In addition, it is important to appreciate the ways in which the data are used within the policy.

So, when Investing in health states that 'life expectancy here improved from 47 years for men and women born in 1900 to 74.5 and 79.6 respectively today' (Department for Health, Social Services and Public Safety, 2002: 22) that seems like solid evidence that health has improved in Northern Ireland since the start of the twentieth century. Of course it does not tell us why this has happened. We might infer that changes in health policy and delivery of health services are responsible since we are reading about it in a health policy document, but in reality it is likely that many other factors are also involved.

Likewise, when the *Better health, better care: Action plan* states that '*over the last 10 years, NHS Scotland's workforce has grown by around 18%*' (Scottish Government, 2007: 13) this might have been seen as support for the idea that there has been great government investment in health services – but again, it does not give information about whether the expansion has been in frontline services or other areas, so it only provides part of the picture.

Consequently, even when research evidence is presented in a fashion that seems difficult to argue with, it is always worth taking a closer look.

- Picking the evidence

It may come as some surprise to learn that evidence is not always viewed in an objective manner, but rather is often deliberately chosen by policy writers to support a particular agenda. All government policy will reflect in some way the ideas and beliefs of the political party which produced it as we have already seen (Naidoo and Wills, 2009). Keeping this in mind, it becomes easier to understand why some evidence will be used and other evidence rejected. Picking the evidence that best suits the chosen agenda is sometimes referred to as 'cherry picking'. To illustrate this point, we will consider an example from one of the key documents (see below), but it should be pointed out that cherry picking is not unique to any one political party – all may make use of it in some manner in order to further their arguments. The document used for this example, *Equity and excellence: Liberating the NHS*, has been chosen as it provides a transparent reference list with additional notes relating to the use of data within the document.

ENGLAND – *EQUITY AND EXCELLENCE: LIBERATING THE NHS* (DH, 2010) – AN ANALYSIS

A key feature of this policy is the focus on choice for patients and carers. It is worth pointing out that choice had been introduced as a focus by the previous government – a fact briefly acknowledged in this document – and this policy promises to widen the scope of choice from that of choosing your provider, to having more control over the 'circumstances of treatment and care you receive' (DH, 2010: 16). What I will focus on here is how the stated desire for increasing choice has been rationalised.

The document is well laid out, with references identified and an explanation of how the evidence was used. To support the idea that people wanted more choice, results from the 2009 British Social Attitudes Survey (NatCen, 2009) are used which are claimed to demonstrate that 'over 95% of people thought that there should be at least some choice in which hospital a patient attends and what kind of treatment they receive' (DH, 2010: 57). That sounds quite compelling, but let's look at the statement a bit more critically.

The claim that over 95% of people thought that there should be a degree of choice in both hospitals attended and in treatment received seems to be based on the answers to four questions (Q581–Q584) within the survey. The first two asked respectively how much choice patients should have in choice of hospital, and how much choice respondents think people actually have. The last two questions were similar but asked about treatment choice instead. Respondents were asked to pick an answer from: 'A great deal', 'Quite a lot', 'A little', 'None at all', or 'Don't know'. At no point is a statement made that 95% of people wanted some choice – that figure seems to come from totalling up how many people responded using one of the first three categories. So that might indeed indicate that the majority thought that some choice should be available, but it does not give an indication of how much choice they wanted. And remember that this statement was being used to support the idea that people wanted more choice (interestingly the survey also points out the dangers of increasing public expectations about choice, unless those same expectations can be met). The same survey also reported that people's level of satisfaction with the NHS was at its highest since 1984 (a fact that the rationale in *Equity and excellence* chooses to omit) which might also lead you to consider that perhaps no further level of choice was actually being sought: it really does depend on how the evidence is presented.

This survey, it should be pointed out, takes in responses from all four countries of the UK, and therefore is not solely based on results obtained from an English population. It is likely that different parts of the UK might place differing degrees of importance on the value of choice in the NHS, and have differing ideas on how much choice is currently on offer. The survey does not discriminate between the four countries.

The statement goes on to say that there is evidence from home and abroad to show that choice improves quality. This statement is supported by a reference linking to an evaluation of the London Patient Choice System carried out by the University of York in 2004. An examination of the project's report points out that any improvements in quality were specific to London and would not necessarily apply outwith that city, thereby weakening the supporting evidence for a national roll-out. Perhaps unsurprisingly, the policy document does not mention this point.

Finally, the document points out that though choice was introduced by the previous government, just under half of patients recalled being given any choice by their General Practitioner. This latter statement links to the Report on the National Patient Choice Survey (DH, 2009) – the explanation of its use states that this survey showed 'only 47% of patients being offered choice' (DH, 2010: 57). Perhaps a more accurate way of putting this would have been to state that 47% of those asked could remember being offered choice: it is actually recall that is being measured here rather than whether or not people were actually offered a choice (which is not quite the same thing). Additionally, the policy writers choose to use one of the less specific results produced by the study – more specific measures of choice seemed to indicate more positive results, for example '67% of patients were able to go to the hospital they wanted' (DH, 2009: 6), but again, including this kind of evidence would not support the agenda of the policy makers.

It should be pointed out that the sources quoted are all credible, and perhaps with the exception of the 2004 evaluation, up-to-date at the time of publication, but questions are perhaps raised by the manner in which each of the sources has been used quite selectively to support a specific agenda. So no matter how sound the support taken from research evidence seems, it will always bear further scrutiny.

At this point it is your chance to consolidate your learning from this chapter as you undertake Activity 5.4. You might want to take the opportunity to consider the policy documents in relation to your field of practice again, so that you can apply your learning to something that is relevant to your everyday practice.

ACTIVITY 5.4

Locate a copy of one of the policy documents used as an example in this section.

1   Select one area from the document which uses some form of research evidence to support it.
2   Try to locate the original sources (or as near to them as you can) for the research evidence used.

Write some short notes on how you think the evidence has been used – is it relevant? Can you find any evidence of 'cherry picking'?

SUMMARY

In completing the learning in this chapter, you should now have a good appreciation of the variety of ways in which research is used in policy.

The critical learning points from this chapter are:

- To act as patients' advocate you need to be aware of their rights and the policy context in which you operate.
- Policy analysis is a way of being able to 'read' a policy document and enables professionals to be critically aware of practice and service developments as part of the policy context.
- It is worth being critical when considering what evidence a policy uses, and how it uses it.

FURTHER READING

The following websites will give you access to current health policy for the four nations of the UK and the World Health Organization.

England: www.dh.gov.uk/health/policy/
Northern Ireland: www.dhsspsni.gov.uk/index/publications
Scotland: www.scotland.gov.uk/Topics/Health/Services
Wales: www.wales.nhs.uk/researchandresources/publications
World Health Organization: www.who.int/topics/health_policy/en/

REFERENCES

Audit Scotland (2007) *Planning ward nursing – Legacy or design?* [online] Available from: www.audit-scotland.gov.uk/docs/health/2006/nr_070125_ward_nursing_followup_km.pdf January 2007, Edinburgh, Audit Scotland (last accessed 27 April 2012).

Bain, H. and Adams, D. (2011) in E. Porter and L. Coles (eds), *Policy and strategy for improving health and wellbeing*. Exeter: Learning Matters.

Buse, K., Mays, N. and Walt, G. (2005) *Making health policy*. Maidenhead: Open University Press.

Cook, R. (2006) Policy: What it is, why it matters, *British Journal of Community Nursing*, 11 (2): 68–69.

Delaney, L. (2009) Descriptive statistics: Simply telling a story, *British Journal of Cardiac Nursing*, 4 (6): 283–289.

Department of Health (2009) *The Report on the National Patient Choice Survey – March 2009 England*. [online] Available from: http://webarchive.nationalarchives.gov.uk/20120503232219/http://www.dh.gov.uk/en/Publicationsandstatistics/Publications/PublicationsStatistics/DH_103479 (last accessed 19 August 2013).

Department of Health (2010) *Equity and excellence: Liberating the NHS*. London: The Stationery Office.

Department of Health (2012) *Liberating the NHS: Developing the healthcare workforce, from design to delivery*. London: The Stationery Office.

Department of Health, Social Services and Public Safety (2002) *Investing in health*. [online] Available from: www.dhsspsni.gov.uk/showconsultations?txtid=10415 (last accessed 19 August 2013).

Fyffe, T. (2009) Nursing shaping and influencing health and social care policy, *Journal of Nursing Management*, 17: 698–706.

Greer, S. (2004) *Four way bet: How devolution has led to four different models for the NHS.* London: UCL.

Health and Social Care Information Centre, Workforce and Facilities Team (2012) *NHS Workforce: Summary of staff in the NHS: Results from September 2011 Census.* [online] Available from: https://catalogue.ic.nhs.uk/publications/workforce/numbers/nhs-staf-2001-2011-over/nhs-staf-2001-2011-over-rep.pdf (last accessed 19 August 2013).

Kunaviktikul, I., Nantsupawat, R., Udomrat, S., Thitinut, A., Bunpitcha, C., Orn-Anong, W., Rawiwan, W., Ratanawadee, C., Pongsri, K., Petsunee, T., Kuladee, A., Cattaliya, S., Summalee, L. and Praneetsin, C. (2010) Knowledge and involvement of nurses in regarding health policy development in Thailand, *Nursing and Health Sciences*, 12 (2): 221–227.

Naidoo, J. and Wills, J. (2008) *Health studies: An introduction* (2nd edition). Basingstoke: Palgrave Macmillan.

Naidoo, J. and Wills, J. (2009) *Health promotion: Foundations for practice* (3rd edition). Edinburgh: Bailliere Tindall.

NatCen (2009) *British social attitudes: The 25th report.* London: Sage.

Nursing and Midwifery Council (2008) *The code, standards of conduct, performance and ethics for nurses and midwives.* [online] Available from: www.nmc-uk.org/Documents/Standards/nmcTheCodeStandardsofConductPerformanceAndEthicsForNursesAndMidwives_TextVersion.pdf \ (last accessed 27 April 2012).

Oberlander, J. (2011) Health care policy in an age of austerity, *New England Journal of Medicine*, 365 (12): 1075–1077.

Scottish Government (2007) *Better health, better care: Action plan.* Edinburgh: Scottish Government.

Scottish Government (2008) *Healthy eating, active living: An action plan to improve diet, increase physical activity and tackle obesity (2008–2011).* Edinburgh: Scottish Government.

Scriven, A. (2010) *Promoting health: A practical guide* (6th edition). Edinburgh: Bailliere Tindall.

Sykes, S. (2011) in E. Porter and L. Coles (eds), *Policy and strategy for improving health and wellbeing.* Exeter: Learning Matters.

Taflinger, R. F. (2011) *The problem with statistics.* [online] Available from http://public.wsu.edu/~taflinge/evistats.html (last accessed 13 April 2012).

Townsend, P. and Davidson, N. (1982) *Inequalities in health.* London: Penguin.

University of York (2004) *Evaluation of the London Patient Choice Project: System wide impacts.* Final Report. [online] Available from: www.york.ac.uk/media/che/documents/papers/london.pdf (last accessed 6 April 2012).

Walt, G. and Gilson, L. (1994) Reforming the health sector in developing countries: the central role of policy and analysis, *Health Policy and Planning*, 9: 353–370.

Weiss, C. H. (1991) in R. Stephenson and M. Hennink (eds), *Moving beyond research to inform policy barriers and strategies for developing countries.* Opportunities and Choices Working Paper No. 2002/05. Southampton: University of Southampton.

Welsh Assembly Government (2005) *Designed for life: Creating world class health and social care for Wales in the 21st century.* [online] Available from: www.wales.nhs.uk/documents/designed-for-life-e.pdf (last accessed 27 April 2012).

Welsh Assembly Government (2006) *Food and fitness – promoting healthy eating and physical activity for children and young people in Wales: 5 year implementation plan.* [online] Available from: http://wales.gov.uk/dphhp/publication/improvement/food/plan/food-fitness-implement-e.pdf?lang=en (last accessed 9 May 2012).

World Health Organization (WHO) (1986) *Ottawa Charter for Health Promotion,* Ottawa, 21 November - WHO/HPR/HEP/95.1. [online] Available from: www.who.int/hpr/NPH/docs/ottawa_charter_hp.pdf (last accessed 27 April 2012).

World Health Organization (WHO) (2002) *Strategic directions for strengthening nursing and midwifery services.* Geneva: World Health Organization.

6

PRACTICAL APPROACHES FOR UNDERSTANDING RESEARCH AND EVIDENCE-BASED PRACTICE

RUTH TAYLOR AND COLIN MACLEAN

Chapter learning outcomes

On completion of Chapter 6, you will be able to:

1   Appreciate the range of tools that are available for your research skills development.
2   Utilise a research journal or reflective diary as a means for personal development.
3   Be clear about the tools that are available for keeping referencing sources.
4   Make the most of your university facilities so that you have the tools for exploring the evidence at your fingertips.
5   Consider how collaborative peer support can assist in your development and the impact on research appreciation.

> ## Key concepts
>
> Research journal/reflective diary, referencing tools, university resources for research development, peer support.

INTRODUCTION

The purpose of this chapter is to shed some light on the many ways in which your life (in relation to learning about research in nursing and healthcare) can be easier! There are lots of practical approaches which will offer you the means to streamline your time, focus your resources, be clear about what you need to achieve, and strengthen your ability to engage with research and evidence-based practice. I asked my students what they found most difficult in relation to undertaking a large piece of work (maybe an essay on a particular topic). I'll tell you what they said later, but first take a few minutes to reflect on your thoughts in relation to Activity 6.1. (Just so that you know, the 'I' in this chapter is Ruth.)

Take some time to think about the following thought-points:

1 What do you find, or think you will find, most challenging about accessing information/ evidence, keeping track of information/evidence, and using that information/evidence effectively?
2 What do you think a 'toolkit' to assist you could look like?

ACTIVITY 6.1

When I asked my students the same questions, here is what they said (see Box 6.1):

> ## Box 6.1   Student voices
>
> What do you find most challenging about accessing information/evidence, keeping track of information/evidence, and using that information/evidence effectively?
>
> *Jo*: It was challenging to find information when I was looking for a specific fact or information that was often buried in the middle of an article that initially didn't sound relevant! Also, choosing the right or most accurate key words when searching a database to get exactly what I wanted to find. It was challenging to keep
>
> *(Continued)*

(Continued)

track of references – writing them down and then losing the piece of paper! It was also challenging to use information effectively so as not to go off on a tangent; fitting the points together while ensuring that it flows smoothly from one point to another.

Pete: I found it difficult to know where to look for evidence and didn't know how to use the databases properly.

Katrina: Finding information is difficult if you don't know where to look.

What do you think a 'toolkit' to assist you could look like?

Jo: A way to keep track of and organise references; an outline for an appraisal table.

Pete: A table for the reference, the information, and something to group together common ideas so it is easier to put things together when writing things up.

Katrina: Having some sort of database like Refworks so you can save the article and then just click on the title and it takes you to the article without having to go hunting for it again. Keeping a table of the reference and the main points you found would help me to keep track of which point came from which article.

Emma: I kept a separate notebook whilst writing my dissertation and used it as a journal, writing down the date and time when I worked on something. In this notebook I wrote down all of my own thoughts, spider diagrams and ideas, lists of what I had to do by when, questions for my supervisor, etc. This helped me to keep everything organised. I also kept an appraisal table to collate my information for my literature review – and would use this for gathering information for chapters of essays as it makes the information far more manageable.

It will be interesting to see if you are thinking the same things as the students I work with came up with. Based on what I know is helpful from my own experience I can imagine what might be useful to you. More importantly I was able to establish what actually *is* important for students through my conversations with my personal tutor group – ways to organise information, to keep track of your thoughts and ideas, and approaches will enable you to collate references and other evidence. So to help you find, use, keep track of, and analyse the evidence, I have come up with a 'toolkit' that aims to contribute to your skills development. I hope that you will find this toolkit to be practical and transferable across all aspects of your learning. What you will need to do is think about how the tools suit your own learning style, and whether you will have to adapt them to suit particular situations.

The resources that are available to you through your university are vital to your learning, but sometimes students can feel overwhelmed by the amount of information, the number of resources, and the scope of the learning requirements, with the result that the tools which are readily available to you go unused or are not utilised to their full capacity. As I write this, I am thinking about all the technology that I have available on this very computer that I am tapping away on. I am reflecting that there is so much on the computer that would make my life easier and more efficient, but I have no idea what these things may be or how to find them. I think my point here is that you don't know what you don't know ... and it is therefore vital that you strategically develop your toolkit to the point where you have pulled together all the valuable resources that will enable you to work most efficiently and effectively.

Having listened to my students, we now have a number of key areas that we would like to explore with you in this chapter. These are:

- The use of a research journal or a reflective journal so you can stretch yourself in the learning process by:

  o reflecting on the use of evidence in practice;
  o demonstrating the development of your learning;
  o considering the different views around particular issues through critical reflection;
  o understanding the ways in which research journals can assist in the research process.

- The way in which you can most effectively keep track of reference sources so that:

  o you can easily go back to the sources you have previously read;
  o you can ensure that your reference list is perfect (without having to frantically run around trying to find a missing reference – we have all been there!).

- The way in which you can make the most of university facilities and resources (for example, the library, online resources, study skills facilities).

- The use of peer support to facilitate:

  o collaborative learning;
  o the sharing of ideas and the development of those ideas through discussion;
  o a focus on particular learning issues.

So, let's get started. Remember that this chapter is just one part of an overall approach to helping you develop a set of skills. There are other tools that will be made available to you as you work your way through the book, and our suggestion is that you drop them into your toolkit as you need them.

JOURNALS AS A TOOL FOR LEARNING

This textbook is not about reflection, but given the importance of reflection in the learning experiences of nurses and other healthcare professionals, I want to take a bit of time to look at the term so that you feel comfortable with reflection for learning in the context of the activities in this textbook. I have already provided a suggested model of reflection in Chapter 1 that you can use to work with (see Figure 6.1 as a reminder). However, as you read around the subject of reflection you will see that there are a number of models available. It is likely that as you gain further skill in

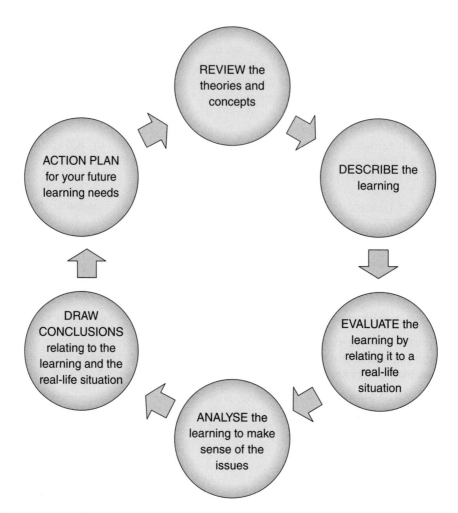

Figure 6.1   Reflective learning cycle, adapted from Gibbs (1988)

reflective learning, you will choose the model that most suits the situation of your learning.

This section now aims to contextualise reflection for learning in healthcare practice. In particular it is worth highlighting that reflexive practice is a crucial component to the practice of research itself. So while you will not be asked to undertake a research project as one of the activities in this book (or possibly even as part of your course), it is important that you get to grips with reflection for learning so that you can take these skills into any research project that you may undertake in the future.

The act of reflection is known to increase learning and to impact on practice when used constructively (Keevers and Treleavan, 2011). A practitioner who is able to reflect in action, and make evidence-based decisions, is one who is able to interact with practice in a meaningful way so that care in that setting can be enhanced. Reflection-in-action is an advanced way of being in the world and one that is challenging to achieve (Bulman and Schutz, 2008). As part of the process of becoming ready for reflection-in-action, we need to develop skills of reflection on our learning – whether that learning is taking place in practice or in the university setting. One way of doing this is to structure reflection in a way that makes it become part of our everyday activity. A reflective learning journal can help in this process.

A notable point to make here is that reflection is a *process* not an outcome. So, while you may be able to point to some outcomes that arise from your reflective practice (for example, you may have developed a deeper understanding of the use of interpersonal skills and been able to put those skills into practice in a particular context), it is the process itself that enables the user to develop as a person and a professional. What I mean when I say that you will develop as a person and as a professional is that your learning on your course will change you in ways that will impact upon you and your loved ones in your life outside your profession, as well as impacting on how you behave as a professional. For me, this is the most exciting part of any learning journey – the development of potential so that we can become the best we can be!

Let's start by jumping in and using the template (see the Appendix at the end of the book) to complete Activity 6.2. Choose to focus on something that will help you with a current concept or situation that is of particular interest to you.

Getting started:

1   Think of an aspect of your learning that you want to explore further (this might be something that you have been doing in the classroom, or something in practice). Use the template for the reflective learning journal to think about the issue or topic critically. Remember that you were introduced to a reflective model in Chapter 1 – the reflective learning journal is based around this model. If you need to, go back to the chapter to refresh your memory before commencing the activity.
2   Once you have completed 1, reflect on how that was for you. Were there any aspects of the exercise that were more challenging or easier than others?

ACTIVITY 6.2

You may have found Activity 6.2 to be straightforward. On the other hand, the process of undertaking the activity may have raised a number of questions. These might include:

- What topics or issues are the right kind to write about?
- What happens if I can't work out what is correct or incorrect?
- What happens if I have a different opinion to someone else?
- What style of writing should I be using?
- How do I make sure that I use what I have learnt in my practice?
- Your own questions.

In answer to these questions, I can really only say that you have to find your own style and that as long as you are constantly questioning yourself and seeking evidence you should be on the right track. In a little more detail though:

- Any topic that impacts on your thinking around your course content and your practice experiences is likely to be relevant for your learning. You will, of course, need to stay focused on particular areas at certain times so that you can positively participate in classroom activities and practice learning experiences. Box 6.2 provides some examples of suitable topics/areas for reflective learning.

Box 6.2   Topics/areas for reflective learning

Here is an article which reported on a research study that was undertaken to explore the health-related quality of life in adults with congenital heart disease. (This is an opportunity to practise your literature searching skills!)

Riley, J.P., Habibi, H., Banya, W., Gatzoulis, M.A., Lau-Walker, M. and Cowie, M.R. (2012) Education and support needs of the older adult with congenital heart disease, *Journal of Advanced Nursing*, 68 (5): 1050–1060.

You can read the article and reflect on its content (using the template in the Appendix) so as to enhance your learning in a way that will enable you to determine ways of being more effective in a practice setting.

The strategy document referenced below provides some key learning for mental health nurses, and whilst the document was written in 2006, it continues to be updated and actively utilised in practice and education.

Scottish Executive (2006) *Rights, relationships and recovery: The report of the National Review of Mental Health Nursing in Scotland* [online]. Available at: www.scotland.gov.uk/Resource/Doc/112046/0027278.pdf (last accessed 17 March 2012).

Using your reflective learning journal should enable you to bring to the forefront the key issues for practice. An example is provided, but you will doubtless have lots of ideas about the kinds of things that are important to you.

A situation in practice occurred as follows:
You were on a 12-hour shift in a children's and young people's ward as a second placement in the first year of your course. You had been asked to admit a 7 year old boy with learning difficulties. His mother was with him. You were very nervous about how to go about the admission procedure, as you had never worked with anyone with learning difficulties and did not feel confident in your communication skills in this situation. What you did was ask the mother to answer all the questions, with the result that the child became bored and tried to leave the environment you were working in. You became flustered but still managed to engage with the boy and brought some appropriate toys across to play with during the admission process. In the end, you got all the information you required and the mother thanked you for your kind approach.

You can use your reflective learning journal to focus on the salient points in order to determine whether there are actions that you need to take forward.

- The use of reflection is often a private activity and therefore you may have some doubts as to whether what you are doing is 'correct'. Reflection works best when you take the opportunity to critically discuss your thoughts with others. You can do this in two ways: firstly, engage in critical discussion with peers; and secondly, read widely around the topic so you have had a 'critical discussion' with the evidence. Both are vital in enabling you to extend your thought processes and come up with new insights. What you will find, I hope, is that you will sometimes hold a different view from that of the literature or your peers. These differences are the stuff of creativity and insight – they will allow you to push past your own personal perspectives towards new ways of thinking.
- Writing for reflective learning is somewhat different from the usual academic style that you would use for essays or report writing. Rather than using an objective approach, you will find yourself adopting a more subjective and conversational tone. Reflective learning allows you to explore thoughts and ideas, developing your opinions, and coming up with a personal perspective on your learning needs. You can therefore use the first person ('I') when you have a particular position on a topic, and your language can be simple and direct (you can even use 'didn't' instead of 'did not'!). If you want to take this informality further, you may find that creative expression will assist your thinking processes (e.g. poetry, drawing). Personally, I find the use of colour and mindmaps useful as ways to think through the issues that occur in a situation.
- Using what you have learnt in practice is crucial to you feeling that you are developing as a practitioner. You will need to feel that what you have learnt is relevant and that you – yes you! – can have a positive impact on practice. The action planning part of the reflective cycle enables you to clearly articulate what it is you want to do following the reflective learning process. You may, for example, simply need to undertake some further reading on recovery-orientated practice in mental health nursing. Alternatively, you may have identified that you need to practise these skills and therefore you will set an objective for your next practice learning situation.

To finish off this section, complete Activity 6.3 – a short activity that aims to help you integrate reflective learning into your everyday learning experience.

Make a promise to yourself – write down three actions that will help you integrate reflective learning into your life.

1

2

3

ACTIVITY 6.3

EFFICIENCY AND EFFECTIVENESS: KEEPING TRACK OF YOUR REFERENCE SOURCES

This section aims to provide you with a straightforward approach to ensuring that you keep track of your reference sources. I am delighted that Colin has produced this section of the chapter as he works with students across Robert Gordon University, including students in the School of Nursing and Midwifery, and has a wealth of knowledge and experience to share.

The huge tide of information you will encounter through your student journey might seem overwhelming and the making sense of it challenging. Tutors will guide you along the way, directing you to key reading and resources, but your goal is to become an independent learner with the ability to find and assimilate information by yourself. In this chapter we offer information about some of the strategies you can adopt around managing information and dealing with some of the issues you face.

While it might seem dispensable, from my own experience I think you will find early adoption of the advice in this section immensely liberating and helpful in building confidence in the subject. Books, websites, academic journal articles, lectures and tutorials will feed your growing knowledge. Don't exclude information sources you use in everyday life because these can all contribute to the whole picture of you both as a person and a professional – a well-informed, highly educated, and capable healthcare professional.

You will be asked to read widely across a range of sources as you work your way through your course. You will need to collect and collate evidence and other information in every part of your learning experience. Some of this evidence and information will be relevant to one aspect of your learning, but more often you will find that much of your learning will impact across the range of theoretical and practice education. You should arm yourself with either an electronic or paper-based 'notebook' that will act as a base for the collection of your thoughts, ideas, analyses and information. As you read take notes, and copy quotes, paragraphs and references to things that seem important, all the while remarking on why. (You may wish to paraphrase some of the ideas that you come across as you go along – remember that you will need to be mindful of plagiarism throughout all aspects of your written work.) Imagine the wonderful store of information and reflection you will gather over time! It is fascinating how things change, some enduring as constants while new themes emerge. Through knowledge comes wisdom and the amazing realisation that everything is connected with everything else in the end.

When you take notes of your reading, it is absolutely crucial that you make sure you also record sufficient information to enable you to find that source again. You might want to use the information in coursework or refer to it in a reflective piece about a placement. Here is a list with one 'don't' and three 'dos', each one an improvement on the one before as far as record-keeping goes:

- Don't just photocopy a page from a book as the copied page alone won't contain enough information to help you find it again.
- People will often describe a textbook by the author's name, e.g. 'Jones, page 66'. That's fine if you will always remember what it refers to, but what if there are other authors called Jones in a reading list (the British Library catalogue lists over 223,000 documents by 'Jones')? If you photocopy, do remember to write on that copy at least the title of the book. That will then give you a fighting chance of finding it again.
- Better still, do write down the author's or editor's name as well as the title on the copy. Figure 6.2 shows you where to find this information.
- Even better, do include the author's name, the title of the book, and the year it was published. The copyright date will usually be the same thing.

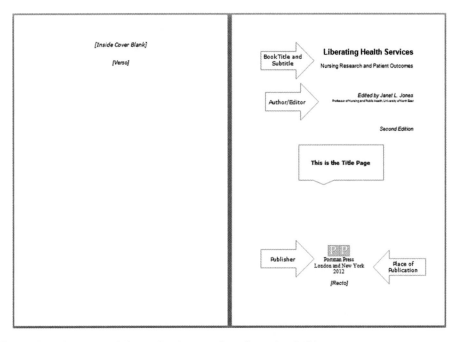

Figure 6.2   Important information from an imaginary book title page

The International Standard Book Number (or ISBN) is a quick way to capture information about a book. On its own it is just a string of numbers (10 digits originally, now 13), but you can find complete bibliographic details by searching using the ISBN in library catalogues, Google and Amazon. Be careful to get all the numbers correct and in the right order for it to have meaning. The International Organization for Standardization (ISO) developed the ISBN format and system and is known as international standard ISO 2108.

The Western tradition of publishing is centuries-old with conventions originating from medieval scriptures. Some of these are still in place today despite electronic publishing and the internet. Pages of a book are described as 'verso' for the left-hand side and 'recto' for the right-hand. The title page is always 'recto' and is the definitive place to find the correct title and subtitle of a book and its authors or editors – what librarians call the 'statement of responsibility' (see Figure 6.2). The title page 'verso' is where to look to find the date of publication, the edition, and the ISBN. The table of contents – where the different sections and chapters are listed with their associated page numbers – will always begins on the 'recto' page, but may also extend over several pages, verso and recto. Chapters will usually start on a 'recto' page. If the chapters have specific authorship, this is where you will find the authors' names (see Figure 6.3).

For journal articles, while a journal title and article title might be enough to find the paper using a search engine or library database, a reference will normally include the author name, the year of publication, the volume and issue numbers, and the beginning and end page numbers as well (see Figure 6.4).

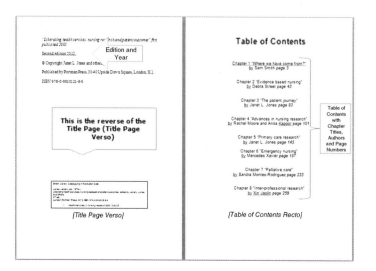

Figure 6.3   Title page verso and the table of contents of an imaginary book

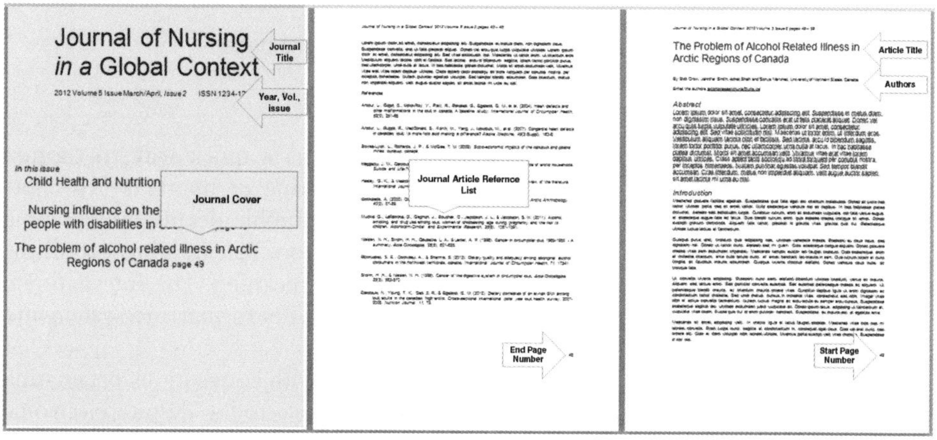

Figure 6.4   Cover and first page of an article from an imaginary academic journal

The information used in these conventions records the elements of what is needed to make reference to a source of information that readers of your work can readily identify. The various elements (author, title, date, publisher) are called 'metadata'.

Publishing, storing, and distributing printed documents involve challenging costs to the businesses concerned, so much so that many organisations (NICE and SIGN, for instance), government departments, NHS, QUANGOS, charities etc. don't do extensive print runs, but instead provide the documents as files that can be downloaded free from the internet. Although the documents are online, the pdf file type that is most often used provides the perfect format for printing, which means that the document actually shares the same publishing conventions of a printed book – with an author, title, date of publication, publisher, place of publication, and even an ISBN, easily discernable. Note that the author may actually be an organisation rather than a person – called a 'corporate author' – and can sometimes be the same as the publisher.

Other kinds of website can be trickier to capture because they can lack the conventions that publishers use for books, but if you dig a bit you will find that in one way or another a person, persons, company or organisation will have been responsible for the website or web page and will be named there. The page will have a title as well as a date and a publisher: this may be the copyright owner, often cited at the bottom of the web page when you scroll down. The most important part of the information is the web address, the URL, and you will need to remember to capture the entire URL (use copy and paste) if you are going to need to find that web page again – unless you rely on Google to find it using keywords from the title, author and publisher. An unfortunate fact of internet publishing is that web pages can be transient, accessible one day and gone the next. Fortunately this is much less likely to be true of authoritative information sources, however it can still occur and prove a problem if you cite a web page that can no longer be found as evidence in your coursework. As a safeguard, and to offer proof that the document existed, you should always record the date when you accessed the information and include this in the reference.

Many people prefer to maintain paper-based systems for recording references. The low-tech advantages to such systems are obvious – all you need is a pen or pencil and a notebook, or a stack of index cards (or you may prefer to use a computer-based alternative, using a Word file for example). However, there are many social network tools that can be used to store and manage bibliographic references (Cite-U-Like, Mendeley, and Zotero are three that you can easily find and make use of for free). These are designed to enable you to easily bookmark and store bibliographic metadata for use in your own personal bibliographic database. The 'social' aspect enables the sharing of references. The information is stored 'in the cloud' (that is, on the web itself) so that you can retrieve it easily. The advantage over a paper-based system is that you can recall the information easily from the database and incorporate the reference into your essay or coursework.

Figure 6.5 is a template or aide memoire that you can use to capture information about books, book chapters, journal articles, and websites for your records. The template could be used in a paper-based system or as a basis for inputting into a personal bibliographic database.

This template can capture the information needed for references and meet most eventualities. An issue arises when incorporating references into course work around the style of reference. Generally speaking, the authors of the books and articles you read will have used one of two styles. The first of these, the author/date or Harvard style, places (cites) the reference to the information source, using the author or organisation name and the year of publication within brackets in the text of the document, like this: (Taylor, 2012). The full bibliographic details are then listed alphabetically

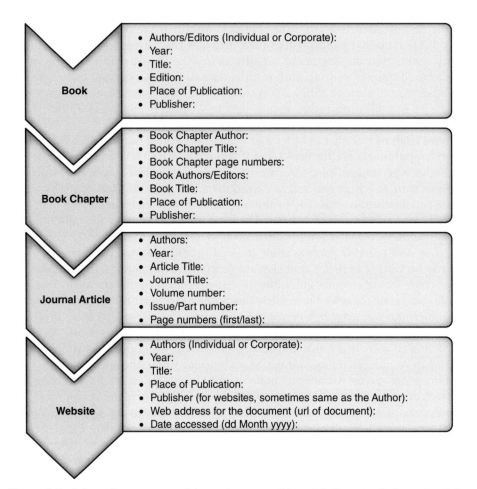

Figure 6.5 Information resource data capture record template for a book, journal article, or website

by author last name in a list of references (sources used) at the end of the document text, like this (for a book):

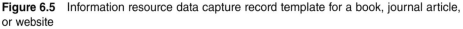

Taylor, R. (2012) Title of the book. Place of publication: Publisher.

Other style conventions used may stipulate the author's name being in capital letters in the reference list, like this: TAYLOR, R. or that the date in the reference list be shown without brackets, or that *the title be in italic characters*. Where the work has multiple authors, only the first named author is given if the number of authors is greater than, say, three or four (although the numbers will vary), in which case the Latin phrase 'et al.' ('*et alia*', meaning 'and others') is used to indicate that other authors were equally responsible in addition to the person or organisation named.

Box 6.3   Practice vignette

The referencing styles that universities require you to follow are examples of codified applications that will often be encountered in healthcare. They may be described as systems, guidelines, recommended practices, conventions, regulations, standards, processes, customs, protocols, norms or rules. The words themselves will have precise meanings but how they are used is actually fairly loosely applied (Girard, 2006). However, they will be documented. Accessing theses documents can usefully provide answers to fundamental questions that occur in most learning and practice situations, for yourself or on behalf of a patient, family member or carer:

- What systems are in place?
- Are there recognised guidelines that can be followed?
- What is the recommended practice for the management of the situation?
- Is there a standard procedure?
- What conventions need to be understood?
- What are the steps in the process?
- Is there a correct protocol?
- What do people customarily do?
- What *norms* do we follow?
- Are there *rules* in place?

Many of these can be embodied in policies and support quality frameworks. Represented within them will be degrees of risk and they may be advisory or obligatory to follow. In healthcare, patient safety is paramount and short-cuts are not permissible. Just having these questions in mind and doing the research, finding the information, evaluating it, using it, and in the process documenting it, are great tools to help reflection.

The second style, sometimes preferred to the Vancouver style, is the numeric style. In some respects it is simpler to apply, because in the text each reference or citation is shown by a running number as it occurs in the text – 1, 2, 3, 4, etc. The full bibliographic details of each reference are given in the list of references at the end of the work, in number order. This style is often referred to as 'Vancouver' and various conventions apply to it as well, in terms of capitalisation, brackets, punctuation, and so on.

The Harvard and Vancouver referencing styles have common characteristics and these, when applied in a consistent way, constitute a system of sorts. However, neither systems are universally applied which means that you will encounter many variations on both these styles in the organisations that you study with or work for. Your best guide is to find out about the style recommended by your university and adopt it. It is likely to be widely used there by students and academic staff and supported by library and study skills. They can usually provide guides or templates about how to apply a style and offer one-to-one help with questions about it.

Universities and organisations will often subscribe to bibliographic management software, similar to Mendeley and Zotero for example, but with the advantage that they will also provide templates in the adopted versions of Harvard and Vancouver referencing styles. You can use this software with a high level of confidence that when you apply the output style to your coursework, the references will display in the preferred format. RefWorks and EndNote are typical examples of the software that is offered and supported. There are clear advantages to using the software your university invests in. While referencing styles will vary according to conventions, the bibliographic metadata that become incorporated into the references are standardised. So if you have previously used one software tool to manage references and wish to adopt another that is being offered, it is usually a simple process to export the data as a formatted file that can in turn be imported to the new tool. Check locally with library staff and ask about referencing styles and software support for using these. At this point complete Activity 6.4 as a way of consolidating your learning in this section.

ACTIVITY 6.4

Now that you have had a chance to consider the ways in which you can efficiently and effectively keep track of your references and other evidence sources, you should practise! Choose a topic – one that you wish to investigate either for the purposes of an assignment or for your own development – and search for five (or more!) relevant sources of evidence. Use one of the techniques/tools described in this section to collate the sources so that you will continue to have easy access to them. (If you would prefer, you could do the same exercise and search for articles about reflective learning.)

You can also make notes on the key learning points for each of the sources – a useful resource for your ongoing learning.

MAKING THE MOST OF YOUR UNIVERSITY FACILITIES

I would be bold enough to say that in every university in the UK (and more widely), there will be departments and resources that are in place to enable your student learning experience to be the best it can be. I don't know about you, but I know that there have been times when I have needed support in something (how to search databases for example) and have struggled to work out what I needed to know, rather than seeking support in the right place. What I want to encourage you to do in this short section is to seek out all the relevant sources of support that are available to you in your own university. If you do this now, you will know the support is there when you actually need it! The other bold statement that I am willing to make is that you will find all the information that you need on your university intranet. So let's move to Activity 6.5 and pull together some resources. I have put together a list of the kinds of things that I think would be useful, but you should feel free to seek out what *you* think you will need. Remember, all of these activities are about *your* learning and *your* needs.

Use this activity to work with your peers (or you can do it alone if you wish) to seek out the sources of support. Write down how you access the support, what the service provides, and when you think you may need it, either now or in the future. Some of the services will not necessarily be directly relevant to your coursework, but the services are there to assist you if you need support to continue working towards the level you wish to reach.

- *Study skills*: Even if you are gaining good grades and/or are confident in the way in which you learn, you may at some point find your study skills support unit useful. All of us can do things better! In addition, these departments usually offer support for people with disabilities (dyslexia, for example).
- *Library facilities*: Libraries and the staff who work there can provide a lot of services – some of which we will be exploring in the book. I am sure that you will become familiar with the physical environment of the library, but you will also find a wealth of support on your library intranet (databases, referencing guidelines, e-books and e-journals, etc.).
- *Academic support for learning units/modules*: Most universities will have a system in place that will allow you to access specific support around the particular learning you are undertaking at different points in the course. For example, a role such as 'academic tutors' who can provide support to student groups and individual students in relation to a particular module.
- *Other academic and/or administrative support*: You may have a personal tutor who can help you in your learning journey. In my university, the personal tutor works with a group of students for the duration of the course in 'learning communities' (see the section on peer support) supporting their general academic learning needs, enabling students to seek relevant assistance if personal problems occur, and facilitating their progress in practice in partnership with our practice education team.
- *Counselling and other services*: You may think that you will never need any support in managing personal situations or coping with challenging problems. I hope that is the case and that you breeze through your course without any challenges (other than the course requirements!). But just in case you need assistance with a problem at some point, it is helpful to know how to access that support quickly.
- Other resources/services that are available for you at your university might include *international student advice*, *medical services*, *student finance*, *childcare*, and *spiritual support*.

Hopefully you will now be able to recognise that there is a wide range of support available to assist you in your learning journey. I would say to you that accessing any of these services early is sensible. As part of my role I help students to deal with complex situations – and my observation is that the last things they need to worry about are some of the practical issues associated with their course. The good thing is that if you talk to someone early, there will always be something that can be done to help you – even if that help simply involves pointing you towards the right service.

PEER SUPPORT: THE KEY TO COLLABORATIVE LEARNING

I have undertaken research in student learning – in particular the first year experience (Taylor, 2009) – and while my research identified a number of crucial aspects that can contribute to a positive learning experience, one of the key areas is the connections that students create with their peers. I have written about 'creating connections' and a theoretical perspective called social capital (Taylor, 2012). Simply put, 'relationships matter' (Field, 2003). In the context of developing a toolkit as part of the way by which you can kit yourself out for your learning journey, I am certain that peer support is fundamental for a positive experience for most people. What peers can do (that others can't) is:

- Understand what you are going through (who else will be able to empathise with you when you have an essay to hand in, some formative work to complete, and you have the kids to pick up from school?).
- Provide a critical perspective to your learning – constructive peer relationships can facilitate the development of enhanced learning through discussion, debate, disagreement, and deliberation (the four 'Ds'!).
- Offer practical support in certain situations – and usually reciprocated in healthy peer support relationships (for example, have you ever been a bit confused about what you need for class the next day and contacted one of your classmates to check on your understanding?).
- Share learning resources so that you both benefit from access to a wider range of information (and allowing you to go on to the four Ds together).
- As well as all these positive aspects of peer support, I am sure that you will already have discovered that your peers can become friends who may be with you for life.

So how do you ensure that you work productively with your peers in this context? There are lots of things that we can do as academics to facilitate peer support. Arising from my research, the School of Nursing and Midwifery at Robert Gordon University made a decision to implement 'learning communities' (Taylor, 2004) within the pre-registration nursing curriculum. The aim of the learning communities, amongst other things, was to provide a way for students to interact and develop relationships with a small(ish) group of students through facilitated learning and other activities. What we have witnessed as we work with students in this way is the strong relationships that students maintain within their small groups (and by way of reward for me, I have wonderful relationships with my learning community!), so we as academics can do a lot to provide an environment in which relationships can flourish. However, it will be up to you to take these relationships and develop them further in order that you then feel you have the support that suits you and your peers as your learning progresses. I am sure that you will have something of what I am describing in place already, but can I suggest that you think critically about how you interact with each other as part of the learning experience so that you may recognise if there is anything else you can do to make the time you spend together more valuable. Below you will see a short overview of some of the principles that lie behind Action Learning Sets (ALS). I am not really suggesting that you set up an ALS, I am simply highlighting some of the principles that may be useful as you move forward with your peers in a purposive way.

ACTION LEARNING SET

- A group of people who come together voluntarily for development.
- A method of exchanging experiences and issues, supporting and challenging each other, and co-creating options for action.
- A process-driven approach that allows for learning and reflection on issues that are important to the participants.
- An opportunity to acquire and improve transferable skills (for example: active listening, skilled questioning/probing, empathy).
- An ongoing process of reflection, co-creation of options, learning, action and more learning.

If you are certain that you want to make the most of your peer relationships, meet together as a small group and complete Activity 6.6. What you will have when you have completed the activity will be an agreed approach to working together – and this can be revisited at any time and changed if necessary. After all, you will be growing as learners and peers and circumstances will change.

As a group of peers who already work together and provide support to each other, you have an opportunity to stretch yourselves in ways that should enhance your overall learning experience. I suggest that you discuss the following thought-points and come up with a group agreement:

- What are the reasons for you coming together as a group?
- How are you going to function as a supportive, confidential, co-creating development group?
- Do you need to develop ground rules? If so, think about how you will go about this, and if you have time you can then develop some ground rules.
- How are you going to make enough time to come together? How often and where do you plan to meet?

Remember the 4Ds – discussion, debate, disagreement and deliberation. Depending on the issues you wish to discuss, you may find these helpful reminders for purposeful and meaningful outcomes from your collaborative efforts. If you are addressing a sensitive situation you may choose not to use the 4Ds and instead utilise skills such as open questioning, reflecting back, and empathy.

ACTIVITY 6.6

SUMMARY

This chapter has started to gather together a range of tools for your use as you develop your skills in research and evidence-based practice. The beauty of these tools is that you will be able to use them in all of your learning situations as you gather evidence for any essay or report, as you consider how you implement evidence in practice, and as you develop as a learner across all aspects of your course. The critical points for your learning so far are:

- Through the collection of a range of tools, you will be able to streamline the ways in which you work with the evidence to support your learning.
- A disciplined approach to reflection on your learning will enable you to grow as a person and as a professional and will contribute to the achievement of your potential as a learner.
- The use of all relevant support – technological support, peer support, university support, family and other support – will offer you the motivation, enthusiasm and purpose at different times.
- Collating your sources of reading at the time you use them will ensure that you have a resource that will be useful throughout your learning on your course.

FURTHER READING

This further reading list offers some suggestions to broaden your knowledge of reflective learning. There is a lot of information out there and one of the activities may have enabled you to collect some of the relevant sources (depending on what you chose to look at for Activity 6.4) – and figure out how to keep track of them!

Bulman, C. and Schutz, S. (eds) (2008) *Reflective practice in nursing*. Chichester: Blackwell. This is a popular book that provides an in-depth overview of the key issues that impact on reflective practice, alongside practical approaches to working towards strength in reflection in and on action.

Freshwater, D. and Johns, C. (2005) (eds) *Transforming nursing through reflective practice* (2nd edition). Oxford: Blackwell. I believe that this book will stretch you to think about reflection as an integral part of the way that you live in the world, so rather than 'deciding to reflect' you will come to a point in your learning where reflective practice is lived. A challenging and innovative book that asks us to consider how we uncover nursing at its core in our daily practice.

REFERENCES

Bulman, C. and Schutz, S. (eds) (2008) *Reflective practice in nursing*. Chichester: Blackwell.
Field, J. (2003) *Social capital*. Oxon: Routledge.
Gibbs, G. (1988) *Learning by doing: A guide to teaching and learning methods*. London: Further Education Unit.

Girard, N.J. (2006) Standards, recommended practices and guidelines, *AORN Journal*, 83 (2): 307–308.

ISO (2005) *ISO 2018:2005 information and documentation: International Standard Book Number (ISBN)*. Geneva: International Organisation for Standardisation.

Keevers, L. and Treleavan, L. (2011) Organizing practices of reflection: A practice-based study, *Management Learning*, 42 (5): 505–520.

Taylor, R. (2004) Creating a connection: Tackling student attrition through curriculum development, *Journal of Further and Higher Education*, 29 (4), 367–374.

Taylor, R. (2009) Creating connections: An investigation into the first year experience of undergraduate nursing students. Unpublished.

Taylor, R. (2012) Social capital and the nursing student experience, *Nurse Education Today*, 32: 250–254.

PART 3

LET'S GET PHILOSOPHICAL

7

THE PHILOSOPHICAL BACKGROUND TO NURSING RESEARCH

ANDREW MCKIE

Chapter learning outcomes

On completion of Chapter 7, you will be able to:

1 Outline the place of philosophy within nursing and healthcare research.
2 Provide definitions of ontology and epistemology.
3 Provide examples of different approaches to nursing knowledge.
4 Outline the place of multi-levelled knowledge in nursing research.

Key concepts

Philosophical enquiry, philosophy in nursing and healthcare research, ontology, epistemology.

INTRODUCTION

The purpose of this chapter is to explore the philosophical concepts that will enable you to appreciate the decisions that researchers make about their approaches to the investigation of a nursing or healthcare issue. The word 'philosophy' may be a bit intimidating, so the chapter presents some foundational theory that aims to assist your understanding and which you can build upon at a later stage in your course or career.

The philosophical perspective impacts upon a researcher over the selection of potential areas or topics to be investigated and inter-related decisions concerning the choice of methodology, design, methods, findings, analysis, presentation and dissemination of data. This philosophical exploration of issues is positioned behind, or prior to, the research enterprise, and is often underestimated, or ignored altogether, by new researchers eager to get started on their 'research journey'.

The briefest of considerations into what we understand by such terms as 'knowledge' and 'methods' will indicate to us that we are dealing with highly complex and intricate issues. Furthermore, when we consider the potential impact of research findings on the practice of nursing itself in terms of the four domains of practice (professional values, communication and interpersonal skills, nursing practice and decision making and leadership/management/team-working: NMC, 2010), we can begin to see how important it is that we take some time to engage in such an exercise.

I am therefore going to start by exploring philosophy broadly, before going on to consider two important concepts – ontology and epistemology (there are several 'isms' and 'ologies' in this chapter!). After that I shall provide some insight into philosophical perspectives (paradigms) while offering examples from nursing and healthcare practice to contextualise the discussions. You will have the opportunity to revisit the terminology and associated concepts as you work through other chapters, but this chapter should serve as a helpful reminder when you need it.

PHILOSOPHY: WHAT DOES IT MEAN FOR NURSING AND HEALTHCARE RESEARCH?

It is important at this stage that we consider what we understand by 'philosophy' and 'philosophical thinking'. The term 'philosophy' derives from the Greek and links two significant terms: *philo*, denoting 'love', and *sophia*, meaning 'wisdom'. Philosophy, then, can be considered in terms of the practice of the 'love of wisdom' and a philosopher as 'one who loves wisdom'. Possessing deep philosophical, religious and psychological roots (McKie et al., 2012), philosophy understood as wisdom is a form of human deliberation which combines different types of knowledge, attention to contextual factors (including time), and the accumulated insights which can be gained from human experience in all its variety.

This philosophical pursuit of wisdom can be contrasted with other forms of enquiry. Many of us over the course of our lives will form variously developed opinions, perspectives and attitudes on a vast array of topics and issues. These can be derived from information gained by our exposure to books, journals, television, film, the internet, and talking to friends, as well as from other life experiences such as employment, raising a family, travelling, participating in sport, or pursuing a hobby or interest. All of these human activities may provide us with considerable accumulated information about many topics of natural and human interest.

By way of contrast, however, the philosophical enquiry is one characterised by a deep, open, and searching pursuit of insight and understanding. Jostein Gaarder, in his very readable novel on the history of ideas, *Sophie's world*, explores this further:

> A philosopher knows that in reality he knows very little. That is why he constantly strives to achieve true insight. A philosopher is therefore someone who recognizes that there is a lot he does not understand, and is troubled by it. In that sense, he is still wiser than all those who brag about their knowledge of things they know nothing about. (Gaarder, 1995: 53)

The philosophical approach, therefore, can be described as a way of thinking about, and being critically questioning of, the established forms and frameworks of enquiry and actions that we take for granted in everyday living itself. This philosophical enquiry, in its deep and critical dimensions, makes little appeal to authority of any kind whether this be political, social, religious, or scientific. Edwards' (2001: 8) definition of philosophical enquiry as a 'second order nature' indicates that it is an activity which allows us to stand back from our everyday concerns to ask critical questions.

If we return to Gaarder's (1995: 53) quotation about the ideal characteristics of the practitioner of philosophy for a moment, the recognition that there are many things about which we know little or nothing suggests the need for philosophical enquiries which are characterised by openness, humility, and a willingness to hold views lightly. The adoption of philosophical approaches can benefit our appreciation of research through a deep, wide-ranging, and critical analysis of the various purposes, assumptions, design guides, and methods of our intended research. It might be helpful for you to take some time to reflect on your understanding of philosophy at this point (see Activity 7.1) and to start some discussions with your friends or peers.

What do you understand by the term 'philosophy'?

- Try to identify ways in which philosophy might have relevance to your everyday life.
- Raise some of these issues in conversation with your friends the next time you see them.
- Note down their responses.
- Do you agree with them?

ACTIVITY 7.1

At this point I will introduce you to some new terms (if you do not know them already). These are:

- *Ontology:* What we understand by reality.
- *Epistemology:* What we mean by our pursuit, or attainment, of knowledge.
- *Aesthetics and ethics:* The particular values which we hold about the world and ourselves.
- *Logic and reasoning:* The ways in which we think and make sense of the world.

Although these four areas of the philosophical approach are closely related to one another, the key linkage which you will explore in this chapter is the one between our understanding of reality (ontology) and the knowledge which we can potentially gain about it (epistemology). But these issues cannot be discussed in a vacuum. We need to consider them alongside what we value, or hold good, in the world (i.e. ethics, sometimes called moral philosophy) and the various means which we use to make sense of it (i.e. reasoning).

Ontology

The term 'ontology' has a wide frame of reference and denotes both theories of 'being' and 'existence'. In respect to the former, it is often used to explore fundamental aspects of people's lives as reagards what it means to be human, the meaning of personhood, self-identity, self-esteem, and the ways in which people relate to one another.

This consideration of ontology can be extended beyond human 'being' terms to incorporate wider 'existence' issues that address questions about what we understand to be real and what is actual. Hughes and Sharrock (1997: 5) suggest that ontological approaches of this sort can be summarised by asking, and finding answers to, this particular question: 'What kind of things really exist in the world?' Such considerations may appear rather abstract and speculative, but remember the earlier point that one of the aims of philosophy is to ask critical and searching questions in the pursuit of insight and understanding. If you accept this, the critical scrutiny of our frequently unexamined assumptions (often called *presuppositions*) about the world we live in may be able to help us towards greater refinement about our ideas, as well as providing us with a rationale for the kind of knowledge which we hope to gain from our research.

The identification of these presuppositions (or assumptions) is important in any philosophical enquiry. These refer to the aims, intentions, and purposes of a discipline or practice, and are often referred to as the ends (or *telos*) of an activity. The Greek philosopher Aristotle (384–322 B.C.) in *The Nicomachean ethics* (1983, Book 1) outlined ends (*telos*) in this way:

> In medicine this is health; in strategy, victory; in architecture, a building – different things in different arts, but in every action and pursuit it is the end, since it is for the sake of this that everything else is done.

In relation to nursing practice itself, you will be able to think about many possible aims, or ends, for nursing: the relief of patients' pain, the alleviation of suffering, the promotion of health, and the fostering of people's autonomy. At this point complete Activity 7.2 which will offer you an opportunity to think more deeply about some of these issues.

ACTIVITY 7.2

- Try to identify some presuppositions (ends) that are particular to your own field of nursing and healthcare practice.
- How do these contribute to your own understanding of the place of values in professional nursing practice? You may wish to refer to the *NMC standards for pre-registration nursing education* (NMC, 2010) which will help you clearly link your thinking to the realities of your education experience.
- In your view, do nurses tend to think about these issues?

One particular way of exploring the place of ontology in our early considerations of research is through the concept of the 'worldview'. Nash (1992: 16) considers a worldview as a 'conceptual scheme by which we consciously or unconsciously place or fit everything we believe and by which we interpret and judge reality'. The 'worldview' framework can help you to consider what views you hold about the world you live in, the place of humanity in it, and the basis (or foundation) upon which researchers make claims for their knowledge.

Exploring these frameworks may help you to uncover hitherto hidden, tacit, or assumed aspects of the ways in which you (and others) understand reality and act in the world. Four different worldviews, amongst many, are presented in Table 7.1 below. Each worldview is presented in categorical terms of its depiction of reality (ontology), its understanding of the nature of humanity (anthropology), knowledge (epistemology), and values (ethics).

Think back to the earlier view of ontology and its concern with 'being' and 'existence'. You can see that even a brief comparison of these worldviews presents us with very different ontological perspectives. Take the categories of 'ontology' and 'epistemology' as an example. Major differences exist between understanding the world in the material terms (one-dimensional, abstract and impersonal) of naturalism compared to viewing it through the material and spiritual terms (personal, sensory, rational and transcendent) of theistic approaches (e.g. Judeo-Christianity).

Now consider the anthropology category. Very different perspectives on the nature of men and women are presented in these worldviews. The human dimensions inherent within, for example, a theistic worldview (personal, spiritual and biological), look quite different from those outlined in the worldviews of pantheism (where absence of the self is prominent) and in post-modernism (where human beings are viewed as socially conditioned).

It may be tempting to consider such 'worldview' perspectives solely in terms of how we *think* about the world. Nevertheless, by giving us insights into different

Table 7.1 Four worldviews adapted from McCallum (1992)

Worldview	Ontology	Anthropology	Epistemology	Values
Naturalism e.g. atheism	Material universe is all that exists; one dimensional; explanation in terms of natural law	Man the chance product of evolution; entirely material	Valid knowledge only through scientific proof	No objective values exist: individual preferences or socially constructed
Pantheism e.g. Hinduism	Only spiritual dimension exists	Man one with ultimate reality; no individuality	Truth beyond all rational description	No real good/evil distinction
Theism e.g. Judeo-Christianity	An infinite God exists; reality is both material and spiritual	Holistic – personal, eternal, spiritual, and biological	Truth gained through revelation, five senses, and rational thought	Objective moral values
Post-modernism	Reality interpreted through language and cultural paradigms	Humans a product of their social setting; no autonomy or freedom	Truth relative to one's culture	Values part of social paradigms; tolerance, freedom of expression, inclusion; provisional nature of knowledge

ontologies, it is possible also to consider the ways in which these worldviews impact upon how men and women *act* in the world. For our purposes, this can centre upon a consideration of the different bases for knowledge in our research. You shall see later in this chapter how these various worldviews can impact upon knowledge that can be used in nursing research. Take a further opportunity here to reflect on your learning so far in Activity 7.3 before you move to learn more about epistemology.

ACTIVITY 7.3

After you have considered the worldviews listed in Table 7.1, try to identify with Jane when she says:

I'm rather confused about all these different categories ... I've never considered these issues before. Philosophy just seems so difficult!

Is this your reaction also? Don't worry if it is – you're normal! But what would you say to Jane if she started to engage you in a 'philosophical' discussion about the 'Big Bang' theory of the origins of the universe, about whether there might after all be an after-life, or about people being merely made up of chemical parts? You would probably have plenty to say to each other.

Personal reflection

- What worldview do you hold?

Try to sketch this out in terms of the ontology and anthropology categories listed in Table 7.1.

- How might these considerations impact on your approach to, and appreciation of, research?

Epistemology

The critical scrutiny that can be provided by philosophical enquiry can be applied to our understanding of knowledge, in particular, what do we mean when we say that we know something? How can we be certain about our claims of knowledge about a category, entity or human action? These are the types of questions that epistemology seeks to address and, if possible, answer. Epistemology is concerned with the theoretical study of knowledge by posing this question: 'How is it possible for us to gain knowledge of the world?' (Hughes and Shurrock, 1997: 5). This question focuses upon:

- The *means* we employ to gain knowledge (e.g. data collection methods).
- The *foundations* upon which such knowledge rests: in other words, the truth claims that address the certainty in what we know.

As you will have seen, there is a close relationship between ontology and epistemology. We are now going to explore several different modes of knowing by locating these within particular worldviews and by showing how certain features of a worldview can influence what can be known (see Table 7.1). Along the way, I will support these points by making reference to examples in nursing research.

Science

The place of science in our contemporary world is so established that we often forget its relatively recent origins in the eighteenth-century Enlightenment. The knowledge, however, that it has provided us about the universe, nature and human life itself is staggering. Moreover, the impact of science on the lives of men and women via industrialisation and technology in employment, transport, home life and healthcare cannot be underestimated. What you need to be able to do is to critically examine key philosophical assumptions, aspects and features of science for the ways in which these can assist your understanding of research.

Schafersman (2012) argues that the scientific method is the most reliable means of gaining knowledge. You will become familiar with the term 'quantitative' as you work through this book which, simply put, refers to the scientific method in which 'quantifiable' data are collected – in other words, numerical data are collected and analysed statistically (more of that in later chapters). However, in emphasising the collection of 'factual' knowledge as the definitive way of investigating reality, the scientific method can be open to the charge of *reductionism*. Robinson (2010: 50) illustrates this reductionist tendency by citing the case of Phineas Gage, an American rail worker who, in 1848, survived an accident when an iron rod passed through his skull. Parascientific interest in Gage's 'recovery' was intense, but this was to the neglect of other significant ontological categories in human values and ethics: '… in these recountings of his afflictions there is no sense at all that he was a human being who thought and felt, a man with a singular and terrible fate. In the absence of an acknowledgement of his subjectivity, his reaction to this disaster is treated as indicating damage to the cerebral machinery, not to his prospects, or his faith, or his self-love'. In nursing, this reductionist tendency can often be noted in certain preoccupations with patients' specific problems (e.g. diagnosis) to the neglect of other potentially relevant factors in patient care (e.g. social, psychological and spiritual perspectives; namely, holism).

Given the prominence of the scientific method in epistemology (how we know about the world), I will now introduce you to some further terminology so that you can come to a deeper understanding of the ways in which knowledge is acquired.

Empiricism

In this method, knowledge is derived from experience (from the Greek *empeirikos* – a trial) and, in particular, from the five human senses of sight, hearing, touch, taste, and smell. Historically, empiricism derives from a late fourteenth-century European Renaissance reaction against religious dogmatism and unquestioning authority, and a later sixteenth-century desire to investigate nature by means of experiment and measurement.

These inter-connected features of the empirical method (observation, experience and experiment) contribute much to popular conceptions of the role of science in both our culture and our professions. You will recall the 'experiment' from your early school encounters with science and that the role of observation as a means of gathering data is a hallmark of many projects deemed to be 'scientific'.

In the practice of nursing itself, it is not difficult to locate the place of empiricism as a means of acquiring relevant knowledge. A key development skill early in your clinical nursing practice as a student nurse centres around observing clinical features such as the patient's skin colour, blood circulation, body posture or mood state. By more precise measurement, nurses record patients' blood pressure, oxygen levels, urinary output and blood sugar levels. In wider epistemological terms, we can note the impact of empirically-derived knowledge on the practice of nursing from the natural sciences (e.g. physics and chemistry), life sciences (biology and physiology), and social sciences (sociology, psychology and economics).

A key assumption of empiricism is that the knowledge gained from experience (via the afore mentioned five human senses) is received objectively by an unbiased human mind. If you consider this for a moment, however, you might wish to question this. To illustrate this last point, consider the issues outlined in Activity 7.4.

- Consider the status of knowledge which you have gained via your senses. How trustworthy do you consider this knowledge to be?
- Consider three areas of your recent practice which involved making decisions. What empirical sources of knowledge were these decisions derived from?
- Try to assess the status of such knowledge and its impact upon your own practice.

ACTIVITY 7.4

Rationalism

The school of philosophical thought known as rationalism asserts that a legitimate source of knowledge lies within human reason itself. According to Lacey (1995: 743), rationalism asserts that 'some of our knowledge, though not all of it, can come to us otherwise than through the senses'. Another source of knowledge may lie within human reasoning itself.

Rationalism has deep roots within the history of philosophical thought. One of its most influential proponents in the modern era was the mathematician René Descartes (1596–1650). By subjecting every aspect of knowledge to radical doubt or scepticism, Descartes posited two forms of reality (or 'substances'), namely that of thought (or 'mind') and extension (or 'matter'). Although adopting a sceptical stance to every knowledge claim, Descartes could not doubt the existence of a mind engaging in such scepticism. Descartes' dictum (*cogito, ergo sum*: 'I think, therefore I am') has become famous for the way in which it has linked human reasoning with ontology itself.

The implications of rationalism for scientific knowledge are extensive. One is to note how human reasoning (or argument or logic) can allow scientific enquiry to proceed via such means as essential truths, theories and frameworks. Another is that by positing two different types of reality in the shape of 'mind' and 'extension' (body or matter), Descartes encouraged a separation (or dualism) between knowledge derived from human reasoning (viewed in 'thinking' or cognitivist terms as abstract, objective and systematic) and knowledge gained from the particularities, uniqueness and concreteness of matter (e.g. the human body) itself. In healthcare, this 'Cartesian dualism' has exerted a major influence in shaping the 'medical' model. This model has viewed knowledge of the person in 'objective' terms of 'cause-and-effect' disease and treatment processes, often to the neglect of so-called 'non-rational' aspects of people's emotions, attitudes, experiences, and life views.

Let's now try to understand the place of rationalism in the pursuit of nursing knowledge through two examples which take the form of rational knowledge. Firstly, the ethical principles have been influential in helping healthcare professionals to address ethical problems, or dilemmas, when they have appeared in clinical practice. You may be familiar with the ethical principles from your ethics sessions in your course and in using them during your clinical practice. The place of ethical principles in ethical decision making is shown in Table 7.2.

Positioned mid-range between generalised ethical theories (level 4) and more specific moral rules (levels 1, 2), ethical principles (level 3) can be used in general

Table 7.2 Hierarchy of ethical principles (source: Beauchamp and Childress, 2009)

Level 4	Ethical theories
Level 3	Ethical principles
Level 2	Moral rules
Level 1	Particular moral rules

and universal ways as action guides to help healthcare professionals address ethical problems in clinical practice. These principles (usually four: autonomy, beneficence, non-maleficence, and justice) contribute to a rational (and logical) approach to addressing ethics in professional healthcare practice. Nurses, for example, will often use this rational way by applying one, or more, of these principles to help them decide how best to care for a patient in any given context. Take, for example, the ethical principle of beneficence which means doing or promoting good. As a principle guiding action, beneficence can act in general ways to remind nurses that they must seek to promote the best for their patients in every situation.

The second example takes the form of rational knowledge used for clinical practice in the shape of 'evidence' derived from 'Best Practice Statements' (BPS). Harris and Bond's (2002) Best Practice Statement for the nutritional care for adults in hospital is based on research evidence suggesting that many hospitalised adult patients are under-nourished. A BPS emerged from the questionnaire responses of ward nurses and chief dieticians across 17 acute hospital trusts in Scotland. The aim of the Statement was to act as a guide for good practice and to stimulate further ideas for research through:

1 Admission to hospital.
2 Nursing management of nutritional care.
3 Screening and documentation.
4 Criteria for nutritional referrals.

It is important, however, for you to consider a number of critical issues around rationalism. The human reasoning aspect (cf. Descartes' 'I think') of rationalism and its influence in many different areas of human life can be noted (e.g. in technology, economics, management, and education). Nevertheless, it might be worthwhile taking time to consider these questions:

- On what basis should a specific aspect of human reason be accepted as valid knowledge for action?
- Should the assumption that human reason is the sole basis for human knowledge go unchallenged?

To return to our first example, on what basis should these four ethical principles and not others be accepted as general, universal and applicable in, and for, all situations in professional nursing practice? The actual promotion, or outworking, of the principle of autonomy (encouraging a person's self-development and independence) for a nurse caring for a person with learning difficulties or dementia may be very complex. It may require additional contextual knowledge by recognising that the most ethical way of promoting this person's wellbeing is by accepting their need for help and assistance. The simple statement 'promote the patient's autonomy' may be a rather 'thin' description of how nurses should act in specific situations. In a similar way, acting upon the principle of beneficence may require a nurse to take account of very specific contextual factors.

Secondly, in returning to the Best Practice Statement (BPS) on nutritional care for hospitalised adults, it may be the case that nurses have to interpret and adapt such (rationally) derived practice statements to take account of varying social, cultural, and religious attitudes to food, nutrition, and health. To return to the link made earlier between epistemology and ontology, nurses using knowledge in nursing practice need to understand, and take account of, the various realities (ontologies) in which such practice is set.

It is vital therefore to critically question the basis of all of the rationally derived tools used to gain knowledge in nursing practice. Take, as an example, the phenomena of the 'checklist'. This tool has become an accepted part of contemporary nursing practice whether it is used in an assessment of wounds, risk, mental state, or behaviour. Ronson's (2011: 255) wry observation, however, is surely worth pondering over: 'a good checklist is useful. But now we're flooded with checklists. You can read them in *Parade* magazine'.

In rounding off this discussion of rationalism, we also need to take account of human values and ethics. It is recognised, for example, that the Nazis between 1930 and 1945 employed 'reasoned', but ethically dubious, means in experimental research with selected patients and prisoners in the pursuit of the 'ends' of societal and ethnic 'cleansing'. In our critical vigilance, we need to ensure that our own research methods do not demean, devalue, or dehumanise those who participate in our research projects. (I shall consider the issue of ethics in research in greater detail in Chapter 13.)

Empirical and rational means of enquiry have a key place in nursing research. The critical nature of philosophical enquiry, however, should help you to recognise the strengths and limitations of each approach. You will then be able to identify specific approaches within a piece of nursing research and critically examine the rationale behind their use. Summarise your learning from this section by working on Activity 7.5.

- Take a Best Practice Statement that you have used in practice recently. Critically examine its key assumptions.
- What implications can you draw for your knowledge in this area of practice?
- Outline key features of a rationalist approach to nursing leadership and management in your own area of practice.
- Can you identify any limitations to this rationalist approach in relation to acquiring knowledge in this area?

ACTIVITY 7.5

Research paradigms

When you are reviewing research relating to your practice, you will find that most research sits within the positivist paradigm or the interpretivist paradigm. Becoming familiar with these two perspectives will enable you to read research in a way that is more meaningful to you. It will also enable you to make judgments about the usefulness of the research itself.

Researchers often refer to, and practitioners frequently look for, use and rely upon, the proven 'facts' about any given topic. This is referred to as 'positivism' in its concern with 'the positive application of knowledge to assist human progress' (Cruickshank, 2012: 71).

Developed by the nineteenth-century thinker Auguste Comte (1798–1857), positivism transferred the insights of the scientific method in its application to the natural world to those of the social sciences. The origins of the discipline of sociology are to be found here via Emile Durkheim's (1858–1917) conception of society being open to scientific investigation and yielding 'social facts' (e.g. European suicide rates). Positivism has significantly influenced professional healthcare practice via the medical model in its focus upon the 'objective' facts of disease aetiology, diagnosis, treatments, and prognosis (outcomes).

An important point here concerns the potential ontological implications of the positivist method. Return for a moment to the 'worldviews' outlined in Table 7.1. Naturalism asserts that scientific knowledge derives from a one-dimensional (i.e. natural) world only, thus excluding knowledge derived from other sources (e.g. a holistic view of people as personal, intentional, spiritual, and biological beings).

Hussey (2011) develops the case for 'naturalistic nursing' and argues that use of the scientific approach should not prevent nurses from understanding the different worlds which their patients inhabit. Nevertheless, you might wish to question whether a researcher's 'objectively' gathered data about a patient's religious views on their suffering would properly put such knowledge into context if the worldviews of both researcher and patient are so markedly different.

It is necessary to consider alternatives to the positivist paradigm. The interpretivist paradigm recognises that the scientific method cannot be the sole means of gaining knowledge about human beings. The diversity of people's lives (in social, historical, political, cultural, psychological, and spiritual terms) may require different modes of enquiry.

The interpretivist paradigm locates the researcher within, rather than outside of, the research enterprise itself. Polanyi's (1962) concept of personal and tacit knowledge recognises the active and embodied role of the researcher in terms of choice of research topic, use of research tools, adoption of strategies, and interpretation of data. This concept of researcher reflexivity represents another key link between epistemology and ontology. This embodied dimension also recognises the interpersonal and collegial nature of the research enterprise. The activity of research usually takes place within communal and institutional contexts of, for example, the National Health Service or university faculties.

The interpretivist paradigm is frequently linked to qualitative research methodologies. Here the researcher employs various methodologies to gather knowledge characterised by its particularity, uniqueness, context, experience, novelty and contingency. Such knowledge stands in sharp contrast to the universal and general data gained by 'objective' means. (Chapter 8 will introduce you to some of these qualitative approaches and how they are important for the investigation of people's experiences, as well as offering an overview of quantitative research in nursing and healthcare research.)

Some contemporary challenges

It is worthwhile at this point for you to consider some contemporary philosophical trends which challenge the claims of positivism and interpretivism outlined in this chapter. If you return to the various 'worldviews' outlined in Table 7.1, you will see the origins of these challenges. By taking account of these trends, you may be able to sharpen your critical understanding of the ontological and epistemological foundations of research.

Post-modernism defies precise definition or categorisation. This is, however, central to its direction as a sceptical, or deconstructing, philosophy. This school of thought challenges the epistemological and ontological foundations of the modern era (hence its appellation of 'post') in its reliance upon scientific knowledge with its objectivist, naturalist, universalist, and theoretical features. By rejecting the 'big story' approaches of such worldviews as Marxism and Judeo-Christianity, post-modernism champions multiple patterns of knowledge that are particular, local, contingent, marginal, and even ambiguous. By focusing upon the analysis of knowledge in speech or written form (discourse), truth is viewed in terms of 'flexible pluralism' (Holmes and Warelow, 2000).

Post-modernism views these forms of knowledge as socially constructed via the media of language and culture. What we might consider as agreed understandings of language (e.g. health, illness, wellbeing) are radically questioned and traditionally accepted ontological pairings (such as health/illness, good/bad and science/art) are decisively rejected. Similarly, post-modernism views reality (ontology) solely through social and cultural terms. No higher, wider, or transcendent view of the human self can exist in its choosing, creating, and knowing ways. If no fixed view of the person exists, then nursing practice may be liberated from previously accepted social and institutional norms to consider other creative and dynamic ways of caring. Several 'post-modern' implications for nursing practice and research are outlined by Holmes and Warelow (2000):

- Rehabilitation of practice to centre stage.
- Disruption of existing discourses.
- Rejection of universals, leading to creative discourse.
- Revision of traditional nursing roles.
- Looking beyond traditional boundaries.
- Acceptance of tensions and differences.

The spirit of philosophical enquiry developed in this chapter, however, might lead you to ask critical questions about post-modernism's own assumptions. These may include:

- Should all knowledge be considered provisional and open to change?
- Are the truth claims of our knowledge solely dependent upon social and cultural factors?
- Are human beings solely dependent upon social and environmental influences?

Social constructionism, in sharing in the deconstructive tendencies of post-modernism, argues that each knowledge claim (epistemology) needs to take account of its social, political, cultural, and institutional dimensions. Foucault (1964), for example, linked this to the exercise of power by noting a 'power-knowledge nexus' in the ways in which European societies historically understood, and addressed, madness and insanity. By developing modes of rationality (via social-control means of setting up hospitals, asylums and prisons), a clear differentiation was made between 'reason' and its opposite.

This 'power-knowledge nexus' can also be seen in contemporary mental health practice in the areas of psychiatric classification of disorders, observation of patients, and legal detention. Similarly, the relationship between knowledge and power might be considered further within professional healthcare practice in the use of 'surveillance' tools for the risk assessment of children and young people and in projects for health promotion in public health. At this point undertake Activity 7.6.

ACTIVITY 7.6

Try to identify possible socio-political issues arising from knowledge derived from nursing research being carried out in one of the following areas (or an area of your choosing):

- Women's health.
- Ethnic groups.
- People with learning difficulties.

Consider these issues in light of Foucault's 'power-knowledge' axis and reflect on how they may impact on the findings from research in the chosen areas. These considerations are important for you as a user of research when you make judgments about the implications of the research for practice.

Critical realism

Bringing together important aspects of your learning from this chapter, the key point that I have been developing centres around the dependency of our knowledge claims (epistemology) upon the assumptions we make about reality itself (ontology). It will not have escaped your attention that many of the ontological, anthropological, epistemological, and ethical implications derived from the worldviews outlined in Table 7.1 may appear incompatible with each other. However, if we accept that there are many different way of looking at the world (multiple realities or ontologies), then it may be possible to accept the legitimacy of knowledge derived from a variety of sources.

By adopting a position of *critical realism*, we may come to recognise reality as an open, rather than a closed, system. By seeing reality in layered or stratified ways, we may be able to recognise the legitimacy of different types of knowledge in research. As a result, our critical and discerning awareness of these ontological assumptions becomes a way of justifying the knowledge claims we make for our own research. Here are some examples.

Firstly, if it is accepted that people can inhabit inter-dependent biological, psychological and social realities, then it may be possible for nurses to derive legitimate 'layered' knowledge about a person's chronic condition, such as diabetes, Crohn's Disease or spina bifida, in ways which will make complementary rather than conflictual contributions to an overall aim (end) of promoting that person's health or wellbeing. Secondly, nurses might be able to acquire research knowledge by noting how individual and social ontologies interact and by considering the ways in which organisational factors within healthcare itself might condition their attitudes and actions. Thirdly, we might consider how nurses recognise, differentiate between, and act upon different types of knowledge in their everyday practice. Carper's (1978) identification of four distinct domains of knowledge in nursing – empirical, personal, aesthetic, and ethical – demonstrates the importance of the dependency of knowledge upon ontology. In Activities 7.7 and 7.8, read the vignettes carefully and consider how a critically realist approach to knowledge can be of help to student nurses practising in these areas.

A senior nursing student becomes interested in critical care as a career option and focuses clinical and classroom time on mastering the knowledge and skills needed to work in this area. During a four-month internship, the student nurse continues to work on mastering the necessary skills for the job: doing a physical examination, knowing complex pharmacology, interpreting laboratory data, and meticulously assessing and responding to rapid changes in the multisystem disease course of patients. But then the disconnect begins. The nurse is well-prepared to assess, monitor, respond, and communicate with colleagues about the physiologic events in critically ill patients, but is ill-prepared to deal with the daily work of responding to pain, anxiety, spiritual crisis, hopelessness, and fear. Most importantly, the nurse has not yet learned how to deal with death in intensive care settings (adapted from Ferrell and Coyle, 2008: 8–9).

ACTIVITY 7.7

'We have a video screen in the room and everyone is watching the video screen, and who is watching the patient? What if the patient is turning blue? We've had the equipment aides suctioning patients rather than the nurses because the nurses are so caught up doing the technical end of things ... What is our priority here?' (Marck, 2000).

ACTIVITY 7.8

Table 7.3   Levels of knowledge (source: Holden, 1996)

Level I	Culturally independent behaviour Subjective/affective knowledge
Level II	Psychomotor skills (practical) e.g. IV infusion, blood pressure
Level III	Non-propositional knowledge, culturally dependent e.g. literature, arts
Level IV	Propositional knowledge from science, mathematics, logic

The different levels of knowledge that can be used in nursing research and practice can be summarised as indicated in Table 7.3. By recognising the existence of different types of 'layered' knowledge, we can see the ways in which a critically realist approach can draw upon knowledge derived from sources as diverse as mathematics and art.

As you complete your learning in this chapter, undertake Activity 7.9 – this activity aims to enable you to consolidate your learning so far.

ACTIVITY 7.9

Student voice

Matthew: This has been a challenging chapter. All those 'isms'! So much to take in. But philosophy is interesting because it forces you to think critically about things that you normally take for granted.

Is your response on completing this chapter similar to Matthew's?

Turn again to the chapter learning outcomes and note down the key learning points from your reading. You may also identify some questions. That's fine – that's what philosophy is all about!

SUMMARY

This chapter has provided you with learning related to key philosophical concepts and terminology. The critical points for your learning so far are:

- Philosophical enquiry adopts a critical approach towards everyday living and the issues themselves are complex.
- Nursing and healthcare practice takes place within rich, multi-layered and complex settings.
- An understanding of philosophy in nursing and healthcare research facilitates greater clarity about concepts, enhanced understanding and a focus upon issues, more appropriate and

carefully constructed methodologies and methods for research, more sensitive approaches towards research participants, and greater clarity surrounding ethical issues affecting all parts of the research journey.

• There are many other philosophical issues to explore in research for there is no end to the pursuit of wisdom.

FURTHER READING

Baggini, J. and Southwell, G. (2012) *Philosophy: Key themes* (2nd edition). London: Palgrave Macmillan. A discussion of philosophical themes in the areas of epistemology, moral philosophy, mind, religion, politics and aesthetics.

Gaarder, J. (1995) *Sophie's world – A novel about the history of philosophy*. London: Phoenix House. A very readable novel about the history of ideas around a complex and exciting plot.

REFERENCES

Aristotle (1983) *The ethics of Aristotle – The Nicomachean ethics*. Harmondsworth: Penguin Classics.

Beauchamp, T.L. and Childress, J.F. (2009) *Principles of biomedical ethics* (6th edition). Oxford: Oxford University Press.

Carper, B. (1978) Fundamental patterns of knowing in nursing, *Advances in Nursing Science*, 1 (1): 13–23.

Cruickshank, J. (2012) Positioning positivism, critical realism and social constructionism in the health sciences: a philosophical orientation, *Nursing Inquiry*, 19 (1): 71–82.

Edwards, S. (2001) *Philosophy of nursing: An introduction*. Hampshire: Palgrave Macmillan.

Ferrell, B.R. and Coyle, N. (2008) *The nature of suffering and the goals of nursing*. New York: Oxford University Press.

Foucault, M. (1964) *Madness and civilisation: A history of insanity in the Age of Reason*. London: Tavistock.

Gaarder, J. (1995) *Sophie's world – A novel about the history of philosophy*. London: Phoenix House.

Harris, G. and Bond, P. (2002) Best Practice Statements: nutritional care for adults in hospital, *Nursing Times*, 98 (31): 32–33.

Holden, R. (1996) Nursing knowledge: the problem of the criterion. In J.F. Kikuchi et al. (eds), *Truth in nursing inquiry*. London: Sage.

Holmes, C.A. and Warelow, P.J. (2000) Some implications of postmodernism for nursing theory, research, and practice, *Canadian Journal of Nursing Research*, 312 (2): 89–101.

Hughes, J. and Sharrock, W. (1997) *The philosophy of social science research* (3rd edition). Essex: Longman.

Hussey, T. (2011) Naturalistic nursing, *Nursing Philosophy*, 12: 45–52.

Lacey, A. (1995) 'Rationalism'. In T. Honderich, *op cit*.

Marck, P. (2000) Nursing in a technological world: searching for healing communities, *Advances in Nursing Science*, 23 (2): 62–81.

McCallum, D. (1992) *Christianity: The faith that makes sense*. London: Tyndale House Publishing.

McKie, A., Baguley, F., Guthrie, C., Jackson, C., Kirkpatrick, P., Laing, A., O'Brien, S., Taylor, R., Wimpenny, P. (2012) Exploring clinical wisdom in nursing education, *Nursing Ethics*, 19 (2): 252–267.

Nash, R. (1992) *Worldviews in conflict: Choosing Christianity in a world of ideas.* Grand Rapids, MI: Zondervan.

Nursing and Midwifery Council (NMC) (2010) *Standards for pre-registration nursing education.* London: NMC.

Polanyi, M. (1962) *Personal knowledge: Towards a post-critical philosophy.* Chicago: University of Chicago Press.

Robinson, M. (2010) *Absence of mind.* New Haven/London: Yale University Press.

Ronson, J. (2011) *The psychopath test: A journey through the madness industry.* London: Picador.

Schafersman, S.D. (2012) An introduction to science – scientific thinking and the scientific method. In S.O. Lilienfeld and W.T. O'Donoghue (eds), *Great readings in clinical science: Essential selections for mental health professionals.* New Jersey: Pearson Education.

8

QUALITATIVE AND QUANTITATIVE RESEARCH APPROACHES

MARY ADDO AND WINIFRED EBOH

Chapter learning outcomes

On completion of Chapter 8 , you will be able to:

1 Identify the key components of qualitative and quantitative research approaches.
2 Understand what is meant by qualitative and quantitative research and their relevance to your practice.
3 Outline the differences between qualitative and quantitative research.
4 Appreciate the importance of the types of knowledge that both research approaches can provide to inform your nursing practice.
5 Discuss the types of topics that can be researched using qualitative or quantitative research approaches.

Key concepts

Qualitative research, quantitative research, research methodologies and methods, nursing knowledge.

INTRODUCTION

With this chapter we aim to illuminate the value of understanding the focus of qualitative and quantitative research approaches, their relevance to nursing and healthcare practice, and the types of knowledge that each research approach provides to enable evidence-based patient care and service delivery. It is therefore important that you do not rest on a particular type of knowledge to inform your understanding of nursing practice regardless of your particular field of specialty, but instead think widely about the sources of evidence to inform your decision making in your practice. (Look back to Chapter 7 to remind yourself of some of the key concepts relating to nursing knowledge that will also inform your thinking as you work your way through this chapter.)

We recognise the depth and breadth of knowledge associated with understanding the concepts associated with qualitative and quantitative research approaches. Considering this challenge, this chapter provides you with an overview of the two key research approaches used in nursing and healthcare research, with examples relating to the kinds of practice experiences you will encounter. You will have the opportunity to get to grips with some of the words that can seem intimidating – phenomenology, quasi-experimental, survey, and ethnography for example. We address these so that you will gain a broad overview of the key approaches, as well as have an opportunity to consider them in more depth later in the book.

Do not worry – you will soon be as enthusiastic as we are about the various approaches to research and your understanding of them will broaden your awareness of the wealth of evidence that exists to help inform your practice. As a registered nurse (and as a student nurse!) you are expected to have knowledge of different types of research and their relevance to your practice (NMC, 2010). Your research literacy will enable you in your decision making processes to utilise research findings that will inform the care you give to patients.

The chapter starts by providing a general overview of qualitative and quantitative research approaches – discussing the purpose of the approaches and the types of research questions that might be answered with those approaches, and demystifying some of the language associated with them. As you use the language of research, you will become more comfortable with its meanings and this will enable you to develop competence in your reading of research. After all, we all want to be able to pick up a research article and determine its usefulness for our practice!

WHAT IS QUALITATIVE RESEARCH?

To make an obvious statement here, as a healthcare professional you must work with people, and as you do so you must also try to understand their experiences so as to offer compassionate person-centred care. Developing an evidence base relating to the human aspects of the patient experience enables us to operate more effectively. Qualitative research seeks to explore human experiences in order to understand the reasons behind the behaviour and meanings embedded in those experiences (Holland and Rees, 2010). The type of knowledge that qualitative research provides for nursing and healthcare practice gives us an understanding of what it is like to have a particular experience: note that quantitative research cannot do this (see Creswell, 2007: there is more discussion on this later in the chapter).

Gaining insights into the world of 'others' – whether patients, their families, carers, or the other professionals you work with – can broaden your thinking and lead to more thoughtful action through the insights gained (Van der Zalm et al., 2000). For example, you cannot measure what it is like to live with or experience emotional distress with a ruler or a tape measure, although various attempts to develop scales to help us measure this sort of phenomenon have been made. According to Myers (2000: 4) 'Conducting research with people who are dealing with personal experiences, cancer or addictions and describing such complex interpersonal investigations are skills that are not possible to investigate with structured instruments. If a researcher were to focus on measuring those phenomena it is likely that he or she would never really come to understand the process that is the real focus of the inquiry'.

Many questions that nurses face in their day-to-day work with patients and others are not just about the numbers (quantity) of incidents that happen (the rate of discharges for example). It is also important for nurses to address questions such as 'What is it like for nurses to work with patients who generate strong emotions in the nurse?' or 'How do patients on admission feel about the communication skills that nurses use to allay their fears?' These sorts of questions relate more to trying to understand the perceived quality of care experiences from a patient perspective, rather than the actual amount (quantity) of care received. Therefore, when we need to understand what it means to have lived a human experience of illness or a disease condition that cannot be measured by predictive instruments (quantitative research) that is when we also need to embrace alternative ways of knowing (qualitative research).

Take a look at Activity 8.1 below. This activity aims to introduce you to the relevance of qualitative research in your own practice.

Think of an area of practice that you are particularly interested in – one that relates to the experience of patients or carers. Undertake a search for one article that relates to this area. We have provided two examples of the types of search terms that you could use to enable you to find an article:

- Patient experience + Pain + Breast cancer
- Carer experience + Epilepsy + Child

(Continued)

ACTIVITY 8.1

(Continued)

Once you have found the article, take some time to read it in detail. Don't worry if you come across words that you are not familiar with as we will come onto these in this and later chapters. Jot down some notes on the following thought-points:

- What is the researcher aiming to find out in the study?
- What tools did the researcher use within the study (e.g. interviews)?
- What are the key findings from the research and their relevance to your own practice?
- Are there any words or concepts (relating to the research approach) that you are unsure about? Make a list of these as learning points to come back to.

While you may not have been able to fully understand all aspects of the article, you will have been able to see that qualitative research does indeed help us understand the experiences of particular people in particular situations or contexts. You can save this article as you may wish to go back to it at the end of the chapter and 'fill in the gaps' in relation to the areas that you identified for further learning (or use it as you work your way through subsequent chapters). You can use the techniques that you have developed through your learning in Chapters 4 and 6 to keep track of your articles and reflect on your learning so far.

We will now move on to examine some further detail on qualitative approaches. As we have already said, you will have an opportunity to expand on your knowledge of these approaches as you progress through the book, so keep in mind that this chapter is an introduction and aims to equip you with an initial understanding of the concepts. Qualitative research has the following properties (Gerrish and Lacey, 2010):

- It is *inductive*, which means that the researcher collects data relating to the phenomenon under investigation (e.g. the inpatient experiences of mental health service users) and develops theory from the data or the situation.
- It is *descriptive* in nature in that the research process allows for a detailed description of the phenomenon (e.g. the experiences of student nurses in clinical practice).
- It is *interpretive* in that the researcher offers one interpretation of the meaning of the data.
- It enables the investigation of human experiences in a diverse range of social contexts.
- It allows the researcher to construct meanings out of people's experiences as lived.

There are different types of qualitative research (see below for a brief overview of the three main types).

TYPES OF QUALITATIVE RESEARCH

Phenomenology

Phenomenology is a term that covers a range of research approaches that are derived from similar, but different, philosophical perspectives. You will come across the works of philosophers such as Husserl, Heidegger and Gadamer, with each offering a view on the way in which the researcher looks at the world. For example, Husserl suggests that the researcher should 'bracket' their experiences, knowledge and attitudes (i.e. set them aside so they do not interfere with the research process). Heidegger, on the other hand, takes the view that the researcher is an inherent part of the research process, and that therefore their knowledge, attitudes and experiences can be taken into the research process (so long as this is clearly articulated within the research itself). Phenomenology aims to investigate the lived experiences of people within the particular context of that experience. The researcher investigates the phenomenon (the particular lived experience) through the people who have had that experience. Data collection methods are normally conducted via in-depth interviews and other verbal or written narratives. Data analysis approaches allow for interpretation of the narratives and would normally be presented as themes and categories. There are various types of phenomenology, including descriptive phenomenology and interpretive or hermeneutic phenomenology.

Example of a research question: What is the lived experience of the daughters of women with breast cancer?

Grounded theory

Grounded theory aims to generate theory by concurrently gathering and analysing data. It is often used to undertake investigations into areas that have not previously been investigated (or are under-researched). Grounded theory can focus on the development of knowledge relating to the ways in which social interactions take place and how these interactions are interpreted within the field, and can therefore shed light on the ways in which these social interactions can be enhanced for the benefit of particular practice situations. Data collection is usually undertaken using in-depth interviews and participants are selected on the basis that they can talk about the phenomenon under investigation. With grounded theory, the people who participate (the sample) will often develop over the course of the research study, with participation sought from those who can describe the issues emerging from the initial interviews. The analytical process is one that is ongoing and results in the development of categories (that emerge as the collection of data progresses).

Example of a research question: What are the perceptions of children's and young people's nurses of their role in caring for patients and their families with cystinosis?

Ethnography

Ethnography aims to study culture and cultural groups through the observation of behaviours, rituals, customs and practice. This observation can take place either overtly (i.e. with the knowledge of the people under investigation) or covertly (i.e. without their knowledge). By this stage you will probably already be thinking about the considerable ethical issues associated with undertaking a research study without the knowledge of the participants – but it has been done! The process of undertaking an ethnography allows the researcher to offer an interpretation of the ways in which the cultural context impacts on people's behaviours and practices within that context. Data collection takes place by the researcher going into the specific 'field', undertaking observations and engaging in discussion/questioning, taking field notes, and potentially undertaking interviews. Data analysis commences with the field notes (where the researcher starts to write down their ideas, interpretations and descriptions of what they see and hear).

Example of a research question: How is patient-centred care enacted in a particular forensic unit?

Each of these research approaches has its own philosophical beliefs and values about doing research. Remember your learning from Chapter 7 when you had to consider the overarching philosophical perspectives relating to research? As you will come to see in subsequent chapters, these philosophical perspectives are important for your understanding of qualitative research approaches – they provide a standpoint from which a researcher views the world and therefore impact on both the type of questions and the investigatory approach that is used for a particular research study. At the heart of qualitative studies lies meaning-making and interpretation of the data collected about the phenomenon under investigation. For example, as alluded to above, one approach that can be used is hermeneutics. Hermeneutics is defined as the science of interpretation of oral or written text and serves the purpose of illuminating our thoughts and understanding by enabling new insights and meaning to be gained about a specific phenomenon. Through this process of illumination and the development of understanding, our previous standpoint may shift in relation to the phenomenon in question to a new and different level (Cohen, 2000).

As you will have gathered qualitative research uses human speech or written data, rather than numbers, as is the case in quantitative research. The sample size (simply put, the number of participants selected from the total population using sampling techniques) is usually small (Cohen et al., 2007) because of the depth and richness of the data generated. Think about when you have conversations with your friends or family about something that is of real interest to you all. If you were to write down the conversation, it would probably run to pages of text. When researchers ask people to participate in their studies, they will invite people who have experienced the phenomenon in question (e.g. domestic violence) and therefore those participants are likely to have a lot to say – thus creating a depth and richness of data (the words). Studies are also undertaken in the research participants' natural environment or settings or in a place of their choosing in order that they are more likely to feel comfortable and at ease in that environment (Denzin and Lincoln, 2005).

As you have seen, data collection in qualitative research requires the researcher to use one or more of a number of different types of data collection methods, such as in-depth interviews, semi-structured interviews, unstructured interviews, focus groups, conversational analysis, participant observations, and videoing. These data collection methods are sometimes termed *subjective* in that the data are open to interpretation and are usually the views or perceptions of each participant. The purpose of qualitative data collection is to gather rich, descriptive data that, once analysed, will enable the researcher to provide a description and/

or interpretation of the phenomenon in question (Green and Browne, 2005). Data analysis for qualitative research can take a number of forms but should always be systematic, rigorous, and appropriate to the philosophical framework. As you will see, the decisions that are made regarding methodology (perhaps phenomenology), data collection method (perhaps in-depth interviewing), and analysis (for example the use of Collaizi's seven steps – you can look that up if you wish, but you will get the chance to consider this and other analytical approaches in later chapters) all come together through a systematic knowledge-based approach to the development of a strong research proposal. You might like to work together in a small group to undertake Activity 8.2.

ACTIVITY 8.2

You may wish to undertake this activity in a group, but you can do it alone if you wish. Go back to the article that you chose to look at in Activity 8.1. Take turns in your group to describe the following:

- The methodology used in the research study.
- The data collection method(s) used.
- The analytical framework used.

Once you have all had a turn, discuss the following thought-points in your group:

- What makes the studies 'qualitative' in nature?
- What kinds of research questions can qualitative research provide 'answers' to?
- How is the qualitative nature of the studies reflected in the methodologies, method and analytical frameworks?
- What are the key features of qualitative research that you have identified so far?

As you will have seen from the studies you discussed as a group, qualitative research can be of a sensitive nature. For example, a study that investigated mental health service users' experiences of sexual and relationship issues uncovered personal information through semi-structured interviews (McCann, 2010). Later in this book you will have the chance to explore the ethical issues associated with undertaking research of any kind (in Chapter 13 which looks at ethics in healthcare research). Here we want to emphasise that the ethical code of practice of the researcher requires special consideration in order not to bring psychological or emotional harm to research participants. In addition, the ethical issues associated with qualitative research require the researcher to make certain that the research is undertaken with rigour which will ensure that the findings are trustworthy and credible. What we mean here is that the research user (for example, the nurse who wishes to implement the findings of a study in practice) can trust that the research has been undertaken in an appropriate way throughout, and that the findings are dependable within the context of qualitative research.

The value and strength of qualitative research lie in helping you to ascertain people's experiences through their exploration in a given social context. It provides thick, rich, and meaningful insights into the phenomenon being studied (Polit and Beck, 2010), and helps in giving a voice to the less articulated knowledge embedded in human experiences (Dunniece, 2002). When you come to Chapter 11 on qualitative research, you will see that the research approach adopted to answer the research question depends on the nature of the topic and the type of data needed.

WHAT IS QUANTITATIVE RESEARCH?

Now that you have considered some of the ways that research can help nursing and healthcare practitioners begin to understand aspects of the human experience, we shall move on to look at quantitative research, which aims to provide evidence relating to clinical interventions and other situations through the collection of numerical data and their subsequent statistical analysis. Quantitative research involves formal *objective* information gathering about the world through the use of measurement tools such as validated questionnaires, to statistically quantify the phenomenon being studied. It can be used to describe and test relationships between various factors in order to examine cause-and-effect relationships (Punch and Punch, 2005). Quantitative researchers will use large samples of participants with the aim of generalising findings to encompass the wider population – what this means in simple terms is that the findings from a quantitative study often aim to be relevant and applicable across the wider population rather than simply those in whom the research was undertaken (the latter is often the case in qualitative research). Quantitative studies involve the use of statistics to describe the findings and enable the research user to make judgments about a study's usefulness in practice. Activity 8.3 aims to give you the opportunity to consider the different kinds of research questions that can be addressed quantitatively (as opposed to qualitatively).

ACTIVITY 8.3

Do another search for a research article that describes a quantitative study in an area of interest (perhaps relating to the qualitative article that you accessed earlier). Consider the following questions and write down your initial thoughts:

- What is the aim of the research (or the research question)?
- What makes the study a quantitative study? For example, is the study aiming to determine the measurable impact of an intervention on the health outcomes of a group of patients?
- Which data collection and data analysis approaches were used? (Do not worry if you feel a little lost with the statistical analysis – later chapters will enable you to engage constructively with the data presented in quantitative studies.)

The most common quantitative research designs include:

- Experimental designs, ranging from:

  - randomised controlled trials (RCTs) in which an experiment is conducted where participants in the study are randomly assigned to the intervention group or a control group;
  - pre-/post-test studies where data are gathered prior to the intervention with the same approach to data collection used to gather data following the intervention – allowing for comparisons to take place between the two;
  - quasi-experiments where it is not possible to undertake a randomised controlled trial – for example, where it would not be possible to introduce an intervention and also have a control group for practical or ethical reasons.

- Surveys including:

  - descriptive – used to describe a population and to determine whether there may be links or trends between variables (a variable is something that can be measured and that can sometimes change over time or in different situations – e.g. blood pressure, age, smoking status);
  - correlation – used to determine whether there are relationships between demographic data (e.g. age, gender) and behaviour (e.g. exercise behaviour);
  - comparative studies – used to determine whether behaviours/variables change over time and in relation to interventions and/or demographics);
  - longitudinal – studies that take place over a longer period of time;
  - cohort studies – studies that follow a particular group of people over a period of time.

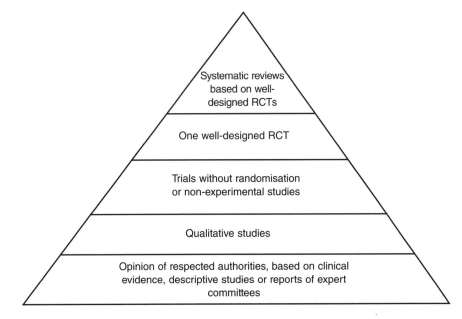

Figure 8.1 An example of a hierarchy of evidence (source: Holland and Rees, 2010)

To some extent all of these designs have a common aim, which is to produce evidence that is tangible, concrete and measurable, justifying why – when considering the hierarchy of evidence – quantitative studies feature high on the list (second to systematic reviews) as shown in Figure 8.1.

This hierarchy of evidence will vary depending on different schools of thought. However, despite these differences of opinion quantitative research remains high on the list of evidence. The rigour of research studies is crucial for all practitioners to consider when selecting evidence to inform practice. Quantitative researchers will use validity (whether the data collection tool, for example, a questionnaire, measures what the researcher says it measures) and reliability (whether the data collection tool consistently measures what it sets out to measure) to measure rigour, whereas (as briefly discussed already) qualitative researchers will use trustworthiness, confirmability, transferability, and credibility (MacNee and McCabe, 2008). The measurements of validity and reliability as considered for quantitative research will be discussed in more detail in Chapter 12.

OBJECTIVE AND SUBJECTIVE MEASUREMENTS IN QUALITATIVE AND QUANTITATIVE RESEARCH

The main aim of quantitative research is to measure or quantify a phenomenon and all data or variables identified to be analysed in numerical form (objective measurements). Making sense of quantitative data requires analysis manually or using a statistical package such as Statistical Package for the Social Sciences (SPSS). There are four types of measurements used to categorise quantitative data. These are listed here with examples of the kinds of data that the terms refer to:

- *Nominal or categorical scales:* Labels (or names) such as gender, ethnicity and religion which have no intrinsic order as such.
- *Ordinal scales:* Data that have named categories and are ordered, such as the honours classifications of an undergraduate degree from 1st class Honours to 3rd class Honours.
- *Interval scales:* Numbers that have a specific order with measures that are equal between each occurring value. An example of this is a Likert scale measuring a respondent's agreement or otherwise which can have values from strongly agree (5) to strongly disagree (1).
- *Ratio scales:* Considered the strongest scale as it has an absolute zero starting-point, enabling the distance between the points to be compared with each other as well as proportionally (e.g. weight, height, blood pressure, pulse rate).

The reason why it is necessary to have some understanding of the types of data that can be gathered quantitatively is that this allows you to determine whether the statistical tests used in a particular study were appropriate for the type of data gathered.

In contrast, qualitative research measurement is subjective in nature and aims to shed light on the hidden meanings attributed to particular human experiences in various social situations. As you have seen, it does this through interpretation and meaning-seeking, by generating categories and themes from the data collected so that the phenomenon being studied can be described (Guba and Lincoln, 2005). Qualitative research measures such as interviews and observations aim to measure, through insight and understanding, unquantifiable concepts such as 'What is compassionate caring'?, and 'How does compassionate caring vary in different nursing situations?'

There will be times when qualitative and quantitative approaches can both be utilised in a single study. For example, the use of standardised measures like questionnaires to collect data relating to the clinical outcomes of a particular healthcare intervention could sit well alongside the use of interviews to investigate patients' experiences of that intervention.

ASSESSING THE QUALITY OF RESEARCH STUDIES

We have already briefly discussed some of the terms associated with the quality of research studies (reliability, validity, credibility). As a research user it is crucial that you really understand the meanings of these terms and how significant these are in your assessment of the usefulness of a particular piece of research for practice. Undertake Activity 8.4 below – this activity aims to consolidate your early understanding of the terms used and help you identify any further learning needs.

Take both of your research articles from Activities 8.1 and 8.3 and do the following:

- List the terms used within each of the articles which indicate that the rigour of the research study has been thought through.
- After doing this define those terms and think about whether they were the appropriate approaches for use within the individual studies.

ACTIVITY 8.4

Many published research studies painstakingly account for the instruments used to gather data. For example, a study may consider whether the data collection tool had been tested in other studies and, if so, whether it was found to be valid and reliable in those other studies. What we are aiming to emphasise here is that the whole research process must be undertaken rigorously (whether the study is qualitative or quantitative) so that the research users (people like yourself who are working in healthcare practice) can be confident that the published research is safe to consider for implementation in practice. A lack of rigour within any study stands the risk of generating unsafe findings which, if used in practice, can put the general public at risk. An example of where published research findings resulted in a risk to the public was research by Dr Andrew Wakefield. Published in *The Lancet* (a reputable medical journal) in 1998, this linked the MMR vaccine with autism, however the study was later found to have major methodological flaws (Godlee et al., 2011). So, we will look at some of these terms in further detail – if you need to, you can go back to Activity 8.4 and fill in any gaps as you work your way through this short section.

Reliability, as discussed earlier, is concerned with the consistency, accuracy and repeatability of the research tool (Moule and Goodman, 2009). Validity, on the other hand, relates to whether a data collection tool does what it professes to do – for example, does an instrument designed to measure depression assess depression? Rather obviously, any data collection tool that does not measure what the researchers aim to measure could produce findings that are at best irrelevant and at worst unsafe. Every aspect of the research process must be transparent and open to scrutiny by those with a vested interest.

The nature of qualitative research means that reliability and validity are not terms that are usually associated with these approaches. Even with a careful description of participants and settings, such research will not facilitate the production of an exact replication of the study because of the uniqueness of the study population and naturalistic settings (Polit and Beck, 2010). As we have said, in qualitative research various strategies are used by researchers to establish methodological rigour. Trustworthiness in qualitative research indicates the level of rigour by looking at:

- *Credibility:* Do we have confidence in the truth of the data and the research findings?
- *Transferability:* What is the degree to which the findings of the study can be transferred to other contexts or settings?
- *Dependability or auditability:* What is the audit trail that demonstrates the procedural routes to decisions made by the researcher at every stage in the research process?
- *Confirmability:* Does the study demonstrate credibility, auditability, transferability? If so, it can be said to possess confirmability.

You may come across other terms that are used within qualitative research to demonstrate rigour. Keep a list of these in your research journal, alongside their meanings, and you will soon build up your confidence with the terminology.

METHODOLOGICAL DIFFERENCES BETWEEN QUALITATIVE AND QUANTITATIVE RESEARCH

In Chapter 10 you will be looking in detail at the research process in order that you are clear about the way in which any research study should be planned and implemented. What is important for this chapter is to highlight one of the early aspects of the research process – the way in which a researcher will choose the methodology for a project. By understanding this key point, you will be able to draw together your growing understanding of qualitative and quantitative approaches before moving on to other chapters that will build on this knowledge.

Selecting the correct approach and design depends on the question posed or the phenomenon under exploration. Given that nursing and healthcare research can

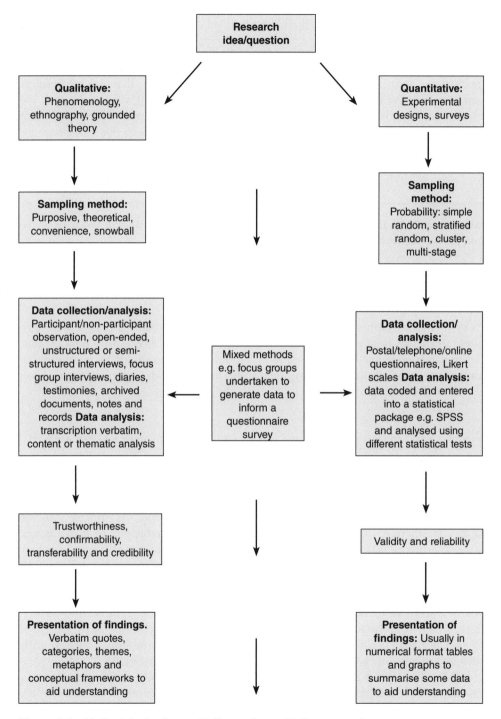

Figure 8.2 Methodologies for qualitative and quantitative research

address many areas of practice including the effectiveness of treatments, or patients' views or experiences of the care they received whilst in hospital, it is important that the methodology fits with the desired aim and objectives of the study.

Figure 8.2 summarises the differences in the methodologies of qualitative and quantitative approaches – already you will be able to see terms that you are familiar with, and we have introduced a number of other terms that you will come across. We have pulled together the key issues addressed in this chapter and represented them in the figure for ease of reference. You may wish to refer back to this in subsequent chapters.

Now complete Activity 8.5 which aims to assist you in consolidating your learning.

ACTIVITY 8.5

Take a few minutes to list some nursing and healthcare-related questions or areas of practice that you feel are worthy of further investigation:

Consider how you would investigate these issues – which methodology would you propose for these investigations and why?

As you will have gathered by now, it is crucial that the approach or design of a study does not dictate how a research question is answered but vice versa – namely, that the research question or line of enquiry should direct the choice of methodology (and subsequent choices regarding data collection methods, sampling techniques, and data analysis approaches).

THE IMPLICATIONS OF QUALITATIVE AND QUANTITATIVE RESEARCH FOR NURSING AND HEALTHCARE

Human experience is complex, and the same goes for the various illnesses and diseases that bring patients to the health and social care services. As nursing involves human interaction, qualitative research approaches will enable you to gain a better understanding of patients' feelings, attitudes and the meanings attributed to their illness, disease and health states or conditions, care, and treatment experience. The quantitative research approach can, for example, demonstrate the benefits (or otherwise) of an intervention that you provide for a patient by doing a pre-test and post-test study to determine what change has occurred. The qualitative and quantitative research approaches will support one another, and help you locate the types of evidence that can inform the care you give to patients, or how you deal with various problems in your practice and the decisions you must make.

Finally, Activity 8.6 provides you with an opportunity to check out your learning thus far and identify any areas for further development. Remember that this chapter aims to give you an overview of qualitative and quantitative approaches and further details will follow in Chapters 11 and 12.

Which of the following are correct?

(Q1) A study of the behaviour of newly admitted patients by observing and recording their day-to-day interactions during their first 72 hours following hospitalisation is:

a. Qualitative research? []
b. Quantitative research? []
c. Both? []

(Q2) Investigating the ways in which nurses are portrayed in the print media by analysing newspapers and magazine articles is:

a. Qualitative research? []
b. Quantitative research? []
c. Both? []

(Q3) Observing whether patients conform to the safety of treatment-prescribed guidelines by counting the number of patients who ignore the guidelines given is:

a. Qualitative research? []
b. Quantitative research? []
c. Both? []

(Q4) Using a written questionnaire with closed (yes and no) and open-ended (information that the person wishes to share in words) questions to survey a large number of victims of domestic violence who may be suffering from post-traumatic stress disorder is:

a. Qualitative research? []
b. Quantitative research? []
c. Both? []

(Q5) Organising a small number of students into a discussion group to study their experience of reflective practice on clinical placement is:

a. Qualitative research? []
b. Quantitative research? []
c. Both? []

(Q6) Testing the relationship between the scores on an intelligence test and scores on a personality test is:

a. Qualitative research? []
b. Quantitative research? []
c. Both? []

(Continued)

(Continued)

(Q7) Observing the effects of using a reward to teach a child to play with other children is:

    a. Qualitative research?   [ ]
    b. Quantitative research?   [ ]
    c. Both?   [ ]

(Q8) Investigating the effects of watching violent films on television by analysing children's drawings after is:

    a. Qualitative research?   [ ]
    b. Quantitative research?   [ ]
    c. Both?   [ ]

(Q9) Conducting an experiment to investigate whether taking regular 15-minute rest breaks during prolonged study sessions in class improves students' performance is:

    a. Qualitative research?   [ ]
    b. Quantitative research?   [ ]
    c. Both?   [ ]

(Q10) Observing the play interactions of nursery school children in the playground using pre-determined items on an observation checklist is:

    a. Qualitative research?   [ ]
    b. Quantitative research?   [ ]
    c. Both?   [ ]

Answers to quiz questions

Q1.	C	Q2.	A	Q3.	B
Q4.	A	Q5.	A	Q6.	B
Q7.	A	Q8.	A	Q9.	B
Q10.	A				

CONCLUSION

This chapter has focused on two research approaches used in nursing and healthcare research. It has served to help you familiarise yourself with qualitative and quantitative approaches, and the differences and similarities that exist. Examples of nursing questions that can be answered with these research approaches have been alluded to, and you have had the opportunity to seek out research articles that relate to both approaches in your area of interest and practice. It is important that you see your development of research literacy as a lifelong commitment to quality enhancement in your professional practice – as a practitioner you will be making decisions about the implementation of evidence into practice in all areas of your work. Qualitative and quantitative research approaches complement each other and the key is in knowing the theoretical underpinnings and which type of research evidence to select to help you answer questions regarding the day-to-day nursing experiences you encounter. We hope that we have demystified any fears and confusion you had about understanding qualitative and quantitative research approaches in reading this chapter.

SUMMARY

The critical learning points for your learning so far are:

- Qualitative and quantitative research methodologies are crucial to the development of different types of nursing knowledge to enhance nursing and healthcare practice.
- Knowledge of the difference between qualitative and quantitative approaches can help you understand research findings and their specific uses for your practice.
- There are different criteria for addressing rigour in qualitative and quantitative studies.

FURTHER READING

The following websites have useful resources that you can access to further enhance your knowledge and understanding of qualitative and quantitative research and related issues. They will help inform your university and clinical placement learning and assessment.

Social Research Methods: www.socialresearchmethods.net/kb/qualmeth.php
A useful website covering all research methods and related issues.
Robert Wood Johnson Foundation: www.qualres.org/
A comprehensive website covering all aspects of qualitative research and related issues.

REFERENCES

Cohen, L., Manion, L., Morrison, K. and Morrison, K.R.B. (2007) *Research methods in education*. London: Psychology Press.

Cohen, M.Z. (2000) How to analyse the data. In M.Z. Cohen, D.L Kahn and R.H. Steeves (eds), *Hermeneutical phenomenological research: A guide for nurse researchers*. London: Sage. Chapter 7.

Creswell, J.W. (2007) *Qualitative inquiry and research design: Choosing among five approaches* (2nd edition). Thousand Oaks, CA: Sage.

Denzin, N.K. and Lincoln, Y.S. (2005) The discipline and practice of qualitative research. In N.K. Denzin and Y.S. Lincoln (eds), *The SAGE handbook of qualitative research* (3rd edition). Thousand Oaks, CA: Sage. pp. 1–32.

Dunniece, U. (2002) Giving voice to the less articulated knowledge of palliative nursing: an interpretive study, *Journal of Palliative Nursing*, 8 (1): 13–20.

Gerrish, K. and Lacey, A. (eds) (2010) *The research process in nursing* (6th edition). Oxford: Blackwell.

Godlee, F., Smith, J. and Marcovitch, H. (2011) Wakefield's article linking MMR vaccine and autism was fraudulent, *British Medical Journal*, 342.

Green, J. and Browne, J. (2005) *Principles of social research*. Reading: Open University Press.

Guba, E.G. and Lincoln, Y.S. (2005) Paradigmatic controversies, contradictions, and emerging confluences. In N.K. Denzin and Y.S. Lincoln (eds), *The SAGE Handbook of qualitative research* (3rd edition). Thousand Oaks, CA: Sage. pp. 191–215.

Holland, K. and Rees, C. (2010) *Evidence-based practice skills*. Oxford: Oxford University Press.

MacNee, C.L. and McCabe, S. (2008) *Understanding nursing research: Using research in evidence-based practice*. Beverley Hills, CA: Lippincott Williams and Wilkins.

McCann, E. (2010) Investigating mental health service user views regarding sexual and relationship issues, *Journal of Psychiatric and Mental Health Nursing*, 17 (3): 251–259.

Moule, P. and Goodman, M. (2009) *Nursing research: An introduction*. London: Sage.

Myers, M. (2000) Qualitative research and the generalizability question: standing firm with Proteus. The Qualitative Report (On-line serial) 4, 3/4 (www.nova.edu/ssss/QR/QR4-1/myers.html).

Nursing and Midwifery Council (NMC) (2010) *The code: Standards of conduct, performance and ethics for nurses and midwives*. London: NMC.

Polit, D.F. and Beck, C.T. (2010) *Essentials of nursing research: Appraising evidence for nursing practice* (7th edition). Philadelphia, PA: Wolters Kluwer Health and Lippincott Williams and Wilkins.

Punch, K.F. and Punch, K. (2005) *Introduction to social research: Quantitative and qualitative approaches*. London: Sage.

Van der Zalm, J.E., Jeanne, E. and Bergum, V. (2000) Hermeneutic–phenomenology: providing living knowledge for nursing practice. Methodological Issues in Nursing Research, *Journal of Advanced Nursing*, 31 (1): 211–218.

9

ALTERNATIVE AND COMPLEMENTARY RESEARCH APPROACHES

RUTH TAYLOR AND SHEELAGH MARTINDALE

Chapter learning outcomes

On completion of Chapter 9, you will be able to:

1 Explore the contexts in which research questions arise.
2 Justify the reasons for using complementary research approaches to answer particular research questions.
3 Understand a range of alternative and complementary research approaches.
4 Explore opportunities for creativity in nursing and healthcare research.

Key concepts

Research questions, action research, evaluation research, case study research, Delphi, mixed methods, creativity in research.

INTRODUCTION

The purpose of this chapter is to consider the range of approaches to undertaking research that are available to investigate nursing and healthcare issues which exist alongside (and complementary to) those discussed in Chapter 8. We are not claiming that the chapter provides an exhaustive overview of these approaches. What we want to help you to do though, is to be prepared to think creatively around the approaches that are available to researchers, and to have an awareness of some of these approaches so that when you read an article which discusses research that has been undertaken less traditionally, you will be able to think critically about the research for your own practice.

In Chapter 8 you had the opportunity to explore the fundamental concepts relating to qualitative and quantitative research approaches and you will have already seen that there are many ways in which a researcher can address research questions or objectives. What we are calling 'complementary' approaches are those that are perhaps not as mainstream as those that you have considered so far. However, we are very aware that some of these approaches are widely and effectively used. For example, one of the authors (Taylor, 2012) used case study research to investigate the experiences of first-year nursing students.

In addition to ensuring that we provide a certain 'coverage' to the approaches that are used in nursing and healthcare research, we are keen that you think about how important creativity is within the research process. As you saw in Chapter 1, one of the ambitions of this textbook is to help you to achieve further enthusiasm for research in practice – creativity is key to enthusiasm in order that we can work towards achieving our potential in practice.

This chapter sets out a number of research approaches that have not been explored thus far. We provide examples of where these approaches have been used in nursing and healthcare practice, and ask you to uncover further examples that have particular relevance to your own practice. We hope you will be able to draw on your developing skills in literature searching that we explored in Chapter 4, so that you can continue to build a portfolio of evidence that will link with your learning at university and your experiences and learning in practice.

HOW DO RESEARCH QUESTIONS ARISE?

Before we look into the various complementary research approaches it would be sensible to think about how we come up with research questions.

Traditionally within the positivist paradigm, as discussed in Chapter 7, research questions arise to test previously generated hypotheses. An example of this is from Martindale's own work where the hypothesis was:

- 'Maternal antioxidant intake during pregnancy can influence childhood susceptibility to asthma and atopic disease' (Martindale et al., 2005:121).

The author set out to test this hypothesis using a research question:

- 'Can antioxidant intake in pregnancy affect the onset of wheeze and eczema in the first two years of life?'

By asking this question not only did it provide the opportunity to test the given hypothesis, but it also directed the researcher to the appropriate design of the research to adequately answer the question (the clue to the appropriate methodology being the word 'affect' within the question). Cause and effect would normally occur as a result of a changed state directly affected by an action or intervention. Going back to Chapter 8, this should remind you about research that relates to measurement and quantity. Therefore the only research approach that would be suitable to answer Martindale's question would be a quantitative approach.

However, as you know, not all research sets out to test a hypothesis. Some research is about the meaning and development of hypotheses. For example:

- 'What are the views of patients, carers and respiratory nurses in relation to what factors influence quality of life in patients with Chronic Obstructive Pulmonary Disease?' (Martindale et al., forthcoming).

Within this question we would want to gather the 'views' of the study groups. Therefore, to ensure that this is achieved, we would need to speak directly to them so they are able to tell us about their lived experience, thereby pointing the researcher in the direction of adopting an inductive qualitative approach to answer the research question as described in Chapter 8. As a reminder from the learning that you completed in the last chapter, complete Activity 9.1.

Review the following research questions and identify whether they should be answered using a qualitative or quantitative approach.

- 'How effective are the screening policies for breast cancer as a public health initiative in Scotland?'
- 'What are the effects of blended learning in research education on the knowledge, attitudes, and opinions of student nurses?'
- 'How do first-year student nurses cope with 12-hour shifts in practice?'
- 'Do families of patients receiving ECT feel stigmatised by the treatment?'
- 'What is the best method for facilitating clinical supervision for remote and rural learners?'
- 'Are children more at risk of developing asthma if they have repeated antibiotic treatments in their first year of life?'

ACTIVITY 9.1

You may have found the above exercise easy and been able to place each question into one of the two approaches. However, don't worry if you were unsure about some of them as a number of the questions could incorporate a range of approaches. You will look into this in more detail later on in the chapter when considering mixed methods research.

In your daily practice it is likely that you constantly ask questions about why or how you are carrying out a certain procedure in a certain way, or compare practice within one area or placement with another. Thinking about your own experiences, complete Activity 9.2.

ACTIVITY 9.2

If you can, get together with some of your peers and consider some questions relating directly to your areas of practice. List these below:

- Discuss how you found the answers to your questions (e.g. through a literature search, discussion with colleagues in practice).
- When you found some answers, did these result in any changes in practice?

It may be that national or local policy is driving change within your area of practice. One example of this was highlighted in Chapter 5 within the Scottish policy document *Better health, better care* (Scottish Government, 2007a), which identified the shifting nature and predominance of chronic diseases rather than acute illnesses (of course, this is true across the UK and more widely). As you will have experienced, healthcare services are changing to take account of the need to ensure that these groups of patients are cared for more effectively and efficiently. As a result, research is often driven by the needs of policy development and implementation – as you have already seen it is vital that healthcare practice is based on evidence and policy, but it is not always developed from an evidence base. Therefore as healthcare practitioners we need to be aware of where the evidence base for practice lies, and work towards the growing development of that evidence base. Within our Master's degree course at our university, students are asked to undertake practice-based projects as part of a drive to grow the evidence base for practice in the students' areas of clinical practice. Box 9.1 below provides an overview of some of these projects, and notes how these originated from policy with the drive to improve practice.

Box 9.1 Practice vignettes

Clinical Question: 'What education and training will a Band 3 Health Care Support Worker require to undertake their role?'

Policy Drivers: *Delivering care, enabling health* (Scottish Executive, 2006); *Better health, better care* (Scottish Government, 2007a); *A guide to health care support worker education and role development* (Scottish Government, 2009).

These policies identified that we are challenged by an ageing population with multiple long-term conditions, as well as an alarming number of qualified nurses approaching retirement age. Therefore, one Health Authority in 2009 developed the Health Care Support Worker Role.

Clinical Question: 'Does the wearing of tabards during drug rounds reduce the number of interruptions?'

Policy Drivers: *Scottish patient safety programme* (Scottish Government, 2007b); *Healthcare quality strategy for NHS Scotland* (Scottish Government, 2010).

It was highlighted within the policies identified above that there was a continual issue about the number of drug errors within practice which inevitably had an effect on patient safety. This project attempted in part to address this issue by piloting the wearing of tabards during drug rounds within a community hospital.

Clinical Question: 'In critically ill patients, are chlorohexidine and tooth brushing more effective to reduce Ventilator Acquired Pneumonia (VAP) compared to other solutions and methods for cleansing the mouth?'

Policy Drivers: *Health care order set: Prevention of ventilator associated pneumonia* (Institute for Clinical Systems Improvement, 2009); *Guidelines for preventing healthcare associated pneumonia 2003: recommendations of CDC and the Healthcare Infection Control Practices Advisory Committee* (Centre for Disease Control and Prevention, 2003).

This project was conducted in an international setting. It was identified from the above documents that the incidence of VAP could be reduced by simple measures. Therefore this project set out to identify from the available evidence the most effective and efficient method of oral hygiene for these patients within an ITU setting. Beyond the constraints of the Master's project, the identified option was to be piloted and implemented into the student's healthcare setting and then evaluated at a later date.

From these examples above, you can see how policy can inform the research agenda and impact on practice. Later on in the book, you will have the chance to learn more about change management, so that you can consider the ways in which you can work with others to implement evidence-based changes in practice.

Finally, in this section we will offer a brief overview of how research questions relating to clinical practice can be developed. The PICO framework is a useful tool (Smith, 2008; Horsley et al., 2009) where:

P = Population or patients

I = Intervention or exposure

C = Comparison or comparator group

O = Outcome

Let's see if we can make sense of this in the real world of research or clinical questions. Once again we have used an example from one of our Master's students, who posed the question 'Is intranasal Diamorphine more effective than Oramorph in the treatment of acute severe pain in children under the age of 12?' Using the PICO acronym:

P= Children under the age of 12

I = Intranasal Diamorphine

C = Oramorph

O= Amount of acute severe pain

Questions developed using the PICO framework often concern enquiries about effectiveness. Relating back to the previous section, questions relating to cause and effect most often adopt a quantitative approach to research and utilise quantitative methods. However, this framework may not always be appropriate for all the questions we will come up with: it may be that the researcher is asking *why* patients feel more relaxed in an anesthetic room when there is music playing; or *how* nurses cope in stressful situations; or *what* are the opinions of relatives about care for their loved ones while in hospital, for example. All of these questions would perhaps make you think that a qualitative approach may be most appropriate for the investigation.

It may be that the clinical or research question is pre-determined by changes already occurring, or about to occur, within the clinical area. An example of this originated from another one of our Master's student projects where it was identified that care plans within a particular clinical area were not being used adequately. It was therefore felt that there was no evidence of patient-centred care. Electronic care plans were implemented for particular areas of patient care which, following a pilot implementation, would then go on to be evaluated. This is an example of 'action research' (Moule and Goodman, 2009) which will be discussed in the following section.

Looking back at some of the questions posed within the practice-based projects displayed within Box 9.1, there are some developments generated within practice that originated from a necessity to change practice which was driven by policy. However, following implementation it becomes essential to evaluate these. A pilot study (in this situation the pilot was the time-bound implementation of the intervention in one particular area) was implemented in the example of:

• 'Does the wearing of tabards during drug rounds reduce the number of interruptions?'

Following on from the pilot study, an evaluation study would allow evidence to be drawn in relation to how effective, applicable, and perhaps acceptable this change to practice has been. The results from the study would assist the service to make decisions as to whether this development should be implemented permanently and perhaps to a wider area (Moule and Goodman, 2009). Again, evaluation research will be covered in more detail later on in this chapter.

At this point we need to talk briefly about audits. There is sometimes a bit of confusion about where audit sits in relation to research. This is likely to be a process that you have had some engagement with, either by undertaking an audit, or by implementing the findings from an audit (see Figure 9.1). Let's start by saying that an audit is not research although it does have a number of similarities with research. An audit in itself is a measured way of improving existing practice. However, prior to any change in practice a baseline audit should be performed (using either quantitative or qualitative data collection methods), the change implemented, and then a further audit must be undertaken to ensure the predetermined objectives and standards have been met. Hopefully this clarifies any confusion relating to audits and research and it is something that you will need to explore more fully in your course, both at university and in practice.

We will now move on to take a look at complementary research approaches – which we have alluded to already – in order that you can build on your knowledge and gain a greater appreciation of the range of approaches that can be used for the investigation of nursing and healthcare practice. Once you have completed the learning within the next section, you might want to go back to Activity 9.1 as you

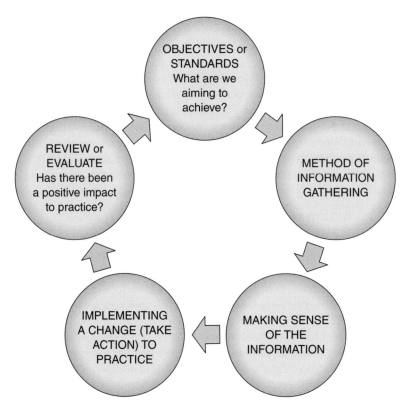

Figure 9.1 The audit cycle

may have identified that some of the research questions did not fit easily into either a quantitative or qualitative approach. For example:

- 'What are the effects of blended learning in research education on the knowledge, attitudes, and opinions of student nurses?'

The words 'effects' and 'knowledge' should make you think that this question would best adopt quantitative methods. However, 'opinion' could sway you towards qualitative methods. Therefore this question may be more suited to a mixed methods study.

COMPLEMENTARY APPROACHES TO RESEARCH

Action research

Action research originated in work by Lewin in 1946 (Cohen et al., 2007) and has since been used within the nursing profession as a means to solving problems in practice situations. Lewin's work focused on organisational learning based on changes within the practice of organisations. Action research aims to impact on practice through the generation of theory in an integrated manner, so that research findings (and the generation of theory) are implemented as part of the overall research process (Moule and Goodman, 2009). The term *action research*, for us, clearly indicates its purpose as a dynamic approach to the development of knowledge in ways that facilitate the improvement of practice. Its focus on changes in practice is through the description of practice, the development of understandings about the practice situation and explanations of the situation, with a focus on improvements for practice (Robson, 2011). Before you go on to look at more of the detail of action research, take some time to review the information in Box 9.2 which provides two examples of action research projects.

Box 9.2　Action research projects

Griffith, S. (2011) Improving practice using action research: resolving the problem of kinking with non-metal cannulae, *International Journal of Palliative Care*, 17: 531–536.

Griffith's article described a research project that aimed to find an alternative cannula device with the result that practice was improved both from a patient and a staff perspective. The steps that were taken to achieve this aim were as follows:

1　Hospice accident books reviewed to provide statistics relating to needlestick injuries over a specified period of time up to (firstly) the point of the introduction of cannula type A and (secondly) the point of introduction of cannula type B. The review revealed that injuries occurred with cannula type A and not with cannula type B. However, it was noted that the cannula type B were kinking.

---

2 Evaluation of the reasons for the kinking of cannula type B and measurement of the frequency of kinking (to allow for comparisons to be made following a change to practice and which took place over a period of two months using a structured data collection tool).

3 A literature search was undertaken which revealed a superior cannula type C for use within the context.

4 Change-over to cannula type C following data collection period 1 (above).

5 Data collection period 2 using the same structured data collection tool for comparison purposes which revealed no improvement in practice outcomes.

6 Reflections of staff who were immersed in the research to identify possible reasons for a lack of improvement in practice outcomes revealed that the giving set type may have been a problem.

7 Search for alternative giving set devices, and a survey of practice in other similar units, revealing alternative cannula type D.

8 Data collection period 3 using the same structured data collection tool for comparison.

9 Findings indicate that the cannula type D is suitable for practice.

Wilson, V., Ho, A. and Walsh, R. (2007). Participatory action research and action learning: changing clinical practice in nursing handover and communication, *Journal of Children's and Young People's Nursing*, 1(2): 85–92.

Wilson et al.'s study investigated ways in which verbal handover processes could be improved in a special care nursery in Australia. Participatory action research is a collective approach to the improvement of practice through the identification of an issue, investigation of the issue, the development of a change in practice, its implementation and evaluation. The steps that were taken within this project were as follows:

1 Nursing staff volunteered to join an action learning set and identified that the nursing handover was an area of concern.

2 Review of current practice through a literature review.

3 Development of a staff survey to determine the views of staff regarding the handover.

4 Development of a handover tool based on the literature review and a survey of findings.

5 Implementation (trial) of the tool on a voluntary basis for three months.

6 Participant observation undertaken to investigate the implementation of the tool over a period of six months.

Findings from the participant observation were used to inform ongoing practice.

As you can see from these two examples, action research enables nursing and health-care staff to answer questions that relate to practice. The characteristics of action research are:

- The research takes place in the 'real world' (Wilson et al., 2007) and is undertaken by those who inhabit that real world.
- There is collaboration between those who are undertaking the research, and those who are being researched (Robson, 2011). Participatory action research (as in the example provided above) in particular emphasises the collaborative nature of the research process.
- It is often small-scale research that focuses on a particular problem in a particular practice area (Griffith, 2011).

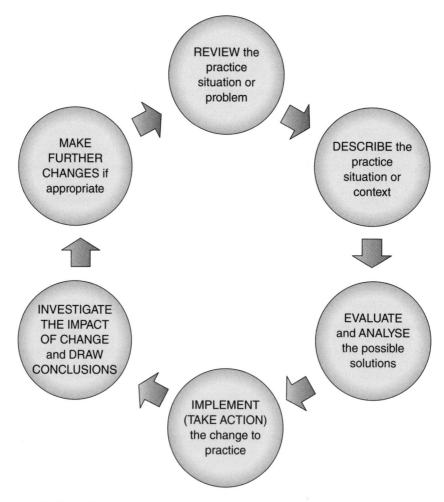

Figure 9.2   The action research cycle

- It is flexible in its design (which can bring problems if the research is carried out in a truly collaborative manner, as those involved may hold a different view to that of the researcher in relation to the best approach to be taken).
- The methods of data collection for action research are varied and include all those covered within our sections on research methods. The key is that the choice of research method is made based on the questions or objectives to be addressed.
- Action research enables practitioners to be empowered within a context of practice change (Streubert and Carpenter, 2011) and gives them the tools to be transformational in their practice.
- Its use facilitates organisational and cultural transformation through a focus on enquiry, learning and enhancement which enables practitioners to meaningfully influence practice.
- The findings from action research directly impact on the area under investigation and can facilitate practice change in a way that addresses some of the challenges of change management (McCormack et al., 2001).

Action research could be viewed as being similar to the reflective process that we have used in previous chapters (see Figure 9.2). A collaborative and participatory approach to identifying the problem, the proposed change, the investigation of the change, and the evaluation of outcomes, are the main components of action research. If you want to have an impact on practice, action research is certainly one of the research approaches that will allow you to do just that. Now undertake Activity 9.3.

Undertake a quick literature search on an area of practice that you are particularly interested in (possibly related to your next placement area), and try and find an example of an action research project. Briefly outline the steps that were taken within the study, and list what you see as the strengths and limitations of action research.

ACTIVITY 9.3

Action research – key steps

Strengths and limitations of action research

Evaluation research

As you will be aware, healthcare providers are under increasing pressure to provide effective and efficient services. As a healthcare professional you will need to be able to demonstrate that your practice is efficient and effective. Evaluation research is one way of determining the impact (or otherwise) of nursing and healthcare practice, with the often explicit aim of assessing the effectiveness and efficiency of a service (Robson, 2011). As Moule and Goodman (2009: 219) state, 'Evaluation research makes use of the tools and techniques of basic research and applies them to research questions about need, efficiency, effectiveness, appropriateness and acceptability.' Box 9.3 offers a short description of one example of evaluation research – one which will be relevant to all nursing and healthcare students in that it focuses on education for the enhancement of healthcare-acquired infections. You may wish to access the article yourself so you can read it in more depth.

Box 9.3   Example of evaluation research

West, B., Macduff, C., McBain, M. and Gass, J. (2006) Evaluation of a national educational programme for healthcare workers on prevention and control of healthcare associated infections, *Journal of Research in Nursing*, 11 (6): 543–557.

The paper presents the findings from an evaluation of a national educational programme (the Cleanliness Champions Programme) that aims to ensure good practice in preventing healthcare-associated infections. The researchers used the following research methods:

- A literature review.
- Large-scale questionnaire surveys of students and mentors.
- 20 key-informant interviews.

The key findings from the research included:

- The Cleanliness Champions Programme was fit for purpose but needed some modifications.
- Two-thirds of those who undertook the programme were nurses.
- Information about the way in which the programme was initially integrated into practice.
- Evidence of the substantial impact the programme had had on personal practice and its influence on others' practice.
- The necessity for other occupational groups to undertake the programme.

The evaluation research aimed to do a number of things, including examining the congruence between what the programme was designed to do and what was actually enacted in terms of programme delivery.

At this stage undertake Activity 9.4. You may wish to do this with one or more or your peers.

Make a list of areas of your own practice that you feel would benefit from evaluation research. These can relate to service delivery, policy implementation, educational initiatives, an innovation, or service organisation (amongst others).

Now choose one of these areas and identify at least one research article that utilises evaluation research to determine its effectiveness, efficiency, outcomes, or quality. Critically review the article and answer the following questions together:

1 What research methods did the research team choose to use to evaluate the area?
2 How appropriate do you think these methods were, and what are your reasons for this?
3 What was it about the research design that made this *evaluation research* as opposed to something else?

The key characteristics of evaluation research are:

- The research is 'real world' research – it is applied research which aims to address issues affecting practice, policy or service (either at a macro or micro level).
- Evaluation research allows researchers to determine why changes occur, what these changes are, and what their impact is (Moule and Goodman, 2009).
- Evaluation research allows researchers to make judgments about nursing and healthcare practice.
- It is usual for evaluation research to take account of the organisational values and purpose, and the evidence that exists about the area under investigation.
- Outcomes from evaluation research enable practitioners to make evidence-based decisions for practice.
- Evaluations can be undertaken formatively (to help with the development of an intervention for example) or summatively (to determine the impact of the intervention).
- Data collection usually focuses on structure (organisational structures and the environment), processes (the intervention activities and the delivery of the service, and outcomes (the impact of the intervention) (Donabedian, 1980).
- The steps that are taken to undertake evaluation research are the same as those for any other research project (see Chapter 10 on the research process) and with a focus on the aims of the evaluation.

Finally, evaluation research is a wide-ranging research area and one which merits further investigation. One way of ensuring that you are comfortable with the topic is to read around the area (further reading is suggested at the end of the chapter), identify some further examples of evaluation research, and then review the articles in light of your theoretical understanding of evaluation research.

Case study research

Case study research (CSR) is variously defined and comes from a number of perspectives. What we aim to do in this short section is capture the key attributes of

CSR, explore the range of issues that can be investigated using CSR, and point you in the direction of further reading as there is a wealth of literature relating to CSR.

Thomas (2011: 3) defines the case study method as 'a kind of research that concentrates on one thing, looking at it in detail, not seeking to generalise from it. When you do a case study, you are interested in that thing in itself, as a whole'. The 'thing' in Thomas's definition can be:

- A person.
- A group.
- An institution.
- An event.
- A period of time.

In truth, it can be anything where you feel that you need to find out the how and why of something. CSR enables researchers to look at a phenomenon (the 'thing') from a number of perspectives and gain a deep understanding which will end with a balanced and rich picture of the subject under investigation. Therefore, when investigating a case, you will need to choose methods that will facilitate its exploration – and these can be varied. Simons (2009: 21) nicely defines CSR as 'an in-depth exploration from multiple perspectives of the complexity and uniqueness of a particular project, policy, institution, programme or system in a "real life" context. It is research-based, inclusive of different methods and is evidence-led. The primary purpose is to generate in-depth understanding of a specific topic'.

There are a number of different types of case study and these are well-described within the literature where you will see differences in viewpoints across the theoretical debate. You don't need to worry about the differences, the important thing is that you get to grips with what a 'case' is (see Box 9.4), the reasons for doing case study research, and the ways in which it can be carried out. If you do these things, you will then be in a position to critically review research undertaken in this way from an informed perspective.

Box 9.4   What is a case?

Taken from Thomas (2011):

- *The case as a container:* The case is 'bounded' and contains everything that relates to the case within it.
- *The case as a situation, event:* The case is a specific situation and the circumstances associated with the situation.

It contains a subject (for example, specialist epilepsy service for adolescents) and an analytical frame or object (for example, an analysis of the reasons for the specialist epilepsy service being an exemplar of good practice).

Case study research does not allow for generalisation. Rather, it is the particular-ness or the uniqueness of the case that is interesting. The boundary referred to before is the way in which the case study is defined – the time/history of the case, and the extent of the case. So why would a researcher choose to undertake case study research? Take a look at Activity 9.5 as this will provide you with some general guidance around the kinds of 'cases' that have been investigated in nursing and healthcare research.

ACTIVITY 9.5

We have chosen some case studies that help to shed light on issues that are relevant to all nursing students, no matter which field of practice they are working in. You should either access the articles that are suggested, or undertake a literature search to locate at least two articles on case study research that are of particular interest to you. As you critically read the articles, answer the following questions:

1 What is the 'case'? Describe its boundaries.
2 How is case study research defined?
3 What is the purpose of the case study research?

Donnelly, F. and Wiechula, R. (2012) Clinical placement and case study methodology: A complex affair, *Nurse Education Today*. Doi: 10.1016/j.nedt.2012.02.010.
   This is an interesting article that describes the potential for the use of case study research in the exploration of clinical placement as a component of nursing education. It is a complex paper but offers some useful insights into case study research methodology.

Cooke, H. (2006) The surveillance of nursing standards: An organizational case study, *International Journal of Nursing Studies*, 43: 975–984.
   Although this paper does not describe case study research, it does provide some nice examples of cases which should emphasise the boundaried nature of the case for you.

As with all research, a case study researcher will utilise the research process (described in Chapter 10). Within the decision making process, the researcher will need to identify which kind of case study approach should be used. Remember that we said earlier that there is a lack of a consensus in relation to some aspects of CSR – this is reflected in the naming of case study research with its attendant purposes. Thomas (2011) – it's a great book! – usefully categorises the purpose, the approaches, and the processes for case study research. We have summarised what he tells us below (see Box 9.5) and we would recommend that you read his accessible and humourous book to gain a greater depth of understanding.

Box 9.5   Purposes, approaches and processes for case study research (from Thomas, 2011)

Purposes: Why do you want to do CSR?

Intrinsic: You are studying the case out of interest.
Instrumental: You are doing the CSR for a reason.
Evaluative: You expect to determine whether something has worked or is working.
Explanatory: You want to explain something.
Exploratory: You want to know more about an issue or a problem so that you will gain a better understanding of the issue.

Approaches

Building a theory: With the aim of explaining the case.
Testing a theory: With the aim of determining the theory's explanatory power.
Illustrative: With the aim of bringing the case to life.
Interpretive: With the aim of developing a deep understanding of the case.
Experimental: With the aim of trying something out.

Processes

Single or multiple: Where one case or a number of cases are investigated.
Retrospective: Where a case is investigated by looking back.
Snapshot: At a particular point in time.
Diachronic studies: Show change over time.
Nested case studies: Looking at how units within a case fit together.
Parallel and sequential studies: Multiple studies where the former looks at a number of cases at the same time, and the latter looks at them one after another.

Key characteristics of case study research include:

- A focus on the context of the research.
- A focus on an holistic understanding of the situation and its related circumstances.
- A focus on the quality of the research to take account of the varied research methods that can be used within CSR.
- A need to be very clear about the purpose of the CSR so that the relevant approach and process(es) can be chosen.
- The opportunity to use a number of research methods so that the phenomenon can be investigated from a number of perspectives and a 'thick' description of the phenomenon can be developed.
- A narrative that 'tells the story' of the case so that others can determine its relevance to their own practice.

Delphi method

The Delphi method is one which, along with other consensus methods, aims to come to a point of common agreement on a particular issue. If you do a quick review of the literature, you will see that the Delphi method is being used in healthcare research quite extensively. Basically, it is an approach which is used where there is a lack of understanding in relation to an identified healthcare issue. An expert group is identified and these people are then involved in a number of Delphi 'rounds' until consensus is identified. The 'rounds' are usually surveys that start with preliminary findings or ideas, and then move into further surveys where the expert opinion feeds into the ongoing questions that are presented to the expert group. Through these rounds it is anticipated that consensus can be achieved, though its main drawback as an approach is that expert opinion may not necessarily be correct. Box 9.6 offers a summary of one Delphi study by way of explanation of the technique.

Box 9.6 Delphi method

Chami, K., Gavazzi, G., de Wazières, B., Lejeune, B., Carrat, F., Piette, F., Hajjar, J. and Rothan-Tondeur, M. (2011) Guidelines for infection control in nursing homes: A Delphi consensus web-based survey.
  Steps:

- Issue identified and a dearth of evidence available.
- A literature review, review of practice guidelines, systematic reviews, and articles or abstracts published in English or French on 'infection prevention'.
- Literature search examined by 23 experts and a list of 301 recommendations made.
- Delphi survey online instrument developed from the recommendations using a nine-point scale from strongly disagree to strongly agree.
- Experts rated their agreement with each of the recommendations (round 1).
- Recommendations developed following round 1 to 130 recommendations.
- Expert group rated the 130 recommendations (round 2).
- Guidelines for infection control in nursing homes developed from the consensus.

Mixed methods research and triangulation

You will have seen that in evaluation research, case study research and action research, it is possible and theoretically sound to use a number of different research methods. You may then be asking yourself – what is the difference between these research approaches and 'mixed methods' research? By now you will have explored a range of literature, reviewed many research articles, and will be coming to a much stronger understanding of the key issues already identified in this book. Therefore, for this section, you are the one who will be coming up with all the answers! We know you can do it. Box 9.7 provides a brief definition and overview of mixed methods research as a starter, and then Activity 9.6 offers you, as a group or individually, the opportunity to pull together an overview of the central points. Once you have captured these points, you will see that you have a resource that will be useful when you are critically reviewing any research article – particularly from a research methods perspective. Thinking about your own practice, you can probably recognise that you already work with a variety of data sources to inform the decisions you must make when providing care. For example, you will take measurements of a patient's vital signs and you will also listen to the patient as you ask probing questions about how they are feeling at that time. In some ways then, you are already familiar with mixed methods!

Box 9.7   Definition

Mixed methods

A mixed methods study is one in which a number of research methods are utilised to address the research questions or objectives within that one study. Usually a mix of qualitative and quantitative methods would be adopted. The use of mixed methods allows for triangulation (where the findings/results from one method sit alongside the findings/results from another method, allowing the researcher to corroborate/validate – or otherwise – the sets of results). The use of mixed methods allows the researcher to seek to address the research questions by utilising a variety of data collection methods (for example, a survey and interviews).

ACTIVITY 9.6

Come together as a group if you can and put together a PowerPoint presentation that addresses the following points:

- Define mixed methods research.
- Provide an overview of why you would use mixed methods research and the kinds of research questions or objectives that you could address using this approach.
- List the strengths and limitations of mixed methods research.
- Identify at least four research projects that have used mixed methods and briefly offer an overview of your critical appraisal of one of these projects.

CREATIVITY IN RESEARCH

This final section is a short paragraph on our view on the need for creativity in research. As part of the book as a whole we are keen to promote how necessary it is for all students to work towards achieving their potential and in so doing impact positively on the patient experience. As part of this achievement of potential, we are certain that the development of creativity across all aspects of the learning experience is one of the key areas that will set you apart from others. When we use the term 'creativity' we do not necessarily mean the use of art (for example) in your work (although this is one way in which you can incorporate creativity into your practice). What we are getting at here is the need for you as an individual to always work towards enhancing your criticality and questioning skills so that you can respond to practice situations in ways that are evidence-based and will lead to the development of better care. In research, the use of creativity allows for the identification of relevant research questions or areas for investigation, and the development of research proposals that will imaginatively allow researchers to seek out greater understandings for the enhancement of patient care. Sometimes it may feel difficult to find a place for creativity in your busy working day, but we will use this book to offer you some ideas about how you can find the time and thinking space to do just that. In the meantime, your learning from this chapter has hopefully allowed you to see that research is a creative activity.

SUMMARY

This chapter has provided you with an overview of some of the alternative and complementary approaches to research that are available for the investigation of research questions that are of relevance to nursing and healthcare. The critical points for your learning so far are:

- The choice of research methodology and methods is the result of a structured decision making process stemming from the research question or objectives that have been identified.
- There are a number of research approaches that are available to the researcher and it is important that as a research user you are familiar with these approaches, as well as their strengths and limitations.
- Thinking of research as a creative activity offers you the opportunity to realise your potential as you continue on your course and move into qualified practice.

FURTHER READING

There are many books and articles that provide detailed accounts of the approaches to research that we have described here. Some of our favourites include:

Cohen, L., Manion, L. and Morrison, K. (2007) *Research methods in education* (6th edition). London: Routledge, Taylor and Francis Group. Cohen et al.'s book is detailed and accessible for students who wish to explore action research and case studies (amongst other areas).
Keeney, S., Hasson, F. and McKenna, H. (2001) A critical review of the Delphi technique as a research methodology for nursing, *International Journal of Nursing Studies,* 38: 195–200.
Moule, P. and Goodman, M. (2009) *Nursing research: An introduction.* London: Sage. Moule and Goodman's book contains very good chapters on evaluation research and consensus methods.
Thomas, G. (2011) *How to do your case study: A guide for students and researchers.* London: Sage.

REFERENCES

Centre for Disease Control and Prevention (2003) *Guidelines for preventing healthcare associated pneumonia 2003: recommendations of CDC and the Healthcare Infection Control Practices Advisory Committee.* Available at: www.cdc.gov/mmwr/preview/mmwrhtml/rr5303a1.htm [last accessed 1 August 2013].
Chami, K., Gavazzi, G., de Wazières, B., Lejeune, B., Carrat, F., Piette, F., Hajjar, J. and Rothan-Tondeur, M. (2011) Guidelines for infection control in nursing homes: A Delphi consensus web-based survey. *Journal of Hospital Infections,* 79(1): 75–89.
Cohen, L., Manion, L. and Morrison, K. (2007) *Research methods in education* (6th edition). London: Routledge, Taylor and Francis Group.

Cooke, H. (2006) The surveillance of nursing standards: An organizational case study, *International Journal of Nursing Studies*, 43: 975–984.

Donnelly, F. and Wiechula, R. (2012) Clinical placement and case study methodology: A complex affair, *Nurse Education Today*. Doi: 10.1016/j.nedt.2012.02.010.

Donabedian, A. (1980) *Explorations in quality assessment and monitoring. Volume 1: The definition of quality and its approaches to assessment.* Chicago: Health Administration Press.

Griffith, S. (2011) Improving practice using action research: resolving the problem of kinking with non-metal cannulae, *International Journal of Palliative Care*, 17: 531–536.

Horsley, T., O'Neill, J. and Campbell, C. (2009) The quality of questions and use of resources in self-directed learning: personal learning projects in the maintenance of certification, *Journal of Continuing Education in the Health Professions*, 29 (2): 91–97.

Institute for Clinical Systems Improvement (2011) *Health care protocol: Prevention of ventilation associated pneumonia.* Available at :www.icsi.org/_asset/y24ruh/VAP.pdf [last accessed 1 August 2013].

Martindale, S., McNeill, G., Devereux, G., Campbell, D., Russell G. and Seaton, A. (2005) Antioxidant intake in pregnancy in relation to wheeze and eczema in the first two years of life, *American Journal of Respiratory and Critical Care Medicine*, 171: 121–128.

Martindale, S., Stephen, A., Addo, M. and Devereux, G. (forthcoming) Views of patients, carers and respiratory nurses in relation to what factors influence quality of life in patients with Chronic Obstructive Pulmonary Disease, *International Journal of Chronic Obstructive Pulmonary Disease.*

McCormack, P., Copper, R., Sutherland, S. and Stewart, H. (2001) The safe use of syringe drivers for palliative care: an action research project, *International Journal of Palliative Nursing*, 7 (12): 574–580.

Moule, P. and Goodman, M. (2009) *Nursing research: An introduction.* London: Sage.

Robson, C. (2011) *Real world research* (3rd edition). Chichester: Wiley.

Scottish Executive (2006) *Delivering care, enabling health. Harnessing the nursing, midwifery and allied health professions' contributions to implementing 'Delivering for Health' in Scotland.* Edinburgh: Scottish Executive.

Scottish Government (2006) *A guide to health care support worker education and role development* (revised 2010). Edinburgh: NHS Education for Scotland.

Scottish Government (2007a) *Better health, better care: Action plan.* Edinburgh: Scottish Government.

Scottish Government (2007b) *Scottish patient safety programme.* Available at: www.scottish patientsafetyprogramme.scot.nhs.uk/programme/about [last accessed 1 August 2013].

Scottish Government (2010) *The healthcare quality strategy for NHS Scotland.* Edinburgh: Scottish Government.

Simons, H. (2009) *Case study research in practice.* London: Sage.

Smith, K.M. (2008) Building upon existing evidence to shape future research endeavours, *American Journal Health-System Pharmacology*, 65: 1767–1774.

Streubert, H. and Carpenter, D. (2011) *Qualitative research in nursing: Advancing the humanistic imperative* (5th edition). Philadelphia, PA: Lippincott, Williams and Wilkin.

Taylor, R. (2012) Social capital and the nursing student experience, *Nurse Education Today*, 32 (3): 250–254.

Thomas, G. (2011) *How to do your case study: A guide for students and researchers.* London: Sage.

West, B., Macduff, C., McBain, M. and Gass, J. (2006) Evaluation of a national educational programme for healthcare workers on prevention and control of healthcare associated infections, *Journal of Research in Nursing*, 11 (6): 543–557.

Wilson, V., Ho, A. and Walsh, R. (2007) Participatory action research and action learning: changing clinical practice in nursing handover and communication, *Journal of Children's and Young People's Nursing*, 1 (2): 85–92.

PART 4

LET'S DO RESEARCH

10

THE RESEARCH PROCESS

DAVE ADAMS AND RUTH TAYLOR

Chapter learning outcomes

On completion of Chapter 10, you will be able to:

1 Understand what is meant by the concept of the research process.
2 Be able to identify the different stages of the research process.
3 Appreciate how the different stages of the research process fit together.
4 Discuss the importance of the research process in relation to critiquing research studies.

Key concepts

Research process, Pyramid Model.

INTRODUCTION

If you are new to research as an academic subject then it can be a little confusing to say the least. The first area of concern to newcomers is probably the language used – but if you have read this book up until this point you should be coming to terms with that (*if not return to page 1 and start again!*).

Another cause of confusion though may well be a lack of knowledge about how a research study is structured. Many texts will assume you are conversant not only with the terminology of research, but also with how it is organised and what is done at each of the different stages of the process.

It's worth pointing out here that the research process is not something external to a research study – in a very real way the research process *is* the research study. Regardless of the methodology and methods used any study will go through the same stages, so even if a study uses an approach that you are unfamiliar with, if you understand the research process you will still be able to make a critical examination of the study itself by attempting to recognise how the study addresses each stage of the research process.

To try and make the process easier to understand for student nurses in a second year research module, a colleague of ours, Elaine Mowatt, had the idea of putting together a model of the process which she and the rest of the module team then went on to develop. The idea was not to reinvent the wheel in terms of the content of the model, rather it was to present the research process in such a way that it would stick in the minds of students and aid their understanding of what the process was and how and why it was sequenced in the way it was. It seemed to work well with them, and hopefully will do the same with you too!

In this chapter then, you will first examine the research process itself, what it is, and what it does. Following this, you will look at what the different stages of the process are, and the sequence they follow, using the Pyramid Model (the importance of this sequencing will also be discussed). Finally, you will consider the use you can make of your new-found knowledge of the process when it comes to appraising a piece of research critically.

THE RESEARCH PROCESS

So before going any further let's look at the research process itself, namely what it is and why you need to know about it. There is no great mystery here – the research process can be briefly summed up as 'a series of steps or stages undertaken by researchers in order to address research questions' (Moule and Goodman, 2009: 28). You can think of it then as a systematic framework for researchers to use when planning their research study, in much the same way as nurses would use the nursing process to design care plans for patients.

As to why you need to know about it (even if you yourself are not planning on carrying out research), it gives you the ability to look critically at and gain an understanding of a research study (and you need to be able to do that to keep up in an evidence-based profession). If you know what the stages of the research process are, you can examine any study, using these stages, to establish how, and why, the research question and design of the study were arrived at.

An understanding of the researcher's rationale behind the design, implementation and reporting of their study can be arrived at in a logical and systematic fashion, which will then allow you to deconstruct (break down) the key stages of the study in order that you can examine them further. In the real world it has long been recognised that the research process is often not as straightforward or linear as the way textbooks make it appear (Moule and Goodman, 2009), but when reading a study it provides a useful and logical manner to go about critiquing it. Our Pyramid Model (Figure 10.1) is explored within the rest of the sections of this chapter and used as a basis to take you through each of the stages of the research process to enable you to become familiar with all aspects of the research process.

THE PYRAMID MODEL

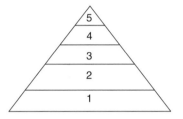

Figure 10.1   The Pyramid Model (source: Mowatt, E., Adams, D., Eboh, W. and Johnson, N. (2013) Unpublished teaching aid used at Robert Gordon University.

The Pyramid Model consists of five stages as shown in Figure 10.1:

- *Stage 1:* Recognise and clarify the problem (including the literature review and the development of the research question).
- *Stage 2:* Discuss and plan the study (including the identification of funding, ethics requirements, and supervision of the research).
- *Stage 3:* Refine the research question and select the appropriate methodology (finalisation of the research question, choice of design and key aspects of the appropriate methodology to be used in the study is made here).
- *Stage 4:* Refine the methodology (a pilot study may be carried out, methodology refined in light of this, and then the main study carried out).
- *Stage 5:* Disseminate findings.

At this point, it is worth including a caveat. You will find that some of the terms within the research process are used differently depending on the researcher's perspective – for example, research approach, methodology, research design. For clarity, we have used the terms in this chapter in the following way:

- *Research approach:* The philosophical underpinning of the research (e.g. qualitative, quantitative or mixed).
- *Methodology:* The methods that are used within the study to collect and analyse the data (e.g. interviews, surveys), the sampling approach, the ethics.
- *Research design:* The approach plus the methodology.

Each of the sections within the model identifies and explains the different stages that make up the various tiers of the Research Pyramid. Just as in a real structure, each tier relies on the tier supporting it for its stability. So, for example, if the literature review in Stage 1 is not properly undertaken, then this will weaken all the tiers above it: the design and methodology may be flawed if all the available information to base them on is not made available through a literature review. Take a look at Activity 10.1 below.

First find a study

Find a published research study, on a topic of interest to yourself, in a relevant professional journal. You will use this study as a basis for the rest of the activities in this chapter (feel free to pick more than one study if you wish to!).

Make sure it is either a full study or a comprehensive journal article, and preferably published in a peer-reviewed journal, which will help ensure the quality of the published material.

Stage 1: Recognise and clarify the problem

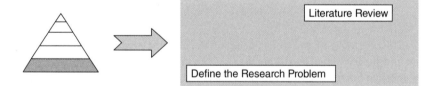

Most studies will start from an idea or an actual or potential problem of some kind, but initially this may well be sketchy and will need to be further defined before the study can go further. For example, healthcare practitioners working in a specific setting may have some key questions relating to how care is delivered and the ways that practice can be enhanced, such as 'Is a particular intervention that we have implemented having an impact on the patient experience?'. You might have had a similar experience if you have been involved in project or group work, where you have to choose a topic and develop a presentation on it. Your first ideas can often be too big and try to take on too much, so the first thing you need to do is narrow things down to exactly what it is you are interested in and sort out exactly what it is you want to do.

For a research study (though it also works well for project/group work) the starting-point for the further development of the research question is a structured and comprehensive search of the literature around the chosen topic (see Chapter 4 for details of the process of undertaking a literature review). The literature search is designed to find out what is known about the topic already, and what studies have been carried out around it previously.

Following on from this search, a review of the literature is undertaken so that the scope and nature of the study to be carried out can be further refined. The parameters of the study (what the researchers have decided to include and exclude within the study) may be clarified, based on what has been found within the literature, and this may then give an initial idea of what kind of approach and design might be best suited to the study.

Look at the literature review within your chosen study and try to answer the following questions, giving a rationale for your answers.

- How comprehensive does the literature review seem to be?
- Does it use material to discuss the rationale for the study? Is the information presented balanced, or is the material presented one-sided?
- Is most of the work reviewed contemporary (i.e. within the last five years) or does it include older work too? And if it does include older work is this relevant for inclusion?
- Does the literature review also inform the research approach and design?

ACTIVITY 10.2

You should now feel able to make a judgment about the comprehensiveness and relevance of the particular literature review for the study you have chosen to use for the activities within this chapter. The skills that you are developing should be used when you review any future research for practice. Remember that as you do these activities you are continuing to develop your critiquing skills further – practice makes the process so much more comfortable and enables you to see things that you might not pick up on when you are just starting out.

Stage 2: Discuss and plan the study

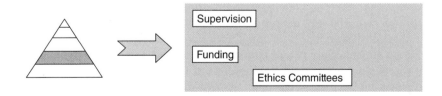

Stage 2 is a bit different from some other descriptions of the research process that you might see in other research textbooks in that we have given these aspects a stage to ensure that they are seen as key components of the research process. It is important that you are familiar with these aspects of the research process as they are certainly relevant for the critique of research.

Thus far, Stage 1 has enabled the researcher to identify the area for investigation and to explore the knowledge that currently exists within that area. In addition, the literature review has provided the researcher with the basis from which to make decisions, regarding the approach to take, in order to answer the research question. Based on the information gained in the first stage, and the subsequent further defining of the research question, the study proposal can now begin to be put together. This part of the process enables the researcher to start to address issues such as supervision for the research, mentorship, funding for the study, and ethical approval through the relevant committees, such as:

- LREC (Local Research Ethics Committee).
- University ethics committees.

The relevant ethics committees would be approached and dealt with at this point. Ethical approval is essential if the research study is ever to get off the ground and actually be carried out. From a critiquing perspective you can gain some insight into a published study by seeing how these factors have been addressed, particularly in relation to the issues of ethical clearance and funding.

Not every published study gives details of all the ethical issues it has considered within an article. In some cases the reader is left to suppose that the study must have gained ethical clearance in view of the fact it was undertaken by a clinical or university-based team. Sometimes there will be only a brief mention made of where clearance was gained, but no further details will be given. However, especially when a study has involved people, it is useful for you to know how, in particular, consent was gained in order for you to gauge if it was indeed free and informed. A lack of information about ethics will make it difficult to evaluate the sampling process in relation to its adherence to ethical principles of research (Macnee and McCabe, 2008).

The lack of free and informed consent is not only unethical (which by itself would mean a study should not take place), it may also have an impact on the veracity (truthfulness) of any information obtained by subjects. For example, if patients within a clinical setting are asked to take part in a study in such a way as to feel they really must do so if they want to receive good care, then their answers to any questions may well be biased towards giving the kind of answers they think the researchers want as opposed to what they may really think. Therefore, when details of ethical issues are given, pay particular attention to how and where the sample population was approached, and any details about how the participants were invited to take part in the study, as well as how much information was given to them. You will read more about ethical issues in subsequent chapters, and particularly in Chapter 13.

Not directly related to ethical issues, but of relevance to them, is the supervision of a research project. It is vital that the research is undertaken by an experienced research team, or that a novice researcher is supervised by someone (or a team) that is able to guide the process so that it is undertaken rigorously. You may not find that the details of the team are discussed within an article, but the authorship of the peer-reviewed article should give you an appreciation of the skill set of the team. At this stage of the research process a team will be pulled together to ensure that the skills and knowledge for the proposed project are such that the project can be carried out to a high level of quality. For all bids for funding, those providing the funding will want to be reassured that the team is able to deliver on the project.

Knowing the funding sources for a study can also be useful (research is expensive to carry out, and all researchers need to have some financial resources to support the running costs of a study), though once again this information is not always given. Funding from commercial sources, government or institutional grants for example, is always worth noting, as perhaps more than other sources this can be open to issues of conflicting interests: in particular, an association has been noted between the pharmaceutical industry's funding of studies and the likelihood of a pro-industry outcome for studies (McGauren et al., 2010; Goldacre, 2012). Any good research study should therefore make any potential conflicts of interest clear from the outset, as this may well have the potential to impact on the validity of any findings that come from the study.

Look at any details on ethical clearance or funding given within your chosen study and try to answer the following questions, giving a rationale for your answers.

- What details of ethical clearance are given?
- Are you able to discern if, and if so, how free and informed, consent was obtained from those taking part in the study?
- Are there any indications of a conflict of interest within the study?

ACTIVITY 10.3

Stage 3: Refine the research question and select the appropriate methodology

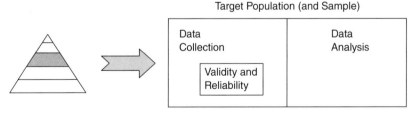

Things may be narrowed down further at this stage, both in terms of exactly what the study will be looking at, and how it is going to go about it. So at this stage of the process the research question/hypothesis may be further refined, based on things such as a consideration of the ethical and/or funding issues; and further thought may be given to the most suitable approach and design to meet the overall aims of the study. Approaches and design in relation to research studies are explored in more detail in subsequent chapters, including Chapter 11 on qualitative research and Chapter 12 on quantitative research.

For example, if a study intends to look at students' attitudes to learning about research then a decision would need to be made as to how best to achieve this. For an overall picture of students' feelings on learning about research, an objective approach using a survey design could be employed. This would tell us how many felt a particular way, but would not give any insight into why they felt the way they did. If feelings were important to the study, a qualitative approach using a phenomeno-logical design might perhaps be considered more appropriate instead (phenomenology was discussed in Chapter 8). If the study was trying to answer both the 'how many' and the 'why' questions, then the researchers might opt to go with a mixed methods design and carry out a survey first, following this up by interviewing some of the participants to find out why they answered the questions as they did.

Choosing the most appropriate approach and design is key to the quality of the research evidence which will be eventually produced (Topping, 2006), so at this stage, when you are critiquing a piece of research, you will need to examine the aim of the study (remember that this might also be expressed as a research question or a hypoth-esis). You might wish to begin here by giving some consideration to how realistic the intention of the study seems to be, and then see if you think the approach and design chosen are the most appropriate to achieve the study's aims. (For details on the nature of qualitative and quantitative approaches see Chapter 8 and Chapter 9.)

ACTIVITY 10.4

Look at the information given within your chosen study in relation to the aim, approach and design and try to answer the following questions, again giving a rationale for your answers.

- How clearly is the aim of the study expressed?
- How well does the approach and design chosen for the study fit with the expressed aim?
- How convincing a rationale is present within the study for the choice of approach and design?

With the approach and design finalised, the appropriate methodology is chosen at this stage in relation to:

- Sampling.
- Data collection methods.
- Data analysis methods.

When considering sampling, you will need to look at the choice of population (everyone or everything which could have been included in the study), the sample (those chosen to represent the wider population) and the sampling technique that was used, in order to decide if these were appropriate to meet the aims of the study.

It is usually not possible to include an entire population in a study (unless you are focusing on a relatively small population to begin with), so a representative selection (the sample) will have to be chosen instead. If either the population or the sample or the sampling technique is not appropriate, then this can be seen as a major flaw in any study.

It's perhaps worth noting that it's not only people that can be considered a population in research – if you were focusing on patient records or health professionals' notes, the total number of these which existed, in the area under study, would also be considered a population (Polit and Beck, 2006).

Therefore, when examining this aspect of a research study, some key things to look for are:

- Has the population chosen been clearly identified and is it appropriate for the aims of the study? For example, if the aim of your study was to find out something about women's personal experiences of childbirth, then your population would be all women who have given birth – you wouldn't include men or women who hadn't experienced childbirth.
- Are any inclusion or exclusion criteria clearly stated, with a suitable rationale given? Sometimes additional criteria will be used to decide who will be included or excluded from a study. For example, the study looking at women's personal experiences of childbirth might add that the researchers were only looking at women who had given birth in the last year and were in a stable relationship. They would need to give a good reason for this of course, so it might be that they wanted the memories to be fairly fresh in the minds of those included in the study, and had a particular interest in those women who had a partner – you should be able to judge from the aim of the study whether or not these criteria were justified, or if the researchers excluded or included individuals who would have been useful for the study.
- Is the chosen sampling technique appropriate for the approach/design of the study? Broadly speaking, sampling can be divided into two main types: quantitative studies will use probability sampling (often called random sampling) and qualitative studies will use non-probability sampling (often called purposive sampling). Random sampling is not appropriate for qualitative studies – you will need to make sure someone has had a particular experience, for example, before you include them in a study about it. Likewise purposive sampling is not appropriate for quantitative studies or you won't be able to generalise from your results.
- Is the size of the sample adequate for the design of the study? Qualitative studies don't for the most part attempt to generalise from their results to a wider population and so small numbers are quite acceptable – the results can only really be applied to those within the sample.

Quantitative studies do want to be able to generalise from their findings, so larger numbers are needed in their samples. How large? Well that depends on the size of the population. Often the size of the sample needed to be statistically significant will be determined by using a tool called a 'power calculation' that will give an indication of the minimum sample size required (Lacey, 2006).

Next you can go on to look at the choices that the researcher has made in relation to the methods for data collection and analysis, and consider their fitness to achieve the aims of the study.

Data collection methods for research studies can include:

- Interviews.
- Focus groups.
- Surveys.
- Observations.
- Documents.
- Diaries.
- Tests and measurement scales.

As you will see when you come on to explore qualitative and quantitative research in more detail, each of these methods serves a particular purpose and is used to address specific kinds of research questions. Decisions relating to the target population and the sampling approach for the research should be congruent with the area under investigation and the data collection methods chosen for the study.

When you critique a research article, you should be looking for evidence that the researcher has given due consideration to the data collection methods and should, for example, not only tell you that they chose to use focus groups to collect their data, but ideally also explain why they opted to use focus groups rather than individual interviews. In the absence of such an explanation it is legitimate for you to be asking questions about why choices were made.

Decisions about the analysis of data also need to be made – these decisions will, of course, relate to the chosen data collection methods and will be qualitative or quantitative analytical approaches. The analysis of the data allows the researcher to identify the findings from the research study (the outcomes from the research process up until that stage that will shed light on the area under investigation). Once these findings have been illuminated, the researcher must then develop a discussion – which will often go back to the literature and other existing evidence – so as to come up with relevant conclusions and recommendations for the study.

Remember that in critiquing a study it is not necessary for you to have all the answers, but you do need to be able to ask the relevant questions that will enable you to make a judgment about the rigour of a particular study.

ACTIVITY 10.5

Look at the information given within your chosen study in relation to sampling, ethics, data collection and data analysis, and try to answer the following questions, again giving a rationale for your answers.

- Can you easily identify the key aspects of the research approach?
- Describe the sampling technique, ethical considerations, data collection and data analysis methods used in the study.
- How well do these fit the approach and design chosen for the study?
- How convincing a rationale is present within the study for the choice of research approach?

Stage 4: Refine the methodology

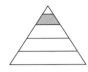

A pilot study may be undertaken, and the methodology of the main study may be refined in the light of the findings of the pilot. The main study can then be undertaken.

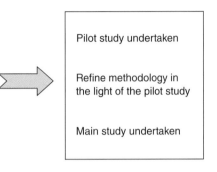

Pilot study undertaken

Refine methodology in the light of the pilot study

Main study undertaken

A pilot study can be described as a smaller version of the proposed main study which is undertaken to test if the components of the main study can all run together successfully (Airain et al., 2010). With the initial methodology decided upon, a pilot study may now be carried out (following ethical approval), primarily to test the data collection instrument/s being used in the study, but also to check a range of other things:

- Assessing the feasibility of a full study.
- Establishing the effectiveness of the sampling technique and recruitment approaches.
- Convincing funding bodies and other stakeholders that the research team is competent and that the study has value (Teijlingen and Hundley, 2001).

This is particularly necessary if such an instrument has been devised or adapted especially for the study rather than using a previously validated tool, as the pilot study allows the researcher to check the tool for its validity and reliability when it is put to use in practice (Smailes and Street, 2011). (For more information about validity and reliability, see Chapter 12 on quantitative research.)

Following a pilot study, adjustments to the study may be made prior to carrying out the main study itself in light of any problems or issues the pilot study may have uncovered.

Stage 5: Disseminate findings

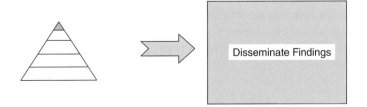

Disseminate Findings

So the main study has been carried out and the data collected have been analysed and discussed and conclusions have been drawn and perhaps various recommendations made – what's next? This is the stage at which the results of the study are disseminated and the process by which any knowledge gained by the study is accurately spread to those who can utilise it to impact on existing practice (Macnee and McCabe, 2008). No matter how good a study is it will be a wasted effort if its findings are not passed on to those who can make best use of them.

The usual way of things following the completion of a research study is for a paper to be written for a peer-reviewed journal. The article will describe the study and its findings, discuss those findings, and perhaps make some recommendations based on them. These papers may then be presented at relevant seminars and/or published in academic and professional journals. However, the researchers will have to have given careful consideration to where exactly they present or publish in order to make sure that the information they have reaches the right target audience. The other thing for you to be aware of is that it can take a considerable length of time to write a paper and get it published, so there is often a time lag between the study finishing and the article being published within a journal – sometimes more than a year or so (and you thought essay writing for exams was hard!). In most cases this is not a problem, but it is worthwhile looking at how long a delay there has been between the study being carried out and it being published, as in some cases things may have moved on in the interim period. This may then mean the study's findings have lost some of their relevance.

ACTIVITY 10.6

In relation to your chosen study try to answer the following questions, again giving a rationale for your answers.

- Who do you think the findings in the study will be most relevant to?
- Was the journal it was published in suitable for reaching this group?
- Is it clear what the potential impact of the findings could be on clinical practice?

CRITIQUING THE LITERATURE

We have talked a great deal about the need for you to understand the research process so that you are in a position to critique the literature. To draw this aspect of the discussion together, we have developed a tool that you may find useful when you are reading articles and research (see Box 10.1). It should allow you to think about all the aspects of the research process in a way that enhances your criticality. It can also provide a useful record of your reading and thinking and you can choose to pull together a collection of these on a particular topic to facilitate your development in this area.

Box 10.1 Literature review source

Using the article that you have found through your search, take about 30 minutes to read this, carefully highlighting the important points. Complete the following questions:

1 What is the title of your article? Does the title inform you of the approach used in the study?

2 What is the rationale or the reason for undertaking the study?

3 Does the literature review give you sufficient information to inform the study? Justify your answer and note down any key points emerging from the literature review.

4 Which approach and design were used? Were they appropriate? Justify your answers.

5 What ethical issues were identified and how were these addressed?

6 What was the sampling frame, sampling technique, and size? Were these appropriate for the study? Justify your answer.

7 How were the data collected, analysed, and presented? Were these approaches appropriate for the study? Justify your answer.

8 List the main findings within the study.

9 How could the findings impact on practice?

10 Did you consider the article easy to read in terms of terminology and presentation? What have been the key learning points for you?

SUMMARY

This chapter has taken you through a particular view of the research process using a framework (the Research Pyramid) which shows the approach to planning a research study, and as you have seen this can be used to deconstruct a study in order to critique it. The critical points for your learning so far are:

- A research study will generally have followed a series of steps or stages in its planning and implementation, referred to as the research process.
- Within this text we have related the stages to a pyramid, starting at the base and working towards the apex. This emphasises that failing to be rigorous at any of the lower stages can undermine the subsequent stages in the process and weaken their integrity.
- From the viewpoint of those learning about research, being able to break a study down into manageable sections should make the study easier to understand.

REFERENCES

Airain, M., Campbell, M.J., Cooper, C.L. and Lancaster, G.A. (2010) What is a pilot or feasibility study? A review of current practice and editorial policy, *BMC Medical Research Methodology* [online], 10 (67). Available from www.biomedcentral.com/content/pdf/1471-2288-10-67.pdf (last accessed 17 January 2013).

Goldacre, B. (2012) *Bad pharma*. London: Fourth Estate. p. 1.

Lacey, A. (2006) in K. Gerrish and A. Lacey (eds), *The research process in nursing* (5th edition). Oxford: Blackwell. pp. 25, 28.

Macnee, C.L. and McCabe, S. (2008) *Understanding nursing research* (2nd edition). Philadelphia, PA: Lippincott Williams and Wilkins. pp.157, 261.

McGauren, N., Wieseler, B., Kreis, J., Schüler, Y.-B., Kölsch, H. and Kaiser, T. (2010) Reporting bias in medical research – a narrative review, *Trials* [online], 11 (37). Available from www.trialsjournal.com/content/11/1/37 (last accessed 3 December 2012).

Moule, P. and Goodman, M. (2009) *Nursing research: An introduction*. London: Sage.

Parahoo, K. (1997) *Nursing research: Principles, process and issues*. Houndsmills: Palgrave Macmillan. pp. 72–75.

Polit, D.F. and Beck, C.T. (2006) *Essentials of nursing research* (6th edition). Philadelphia, PA: Lippincott Williams and Wilkins. p. 259.

Smailes, S. and Street, C. (2011) *The health studies companion*. Houndmills: Palgrave Macmillan. p. 282.

Teijlingen Van, E. and Hundley, V. (2001) The importance of pilot studies, *Social Research Update* [online], 35. Available from http://sru.soc.surrey.ac.uk/SRU35.html (last accessed 17 January 2013).

Topping, A. (2006) in K. Gerrish and A. Lacey (eds), *The research process in nursing* (5th edition). Oxford: Blackwell. p. 157.

11

QUALITATIVE RESEARCH
MARY ADDO

Chapter learning outcomes

On completion of Chapter 11, you will be able to:

1 Identify the key sampling strategies used in qualitative research.
2 Describe the major data collection and analysis methods used in qualitative research.
3 Understand specific ethical issues in qualitative research.
4 Discuss the presentation of qualitative research findings, and the potential impact of qualitative research in healthcare practice.

Key concepts

Qualitative research, sampling, data collection and analysis, ethical issues, methodological rigour.

INTRODUCTION

As you will have gathered by now, in any kind of research enterprise the researcher must identify the research question prior to deciding on the most appropriate approach for undertaking the investigation. The aim of this chapter is to provide a summary of the key issues associated with qualitative research – building on the *Qualitative and quantitative research approaches* chapter (Chapter 8). You will remember from that chapter that qualitative researchers use approaches that enable the exploration of phenomenon through the collection of non-numerical data (for example through interviews). Examples drawn from the literature to illustrate the key concepts and reflective activities should allow you to deepen your understanding and explore areas of practice that you have a particular interest in. Being able to critique qualitative research studies as a healthcare professional is important so that you are in a position to determine their relevance for evidence-based practice.

SAMPLING APPROACHES IN QUALITATIVE RESEARCH

When the research topic and questions have been established, explicit decisions must be made about which sample (individuals or groups) will offer researchers an opportunity to gather the appropriate data. Sampling in qualitative research involves decisions about:

- The types of people that should be included in order to allow researchers to explore the phenomenon.
- The relevant approach to selecting the sample.
- The sample size.

A qualitative researcher will develop inclusion and exclusion criteria (i.e. those who are, and those who are not, eligible to be included in the study). Sampling necessitates the identification of a target population (for example, 'all registered nurses' is a population). However, in qualitative research a researcher could not possibly access the whole of the population due to cost and feasibility and so will formulate an approach for the selection of a portion of the population. A key aspect of sampling within qualitative research is that the participants must be those individuals who have experienced the phenomenon (or are experiencing the phenomenon). Examples could include:

- Children's nurses working with asthma patients in a particular health centre.
- Mental health nurses working with offenders in organisations across Scotland.
- Adult nurses working with people with dementia in care home settings across the UK.
- Learning disability nurses working with clients in community settings in a specific town.

In general, small sample sizes are used in qualitative research to allow for richness, depth and detail in the data collected (Parahoo, 2006). Remember that the research question, methodology and design will all influence the sampling process. You will find some commonly used sampling methods that were used in particular qualitative research studies in Box 11.1. You can refer to these as you work your way through the information about sampling approaches – the examples may help you to understand the different approaches better.

Box 11.1

Zurcher et al. (2011) used *convenience sampling* to identify 78 elderly in-patients in a Swiss hospital who had been screened for urinary infection, and who were willing to be questioned about urinary infection during hospitalisation.

Gass (2008) used *theoretical sampling* to conduct a grounded theory research study into electroconvulsive therapy and the work of mental health nurses.

Addo (2006) used *purposive sampling* to recruit and study nine registered nurses' experiences of working with sex offenders in two maximum secure settings in the UK.

Sissolak et al. (2011) used *quota sampling* in a phenomenological study which aimed to investigate the tuberculosis infection control experiences of South African nurses.

Sulaiman-Hill and Thomson (2011) used *snowball sampling* to recruit 193 former refugees to investigate refugee resettlement in Australia.

Convenience sampling refers to the ease of accessibility with which the recruitment of participants can take place in a study. It is sometimes referred to as opportunity sampling, reflecting the way in which the researcher selects those participants who are most easy to access until the required number of participants for the study is reached. Remember that the findings from a study that uses convenience sampling (and most other qualitative research sampling strategies) will be unrepresentative of the wider population. However, there is usually no aim to generalise the findings from a qualitative study.

Theoretical sampling is based on selecting research participants for their potential representation or manifestation of important theoretical constructs (Patton, 2002). It is the principal strategy for grounded theory research, which is described by Glaser and Strauss (1967) as an iterative sampling process that is based on the emergence of theoretical concepts. In this sampling approach, a few participants who are likely to be able to provide the relevant data are interviewed, with data analysis following in which themes and categories are generated. Further participants are then selected until the point at which data saturation is achieved (i.e. the participants are no longer providing different views or information through the interview process) (Gerrish and Lacey, 2010).

Purposive sampling allows the researcher to select information-rich cases (participants and settings) for an in-depth exploration and illumination of the research topic based on their specific characteristics (Robson, 2011). The sample therefore suits the needs of the specific research study – those who can discuss a particular experience rather than those who have no experience of the specific situation.

Quota sampling involves the selection of individuals from specific sub-sections of the general population based on common characteristics such as gender, age, class or marital status, in proportions that are representative of the wider target population. However, it is challenging to demonstrate that any sample is representative of a particular population where there are a number of variables in play as the sample can become too large for a qualitative study.

Snowball sampling involves requesting that well-informed individuals identify informants who know a lot about the phenomenon under investigation. This approach is useful where the potential participants are in hard-to-access groups such as the homeless. By following contacts researchers can identify and gain a critical mass of individuals for a study.

So, you have now had the chance to gain an overview of the sampling techniques and approaches that are appropriate for qualitative research. Activity 11.1 provides an opportunity for you to consolidate your learning.

ACTIVITY 11.1

What factors would the researcher need to consider when choosing their sampling approaches for the following studies?

- An investigation into the lived experiences of nurses caring for people with dementia in acute ward settings.
- An exploration of the experiences of children and young people with epilepsy.

ETHICAL ISSUES IN QUALITATIVE RESEARCH

In all research there will be ethical principles to follow in order to ensure the rights, safety and wellbeing of participants. Research studies should generate knowledge that has the potential to benefit the participants, other individuals and/ or wider society (Polit and Hungler, 2010). A detailed discussion of ethical issues is presented in Chapter 13, so you may wish to look at some of the key issues there as you read through this discussion on those ethical issues that are of particular relevance to qualitative research (see Table 11.1 which also offers suggested ethical resolutions).

In all research, the researcher has a duty of care to the participants to ensure that no harm is done. However, where abuse or crime of any kind is reported or witnessed in the course of a study, the researcher has a legal and professional responsibility to address this (Wiles et al., 2008). You might want to think about some of the studies already referred to when vulnerable people have participated in studies where there is the potential for wrongdoing to be identified (see Box 11.1). Now complete Activity 11.2 – although you are not expected to complete a research study at this stage in your learning, this activity asks you to put yourself in a researcher's shoes so that you can think deeply about the ethical issues in qualitative research.

Table 11.1 Ethical issues in qualitative research

Ethical risks	Ethical resolutions
Anxiety and distress due to the research subject matter.	Provide a robust referral process for relevant services such as counselling.
	Consider the conduct of the data collection and the ways in which the researcher can reduce anxiety and distress.
	Utilise supervisory support for novice researchers.
Exploitation of power in the researcher/participant relationship – especially in the context of vulnerable groups, and perceptions of coercion.	The researcher must:
	• Tell the participant who they are and what the purpose of the research is.
	• Provide full details of the research prior to the data collection episode, with the opportunity for further discussion, raising concerns and asking questions available.
	• Seek and gain informed consent.
	• Demonstrate respect for others.
	• Ensure that participants understand their right to withdraw from the study at any time without any negative impact.
	• Ensure that participants understand their right to withdraw consent for the use of the information provided.
Misrepresentation and/or misinterpretation.	The researcher can seek participant validation (e.g. through member checking where the participant checks the transcript of an interview for accuracy).
	Novice qualitative researchers should be supervised.
	The researcher could use a reflexive journal to reflect on personal biases and on the research journey overall.
	The researcher needs to state the theoretical stance of the topic.
	The researcher should consider how professional and personal characteristics may affect data interpretation.
Identification of participants in a published report and/or data transcripts contains multiple clues about the sources of information (places or participants).	Practise anonymity and confidentiality.
	Secure storage of data.
	Use of pseudonyms or codes for participants and other identifiers.

You are conducting a series of focus group interviews with eight women from different ethnic backgrounds who have experienced domestic abuse. You are interested in asking these women to describe their experiences and what they are doing to keep safe.

1 What possible risks may occur to these women as a result of their participating in your focus group interviews?
2 How could you minimise these risks?
3 As a member of an ethics committee what are your concerns about focus group interviews, and what are your concerns about this one in particular?

METHODS FOR DATA COLLECTION

Interviews, focus groups, observations, diaries and documentation are examples of qualitative data collection methods (Whittaker and Williamson, 2011). Let's consider these approaches and the ways in which researchers could use the methods. Remember that as a user of research you need to be sure about the appropriateness, or otherwise, of research methods in particular studies.

Interviews

Interviews allow researchers to gather data through conversations with research participants: they are often recorded and then transcribed into text for analysis. The interviews will focus on the phenomenon under investigation (for example, the experience of having breast cancer), with interviewing being a highly skilled activity involving the following skills (Le May and Holmes, 2012):

- Active questioning and listening.
- Reflecting on responses and non-verbal cues.
- Ability to probe, clarify and summarise in order to ensure understanding.
- Ability to interpret responses in order to appropriately frame the next question.

Interviews are time-consuming, laborious and challenging to analyse due to the volume of data generated and the need to synthesise understandings across participants' narratives. However, interviews enable researchers to collect detailed information on (sometimes) sensitive issues and experiences. As you have already seen in Chapter 8, qualitative research seeks to investigate phenomena in depth. Interviews can be undertaken face-to-face, by telephone, or through video-conferencing (or other electronic means). They can be one-to-one or group interviews – depending on their purpose. The format can be unstructured, semi-structured, or structured (see Table 11.2).

Table 11.2 Interview characteristics

Unstructured interviews
Also called in-depth interviewing.

- Useful when little is known about the topic.
- Allows participants to respond and express views freely.
- Direction of the interview is determined by both interviewer and interviewee.
- Yields rich data with issues emerging within the interview process.
- Lack of a formal structure.
- Can be challenging to analyse data due to the lack of structure.

EXAMPLE
I used in-depth interviewing to collect data from a purposive sample of nine registered nurses working with sex offenders in two maximum secure settings in the UK (Addo, 2006). The central finding suggested that the nurses experienced a complex interplay of personal and professional difficulties and emotional reactions in working with sex offenders that went beyond their professional life.

Structured interviews

- Utilise a pre-determined and standardised set of clearly worded questions.
- The goal of the research is clearly defined.
- Allows for an efficient approach to the conduct of the interview.
- Can produce consistent data across the participants in the study.
- Best suited to studies in which what is known on the topic is highly developed.

EXAMPLE
Newcommon et al. (2003) used structured interviews with 34 patients with a discharge diagnosis of stroke. The research team interviewed them three to six months from the day of admission in order to assign grades on the modified Rankin Scale (which relates to an assessment of the outcome in strokes). They were able to show that using a structured interview approach improved the reliability between observers, and the importance of physicians and/or qualified nurses scoring patients in person rather than relying on telephone interviews.

Semi-structured interviews

- The researcher uses a list of key themes, issues and/or questions to be covered within an interview.
- Discretion is used around the order of the questions, depending on interviewee responses.
- Probing questions allow the researcher to explore the topic, thus allowing for flexibility within the interview.
- Semi-structured interviews provide reliable, comparable data and structure.

EXAMPLE
In order to understand healthcare professionals' and mothers' knowledge of, attitudes to, and experiences with, baby-led weaning, Cameron et al. (2012) used semi-structured interviews. Their findings indicated that healthcare professionals had limited direct experience with baby-led weaning, and that the main concerns for participants were perceptions related to increased choking risk, iron deficiency, and inadequate energy intake.

Focus group interviewing

A group interviewing approach, the use of focus groups allows researchers to explore the general nature and comments of individuals, while also allowing rich data to emerge through the interactions within the group. In focus groups it is possible that the topic under investigation is further illuminated as individuals develop and express their thoughts in ways that may not have occurred in individual interviews. Onwuegbuzie et al. (2009) cite the benefits and limitations to the use of focus groups. The benefits are:

- An efficient and economical approach to the collection of interview data.
- Creates opportunities for the sharing and development of thoughts, ideas and views.
- A transparent approach to data collection (all focus group members can hear what has been said).

The limitations are:

- Some members of the focus group may find the group discussion intimidating.
- Operational challenges associated with the organisation of a focus group (e.g. arranging for all members of the focus group to come together).
- Potential issues with power and dominant relations in the group.
- The need for skilled facilitation.

EXAMPLE

Hasson et al. (2012) explored the impact of student nurses working part-time as healthcare assistants using focus groups. The study findings indicated that the key issues affecting students were:

- Confidence and experience.
- Preparation for the realities of nursing practice.
- The way in which members of staff treated the students/healthcare assistants.
- Questioning the value of a placement.
- Role confusion.

Observations

Observations can be participant or non-participant, and are used to collect data through the prolonged immersion of researchers in the participants' natural setting – observing how the participants relate, interact, and go about their daily social activities in order to develop an understanding of the topic under investigation (Petty et al., 2012). Participant observation requires that the researcher becomes an active participant in the same context and culture as that of the participants under observation.

Non-participant observation is when the researcher takes a detached observer role in the context of the participants' natural setting. Observations are utilised in ethnographic research, allowing for a description of what is observed and then the development of a theoretical framework which aims to explain what is taking place in that setting. The researchers' presence among the participants may influence their behaviour – as you can imagine this is a limitation for the method, but one which is taken into account within the interpretive process.

EXAMPLE

Murphy and Philpin (2010) used observations in an ethnographic study based on early miscarriage as 'matter of place' in nursing practice. The researchers aimed to capture the everyday practices of the social world, meanings, and ordinary activities of those involved in their study. Their findings illustrated the ambiguous nature of miscarriage and supported the position that miscarriage may be construed as an atypical bereavement, with the need to raise this awareness in helping nurses to provide sensitive care.

Documentary

Documentary research refers to the use of existing documents or records of any kind and can include newspapers, photographs, policy documents, historical documents, and patient care planning documents. The use of documentation for research can be helpful in providing the context to a particular study, or it can be a study in itself (for example, an investigation into the life of an influential nurse academic). The content analysis of documents can enrich the understanding of important issues on the political, economic, and social aspects of healthcare and nursing that are not easily captured through other forms of data collection methods. The kinds of research questions that can be investigated through documentary evidence include:

- How do media representations of nursing practice differ from the representations of other professions?
- How do internationally registered nurses working in the UK experience anti-discriminatory practices in their day-to-day nursing practice?

Questions of these kinds are vital for providing insights into both the styles of argumentation that are made in relation to healthcare issues and the reasons why such representations or accounts differ over time.

EXAMPLE

In order to explore and interpret constructions of difference within mentorship relationships that involved internationally-registered nurses and white English nursing students, Scammell and Olumide (2012) used four data collection approaches that were inclusive of documentary sources such as a pre-registration adult nursing curriculum, the revised curriculum for subsequent students, practice assessment tools for nursing students, curricular and mentor documents, and Nursing and Midwifery Council documents. Their findings highlighted the importance for nursing students to be well-informed of the societal structures and networks of power and the ways these can influence individual experiences. In addition, the need for students to consider why discrimination and prejudice can occur and their potential part in these constructs was highlighted.

Diaries

Solicited diaries from research participants are excellent sources of data collection as their use can approximate the real activities of, and enable a better understanding of, the lifeworlds of research participants (Nicholl, 2010). The diary as a data collection tool is advantageous as it allows for the collection of data in real time and can be used as an independent data collection method or combined with other methods. Diaries are also useful in the area of nursing care as the viewpoints of patients can potentially be accessed where interviews may not be possible.

EXAMPLE

In order to explore strategies used by older adults to manage their chronic health problems, Jacelon and Imperio (2005) used diaries to collect data. The diaries were guided by a set of open-ended questions which were designed to encourage participants to focus on their daily activities. They provided a rich source of data and were a useful strategy in this case for when periods of prolonged participant observation were not practical.

ACTIVITY 11.3

Find a research article that describes a qualitative study in an area of interest (you may wish to use one of the articles that you have used for previous activities). Now consider the following questions:

1   Which data collection method(s) was used and what was the rationale for its use?
2   Identify the strengths and limitations of the data collection method(s) used in this study and consider why other approaches were not utilised in this case.

APPROACHES TO DATA ANALYSIS

As you will have realised by now, qualitative research encompasses a wide range of approaches. What this means is that there are a number of ways in which data should be analysed. Analysing qualitative data is a complex, creative, iterative, interactive, inductive and reflexive activity. As you will have gathered, rigour and transparency are important to the analytical process. Morse (1994 – a seminal text) provided a summary of how the researcher's cognitive processes interact with qualitative data to construct findings and to generate new knowledge, regardless of the specific approach adopted:

- Comprehending the phenomenon under investigation.
- Synthesising the data that account for the relationships and linkages across the findings.
- Theorising about how and why these relationships appear as they do.
- Recontextualising the new knowledge to facilitate the evolution of the knowledge associated with the phenomenon.

I now present an overview of a number of approaches to data analysis. What is important for you to understand is that this is a snapshot of the approaches that are available to researchers, and therefore you will need to keep an open mind (and possibly do some further reading) when confronted with analytical approaches for qualitative research. Table 11.3 provides this overview.

Table 11.3   Approaches to qualitative data analysis

Content analysis

- The process of organising narrative qualitative information according to categories, themes and concepts with the aim of building a model to describe the phenomenon in conceptual form.
- Requires the systematic coding of responses and the examination for meaning through the frequency of words and/or phrases.
- The main line of enquiry is used as an initial guide within this examination.
- The stages include:

✓ Becoming familiar with the data through transcription of the data, reading and rereading, making brief notes in the margins when interesting or relevant information is found.
✓ Listing the information found in the margins, reading through the list, and categorising each item in a way that offers a description of what the information relates to.
✓ Identifying whether or not the information can be linked in any way and listing major and minor categories/themes.
✓ Comparing the categories and contrasting across the categories.
✓ Repeating this process across all the transcripts.
✓ Collating all the categories and conducting a detailed examination of their relevance.
✓ Reviewing all minor and major categories to establish relevance and having the opportunity to merge categories.
✓ Returning to original transcripts to ensure that all the information has been categorised appropriately.

(Continued)

Table 11.3　(Continued)

Thematic analysis

- Focuses on the identification of behaviours, patterns and themes in participants' experiences from interview data. The stages include:

✓ Becoming familiar with the data through immersion by transcribing the data (if necessary), reading and rereading the data, and noting down initial ideas.
✓ Generating initial codes by the identification of interesting features of the data in a systematic fashion across the entire data set, and collation of the data relevant to each code.
✓ Searching for themes through the collation of codes into potential themes gathering all relevant data to each potential theme.
✓ Reviewing themes in relation to the coded extracts (level 1) and the entire data set (level 2), generating a thematic map of the analysis.
✓ Defining and naming themes through ongoing analysis of each theme generating clear definitions for each theme.
✓ Producing the report where the final opportunity for analysis lies – including the selection of vivid and compelling extracts from the raw data.

Hermeneutic analysis

- Can be treated as both an underlying philosophy and a specific mode of analysis.
- A way of understanding textual data through its interpretation.
- The aim is to illuminate the concealed meanings and interpretations embedded within narratives of lived experiences in order to inform previous understandings of a phenomenon.
- The stages include:

✓ Immersion in the data through transcription of the data, reading and rereading.
✓ Summarising each interview and comparing pre-understandings of the phenomenon to the understanding of the text as a whole.
✓ Screening transcripts for expressions and patterns of meaningful quotes of the lived experience and clustering into themes.
✓ Searching for constitutive patterns where themes are compared with the understanding of the text as a whole, with contextual notes included.
✓ Selecting quotes to illustrate the different experiences that illuminate the phenomenon under investigation.
✓ Creating a metaphor to describe the experience while staying true to the participants' narratives.
✓ Seeking the validity of the interpretation of the experience from participants and others.
✓ Constructing a written account of the whole lived experience.

Constant comparative analysis

- Developed by Glaser and Strauss (1967) and mostly used in grounded theory research.
- Involves taking one piece of data such as one interview, one theme, or one statement, and comparing it with others that may be similar or could be different, so as to develop conceptualisations of the possible relationships between various aspects of the data.
- Stages include:

✓ Examining the interview data.
✓ Identifying indicators of events, behaviours, views.
✓ Coding early analysis.
✓ Comparing codes to find consistencies and differences and reveal emerging categories.
✓ Category saturation occurring when no new codes relating to a category are found.

Phenomenological analysis

- Requires the preservation of the uniqueness of each lived experience of the phenomenon under investigation.
- Colaizzi's (1978) seven-stage approach is well known and can be summarised as follows:

- ✓ Transcription of interview data.
- ✓ Identification of significant statements relating to the topic of the study.
- ✓ Formulation of meanings from participants' narratives.
- ✓ Organisation of meanings into clusters or themes.
- ✓ Use of themes to describe participants' lived experiences.
- ✓ Confirmation of validity through participant validation.
- ✓ Incorporation of relevant data acquired from participant validation into the final description.

Ethnographic analysis

- Focuses on the cultural ideas that arise during active data collection which are transformed, translated, or presented in a written document.
- Stages include:

- ✓ Sifting and sorting through data to organise material.
- ✓ Reading and thinking about the data.
- ✓ Coding data to detect and interpret thematic categorisations.
- ✓ Searching for inconsistencies and contradictions.
- ✓ Generating conclusions about what has happened and why.

Narrative analysis

- Focuses on how participants give order to the sequence of experiences in their lives, making sense of the events and actions in which they have participated.
- An umbrella term for an eclectic mix of approaches informed by many theoretical orientations, including hermeneutics, phenomenology or interactionism.
- Focuses on meaning-making.
- Models of narrative analysis is:

- ✓ Thematic analysis – emphasis on the content of the text, paying attention to the sequence of themes within the narrative.
- ✓ Structural analysis – the way the story is told with a focus on form and content.
- ✓ Interactional analysis with an emphasis on the dialogic process between the teller and the listener.
- ✓ Performative analysis – story telling seen as a performance.
- ✓ Presentation of findings in the form of case studies.

Discourse analysis

- A range of analytical approaches that focus on the use of language as a way of understanding the complexities of taken-for-granted ideas and practices.
- Has been used to understand a wide range of texts including natural speech, professional documentation, and interview materials.

Given the wide range of approaches, you will find it most useful to access relevant literature at the time of reading of research articles – the scope of this chapter does not allow for an in-depth discussion, rather it raises awareness for your understanding.

Using the article that you found earlier for Activity 11.3, do the following:

1 Describe the analytical process used within the study.
2 Explain why the approach was appropriate or otherwise.

As you can see by now there is a wide range of approaches to qualitative analysis. What they have in common is a need for immersion in the data (for example, through reading and rereading the texts), a going backwards and forwards between and across the data, and a rigorous approach to the thinking associated with the development of categories and themes.

RIGOUR, TRUSTWORTHINESS AND CREDIBILITY IN QUALITATIVE RESEARCH

Rigour in research refers to the strength of the research study in terms of its adherence to procedures, accuracy and consistency (Gerrish and Lacey, 2010). Trustworthiness in qualitative research is about the quality of the data collection and analysis, and their interpretation and presentation by the researcher. In addition it relates to the credibility of the findings. (Trustworthiness has previously been discussed in Chapter 8 and you may wish to refer back to that chapter.)

Credibility refers to the confidence in the 'truth' of the data and the interpretations provided, and is accomplished by:

• A faithful description of the research process and of the participants' experiences.
• The use of participants' own words as quotes to describe their experiences and to give their voice.
• Seeking participants' validation to provide internal checks by taking data (for accuracy) and interpretations to the source from which the data originated.

Dependability refers to procedural processes where an audit trail is outlined in order to check the routes for decision making at every stage of the research process. If you think about reading the outcomes from a piece of research, it is important that you are confident that decisions have been made that are based on evidence (which can be derived from the literature or from the ongoing data analysis, for example). An audit trail can include:

• The raw data, the data analysis and reduction processes, data reconstruction and synthesis processes through notes and other approaches (e.g. mind mapping).
• Records of decisions made and experiences encountered at each stage of the research process through a reflexive journal.
• Records from validation checks – e.g. member checking, which is the process through which participants are asked to ensure that the data transcription is accurate, for example.

Transferability relates to the degree to which the results of the qualitative research are applicable to others in comparable situations. So if you are reading a piece of qualitative research it is likely that you will be asking yourself how relevant the findings from the research are to your own area of practice. The extent to which you can determine this relates to the degree of transferability that exists within a research project. Transferability is achieved when the researcher provides a thick description of the research setting, location and context, as well as the participants. This information allows the reader to see if the results can be transferred to a similar and/or different setting.

Confirmability refers to the degree to which the results of a study may be collaborated or confirmed by others and can be accomplished by:

- Participants' validation or member checking as previously discussed. This practice reflects the perspective that research participants are not 'subjects' who are acted upon but are instead 'expert informants' who can help the researcher to better understand the phenomenon under investigation (Creswell, 2007).
- The provision of a balanced approach to the reporting of results/findings.
- A clear audit trail to help establish that the results and interpretations are clearly derived from the data.
- Evidence of reflexivity in the research process.

In order to consolidate your learning in relation to the rigour of qualitative research, using the article from the previous activities, do the following:

1 Describe the processes within the study that were used to ensure trustworthiness and rigour.
2 In your opinion, was the study undertaken in a rigorous way? Provide a rationale for your answer.

ACTIVITY 11.5

PRESENTATION OF QUALITATIVE RESEARCH

By now you will have had the chance to read a number of research articles where the findings from a qualitative research project are presented. You will have seen, I am sure, that the general approach to the presentation of the study for publication fits into a format that encompasses the following:

1 Abstract.
2 Introduction and background to the project.
3 Literature review.
4 Study design (sometimes called methodology and methods).
5 Findings.
6 Discussion.
7 Conclusion and recommendations.

As you will have probably gathered, this structure is similar to that of quantitative studies. The differences between their presentation lie in the nature of the data and the way in which the findings from the studies are laid out for the reader. As I discussed earlier, the researcher needs to ensure that the outcome of the research has transferability and credibility. Some of the ways that these are achieved are through the presentation. Some key points which are of relevance are as follows:

- The richness of the data should be evident within the presentation. So, for example, the researcher will provide a number of quotes that aim to give the reader a sense of the findings. These quotes will be used to illustrate the differences between participants within a study and also as examples to illuminate particular findings where there are thematic similarities.
- Participants' anonymity must always be protected through the use of pseudonyms.

The trick for the researcher is in telling the story of the research through its appropriate presentation. To give you a glimpse of what I mean by this, Box 11.2 contains an extract from one of the studies that I completed (Addo, 2006).

Box 11.2

I conducted an in-depth study using hermeneutic phenomenology to generate a description and an understanding of registered nurses' experiences of working with sex offenders in two maximum secure settings in the United Kingdom. My focus was on seeking to illuminate and understand 'What is it like for nurses in their day-to-day work with sex offenders?' Ethical approval was granted, and a purposive sample of nine nurses participated following informed consent. Data were collected through in-depth recorded interviews in the participants' place of work. These were transcribed and analysed manually using an interpretive approach (hermeneutics). The question that I asked at interview was: 'Could you share with me what it has been like for you in working with sex offenders?' From there, I probed and sought clarification on issues in order to gain a depth and breadth of coverage relating to their experiences. Eleven themes emerged from the analytical process. One theme – 'Feeling unsupported' – is exemplified by the following excerpt:

> We need someone independent that we can just offload to ... we do need something ... This is like a counselling session for me [referring to research interview]. You need somebody that is independent to the secure setting who is attached to the organisation as a support mechanism. Quite frankly we don't have any support mechanisms. We have an employee assistance programme where we can phone up and speak to counsellors and things but what do these people know about working with sex offenders ... [Nora]

I concluded that the nurses' narratives provided a thick description of the participants' work with sex offenders, and highlighted their need for effective specialist education and support for such practice.

I hope that you can see how the use of just one quote illuminates an aspect of the experience in a way that allows the participants to tell their own stories.

STRENGTHS AND LIMITATIONS OF QUALITATIVE RESEARCH

As you will have gathered through your reading and engagement with some of the other activities, all research approaches have their strengths and limitations. Table 11.4 offers a summary of these for qualitative research. What you will need to do when considering using the findings from a research project is consider the ways in which a researcher has addressed the limitations and the appropriateness of the chosen approach (bearing in mind the strengths).

Table 11.4 Strengths and limitations of qualitative research

Strengths	Limitations
• Useful for the study of human experiences. • Increases understanding of a given topic and can evoke recognition. • Useful in elaborating on quantitative research findings. • Offers the ability to empower participants and 'give voice' to human experiences. • Helps to humanise the understanding of professional practice – crucial to ethical practice. • Can alter healthcare professionals' ways of working with patients and others. • Enables a broader understanding of clinical realities. • Promotes holistic decision making based on a rounded perspective of the issue under investigation. • Allows the researcher to enter into the research process – and the coming-together of worldviews in certain approaches.	• There are specific ethical issues, particularly with vulnerable groups. • There is a risk of bias occurring within the sampling approach (particularly with convenience and snowball samples). • Data collection methods can be intrusive and put demands on participants' time. • Generates copious amounts of data with the associated data management challenges. • Labour intensive (e.g. in relation to transcription and analysis). • Can arouse feelings of distress among participants and the researcher. • Anonymity and confidentiality harder to maintain. • Research quality is heavily dependent on the skills of the researcher. • Possible misinterpretation or misrepresentation. • Limited transferability of findings to the wider population. • Seen as subjective.

IMPACT OF FINDINGS ON PRACTICE

I have offered an overview of the key concepts that are vital for your understanding of qualitative research. What you should now be in a better position to do is critique qualitative research and determine its applicability for practice. I cannot put it better than Kearney did in 2001 with statements regarding the impact of qualitative research in practice, as follows:

- By leading to new clinical insights nurses can learn and appreciate 'what it feels like' from a patient's perspective to live daily with the health conditions and challenges endured, and the different ways that patients view an illness.
- With this understanding healthcare professionals can begin to be more attentive to patient needs in the caring process (be more empathic), and thereby give support and attention in a more informed way.
- Can be useful as an interventionist approach with nurses sharing the evidence directly with patients and having an opportunity to explore the issues raised within the evidence.

SUMMARY

The critical learning points within this chapter are:

- There is a need to understand the various approaches taken in the design of qualitative studies so that you are in a position to critique studies for your practice.
- Qualitative research contributes to the development of evidence-based practice by providing a holistic view of phenomena that impact on healthcare.
- Knowledge of specific ethical issues in qualitative research, alongside the approaches that can be taken to ensuring rigour, are vital for your decisions on the trustworthiness and credibility of research and their relevance to your practice.

FURTHER READING

http://onlineqda.hud.ac.uk/Intro_QDA/phpechopage_titleOnlineQDA-Examples_QDA.php

Examples of qualitative research

www.public.asu.edu/~ifmls/artinculturalcontextsfolder/qualintermeth.html# typesofinterviews.
An understandable and useful insight into interviewing as a methodology.
http://onlineqda.hud.ac.uk/intro_qda/what_is_qda.php
A short but useful introduction to qualitative research data analysis.

REFERENCES

Addo, M. (2006) The UNSEEN ABYSS: registered nurses' experience in working with sex offenders – a hermeneutic phenomenological study. [online] Available from: www.researchgate.net/publication/215784229_THE_UNSEEN_ABYSS_Registered_Nurses'_Experience_in_Working_with_Sex_offenders_-_a_Hermeneutic_Phenomenological_Study (last accessed 19 August 2013).

Cameron, S.L., Heath, A-L.M. and Taylor, R.W. (2012) Healthcare professionals' and mothers' knowledge of, attitudes to and experiences with, baby-led weaning: A content analysis, *BMJ Open* 2, doi: 10.1136/bmjopen-2012-001542

Colaizzi, P.F. (1978) Psychological research as the phenomenologist view it. In R. Valle and M. King (eds), *Existential phenomenological alternative for psychology*. Oxford: Oxford University Press.

Creswell, J.W. (2007) *Qualitative inquiry and research design: Choosing among five traditions* (2nd edition). Thousand Oaks, CA: Sage.

Gass, J. (2008) Electroconvulsive therapy and the work of mental health nurses: a grounded theory study, *International Journal of Nursing Studies*, 45 (2): 191–202.

Gerrish, K. and Lacey, A. (2010) *The research process in nursing* (6th edition). Chichester: Wiley-Blackwell.

Glaser, B.G. and Strauss, A.L. (1967) *The discovery of grounded theory: Strategies for qualitative research*. Aldine: New York.

Hasson, F., McKenna, H. P. and Kenney, S. (2012) A qualitative study exploring the impact of student nurses working part time as a health care assistant, *Nurse Education Today*, 14. Available at: http://dx.doi.org/10.1016/j.nedt.2012.09.014 (last accessed 28 November 2012).

Jacelon, C.S. and Imperio, K. (2005) Participant diaries as a source of data in research with older adults, *Qualitative Health Research*, 15 (7): 991–997.

Kearney, M. (2001) Levels and applications of qualitative research evidence, *Research in Nursing and Health*, 24: 145–153.

Le May, A. and Holmes, S. (2012) *Introduction to nursing research: Developing research awareness*. London: Hodder Arnold.

Morse, J.M. (1994) Emerging from the data: cognitive processes of analysis in qualitative inquiry. In J. Morse (ed.), *Critical issues in qualitative research*. Menlo Park, CA: Sage. pp. 23–43.

Murphy, F. and Philpin, S. (2010) Early miscarriage as a 'matter out of place': An ethnographic study of nursing practice in a hospital gynaecological unit, *International Journal of Nursing Studies*, 47: 534–541.

Newcommon, J., Green, T.L., Haley, E., Cooke, T. and Hill, M.D. (2003) Improving the assessment of outcomes in stroke: Use of a structured interview to assign grades on the Modified Rankin Scale, *Journal of the American Heart Association, Stroke*, 34: 377–378.

Nicholl, H. (2010) Diaries as a method of data collection in research, *Paediatric Nursing*, 22 (7): 16–20.

Onwuegbuzie, A.J., Leech, N.L. and Collins, K.M.T. (2009) Innovative data collection strategies in qualitative research, The Qualitative Report, 5 (3): 696–726.

Parahoo, K. (2006) *Nursing research: Principles, process and issues* (2nd edition). Houndsmill: Palgrave Macmillan.

Patton, M. (2002) *Qualitative research and evaluation methods*. Newebury Park, CA: Sage.

Petty, N.J., Oliver, P.T. and Stew, G. (2012) Ready for paradigm shift? Part 2: Introducing qualitative research methodologies and methods, *Manual Therapy*, 17: 378–384.

Polit, D.F. and Hungler, B.P. (2010) *Essentials of nursing research: Appraising evidence for nursing practice* (6th edition). Philadelphia, PA: Lippincott Williams and Wilkins.

Robson, C. (2011) *Real world research* (3rd edition). Chichester: Wiley.

Scammell, J.M.E. and Olumide, G. (2012) Racism and mentor–student relationship: Nurse education through a white lens, *Nurse Education*, 32: 545–550.

Sissolak, D., Marais, F. and Mehtar, S. (2011) TB infection prevention and control experiences in South African nurses – a phenomenological study, *BMC Public Health*, 11, 262.

Sulaiman-Hill, C.M.R. and Thompson, S.C. (2011) Sampling challenges in a study examining refugee resettlement, *BMC International Health and Human Rights*, 11, 2.

Wiles, R., Crow, G., Heath, S. and Charles, V. (2008) The management of confidentiality and anonymity in social research, *International Journal of Social Research Methodology*, 11 (5): 417–428.

Whittaker, A. and Williamson, G.R. (2011) *Transforming nursing practice: Succeeding in research project plans and literature reviews for nursing students*. Exeter: Learning Matters.

Zurcher, S., Saxer, S.M. and Schwendimann, R. (2011) Urinary incontinence in hospitalised elderly patients: do nurses recognise and manage the problem? *Nursing Research and Practice*. Article ID 671302.

12

QUANTITATIVE RESEARCH

SHEELAGH MARTINDALE AND WINIFRED EBOH

Chapter learning outcomes

On completion of Chapter 12, you will be able to:

1 Decide on the appropriate quantitative methodology for particular research questions.
2 Determine the most appropriate methods for sampling/data collection/analysis for a chosen study.
3 Assess the quality of the methods chosen for a particular study, taking into account areas such as validity, reliability and ethical issues.
4 Identify the strengths and challenges of quantitative research methods.
5 Appreciate the use of quantitative research methods in practice.

Key concepts

Quantitative methods, experimental research, survey, questionnaire, validity, reliability.

INTRODUCTION

For the purpose of this chapter, quantitative research methods are discussed under two main headings: 'experiments' and 'surveys'. From there we will take you through the research journey, deciding on how samples will be selected from a given population, the way data will be collected and analysed, and in so doing considering issues around ethics, validity and reliability. By the end of the chapter you should be able to identify the strengths and challenges associated with quantitative research. Having reached this point, it is important that you can recognise how quantitative research can be applied to real practice situations. Embedded activities will help you build on your knowledge and how best to apply this methodology to a given research question.

ASKING THE RESEARCH QUESTION

Most research starts with a question. (The development of the research question using the PICO framework was discussed in Chapter 9 so you may wish to refer back to that section as a reminder.) Once the question has been formulated, this informs the design of the study. Within each design, the most appropriate sampling frame and approach, data collection and analysis methods are chosen. The two main methods employed in quantitative research as stated earlier are experiments and surveys: although there are overlaps in sections such as sampling, data collection and analysis, there are distinct differences that need to be explored.

EXPERIMENTS

Although there are similarities in relation to research methods for all experimental research designs, there are unique features which set the different designs apart. Questions of effectiveness will normally point researchers in the direction of designing an experimental study. In Chapter 8, the 'hierarchy of evidence' (Holland and Rees, 2010) pyramid shows the randomised controlled trial (RCT) as top of the hierarchy of evidence. Therefore to discuss research methods in relation to experimental research an RCT is the main focus of this section.

Whether an RCT is the right design for a study or not should be given due consideration prior to continuing with the selection of the study methods (Petticrew et al., 2012). An RCT is an experimental study which tests a given hypothesis in comparison with what is already known. This can often be to test how effective a new drug or treatment is on a known condition or outcome, or it may be used to see how effective a change in service is compared to the standard service, for example. Before looking into this design in more detail, Activity 12.1 will enable you to think about the type of scenarios that will fit with this design.

In your area of practice or learning consider the type of questions that an experimental design may be suited to. Identify two questions and give the reasons for your choice.

ACTIVITY 12.1

Definition of groups

Prior to embarking on an RCT, the groups in which participants will be placed should be clearly detailed. A simple RCT will have one *intervention group* and one *control group*. However other studies may have two or more intervention groups and one control group (Uijen et al., 2012) where each intervention group will test the effectiveness of a different treatment type and this will then be compared to the standard control treatment in which all groups will be assessed for the pre-determined outcome. For example, if a researcher wishes to determine whether increased amounts of vitamin E during pregnancy would prevent the onset of asthma in the baby during childhood, one intervention group may be identified to receive vitamin E supplements while another intervention group will receive regular dietary advice from a dietician to increase their dietary vitamin E intake. The control group would have no form of intervention (see Box 12.1 below).

Box 12.1   Working example of a randomised controlled trial

Within this section to apply the theoretical methods of an RCT, a hypothetical example will be referred to. An overview of this hypothetical study is provided below.

Previous research into relationships between the in utero environment and atopic disease in childhood suggests that increased dietary vitamin E intake during pregnancy was associated with a reduced prevalence of asthma and wheeze in children within their first two years of life (Martindale et al., 2005). One way of testing this hypothesis would be to undertake an experimental or interventional study.

Hypothetical working example

A sample of pregnant women between 8 and 16 weeks of pregnancy were recruited from an antenatal clinic to take part in an RCT to test whether increased intake of vitamin E during pregnancy protected their baby from developing asthma during childhood. They were allocated to one of three groups: Group 1 Intervention – participants will receive vitamin E supplements; Group 2 Intervention – participants will receive regular dietary advice from a dietician to increase their dietary vitamin E intake; and Group 3 Control – participants will receive no form of intervention. Blood levels will be collected from the participants whilst in labour to assign their levels of vitamin E. The participants will be asked to complete a questionnaire when their baby is 12 months and again at 24 months to assess for asthma and eczema.

Sample and population

Within experimental research, it is important to ensure that the sample that is recruited is fully justified (Turton et al., 2010). If this is not the case it opens up the study to weaknesses in relation to bias. One of the most crucial considerations is that of sample size. The main areas of consideration when deciding the size of sample are in relation to the population of interest, the size of difference or effect anticipated, and the expected variability in the outcome variable. The overall sample size should be large enough to ensure that once the group is split into the intervention and control groups, the expected effect from the intervention has adequate statistical power and is unlikely to have occurred by chance (Neale, 2009).

Another consideration of the sample is that of the type of sample. A probability or random sample is the ultimate sample for RCTs and one in which any individual within the population of interest can be selected to be part of the study. Keeping within the example mentioned above and as illustrated within Figure 12.1, the population for which the study has relevance is pregnant women (see Figure 12.1, first level box, page 217), therefore selecting any woman during her pregnancy would be a random selection. However, it may be that researchers would want to place some rules around this: for instance, the recruitment of women who have no underlying medical condition (for example, diabetes); the recruitment of women within a particular stage of their pregnancy (for example, within 8–16 weeks); the recruitment of women who have had previous children, or importantly in this example, women who are on any form of dietary restrictions. Thus what has been developed within the sampling frame are the 'inclusion and exclusion criteria' (see Figure 12.1, second level box).

Randomisation

Another major consideration in the design of an RCT is that of randomisation (Neale, 2009). This is different from the random sample described above. Randomisation is the term used for the process by which the participants who have been recruited into the study (the sample) are then directed into the 'defined groups' of the study. If this is not performed in a pre-determined manner, it is another area where bias may be introduced into the study. Simple forms of randomisation include tossing a coin or throwing a dice from which the participant will then go into the control or intervention groups. However, the most common method for larger RCTs is computer-generated randomisation. By using this method, the researcher can ensure that equal numbers are assigned to each defined group, although they will not at this point know which group each allocated participant belongs to – thereby ensuring that the numbers cannot be tampered with.

Some RCT studies may not be able to use a computer-generated system, for example, if they have smaller sample sizes or if the groups they are using have more determined criteria. Such studies may adopt a stratified randomisation approach which will ensure that equal numbers of participants are assigned to each group, with similar characteristics that may affect the outcome. Going back to the example of increased vitamin E intake in pregnancy preventing the onset of asthma in childhood, it could be worthwhile to ensure that equal numbers of pregnant women who have asthma themselves are recruited into each group. That way, this factor would not interfere with the results within the study (see Figure 12.1, third level box).

Blinding

Another essential consideration of an RCT is that of blinding. Single blinding is when either the researcher or the participant is unaware of whether the participant is in the intervention or control group. Double blinding is when both the researcher and participant are unaware of the grouping: this is the best technique for reducing bias in a study. Double blinding may be utilised in studies that involve testing the effectiveness of new drugs where the control groups can be given placebos. All the participants within such a study will be unaware of whether they are taking the actual drug or the dummy (placebo) drug. However, it is not always possible to achieve double blinding with an RCT design such as in the example we have used so far, as the participants within both intervention groups would know that they were either receiving increased dietary advice from a dietician about eating more foods rich in vitamin E, or that they were taking a vitamin E supplement (see Figure 12.1, fourth level boxes).

Outcomes

The primary outcome of an RCT should be determined at the beginning of the study design and will relate to the main area of interest identified within the hypothesis or research question. The outcome will allow the definition of the intervention and control groups to be made, ensuring that whatever the intervention is, it should (as the hypothesis would state) make a difference to the outcome. The sample size cannot be calculated without knowing what the size of the desired effect has been on the primary outcome. There may, however, be secondary outcomes related to the primary outcome, but these should not be given the same importance as the primary outcome. Within the working example the primary outcome is 'asthma'. However, secondary outcomes may be 'infant wheeze', 'eczema', 'hay fever', etc. Knowing what the primary outcome is within the study of interest should then direct the researcher towards the most appropriate methods of data collection and analysis of these data.

Data collection

The method of data collection within an RCT design is normally determined by the primary outcome. If the study aims to assess the effectiveness of a new drug on a disease, it may be that biochemical markers within the blood may be required to detect any changes during the course of study. Other measurement apparatus may also be used (for example, blood pressure monitors, spirometers, etc.). Other forms of data collection within this study design could be questionnaires which could collect data to assess whether a disease (or condition) is present or not at the end of the study period. Questionnaires also allow researchers to collect demographic data and additional data which may interfere with the primary outcome. The data can then be added to the final analysis to ensure that researchers have an accurate interpretation of the tested hypothesis. The questionnaire used for data collection in studies such as the one suggested here (see Figure 12.1, fifth level box) are often structured or checklists with closed questions. This approach differs from the semi-structured questionnaires preferred in surveys.

Data analysis

Within experimental research it is likely that the research team will aim to gather information that will allow them to make comparisons within the sample. However, to then go on and state that their findings are generalisable to the wider population, the researchers will need to have a level of confidence with their results – referred to as 'inferential statistics' (Watson et al., 2006). As previously stated, experimental research sets out to test a given hypothesis. Within the working example, the hypothesis is 'an increased intake of vitamin E in pregnancy will prevent the onset of asthma in childhood', and therefore the aim of the research is to confirm this hypothesis or reject it. If the results confirm the hypothesis, the researchers will need to determine whether the results simply occurred by chance.

There are various types of statistical tests that can be calculated to answer different hypotheses, however it is not the purpose of this chapter to discuss statistical tests in depth and you may wish to access a statistics textbook to take your learning further. From the example, the primary outcome is 'asthma', which within the dataset would be known as the *dependant variable* which would entail assessing from the study population whether there was 'asthma present' or 'asthma not present'. The variable type would be a nominal variable. Vitamin E level would be the *independent variable*. However there may be other factors present which could skew the result and therefore we should not be confident that the result would only come from this variable. Other factors may be 'pets in the home' or 'family history of asthma' or 'passive smoking', for example. Therefore the researchers would need to ensure that any result would take account of these factors – the *confounding variables* – which would involve using a logistic regression technique from which an 'odds ratio' test could be generated (see Figure 12.1, sixth level box). An 'odds ratio' is predicted where the odds of an event occurring are divided by the odds of that event not occurring.

Therefore, data analysis within experimental designs requires sophisticated statistical analysis. During the planning stage of the study, the methods of analysis should be decided to ensure the correct type of data are collected to answer the main hypothesis.

In summary, what has been presented in this section has related to the simple RCT study design which is illustrated in Figure 12.1. However, there are other RCT designs such as 'crossover', 'multi-arm' and 'complex intervention', to name but a

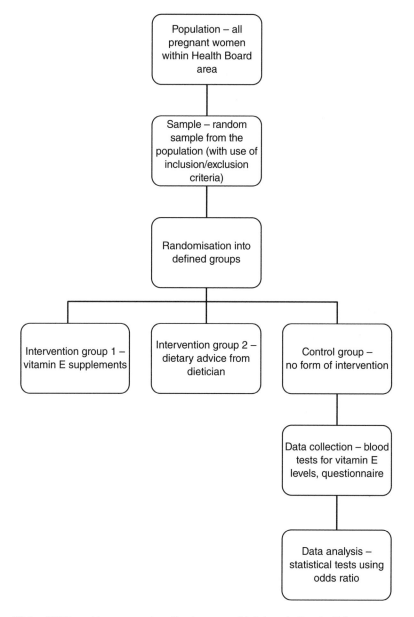

Figure 12.1   RCT working example – 'An increased intake of vitamin E in pregnancy will prevent the onset of asthma in childhood'

few. Due to the complex nature of RCTs they can often be time-consuming and costly. There are numerous issues relating to bias, which if not addressed could lower the credibility of the study, but if contingencies are implemented to ensure bias is minimised at all stages, the RCT design will reach its position at the top of the 'hierarchy of evidence' (Holland and Rees, 2010).

QUASI EXPERIMENTS

A quasi experiment is one in which the 'rules' of a true experiment (RCT) are not always followed – often the case in nursing research. For instance, it may be that the hypothesis is 'the wearing of drug tabards reduces medication round interruptions', as discussed in Chapter 9, but it would be difficult within one ward to have two systems running concurrently. Therefore it would make more sense to test the system in one ward and compare it to another ward where the system is not in place, which means that there is no true randomisation happening for participants in this study and the researcher cannot control for any extraneous factors between the groups. These aspects are what make this experimental study a *quasi* experiment rather than a randomised controlled trial. They are not rated as highly as RCTs in the 'hierarchy of evidence' (Holland and Rees, 2010).

SURVEYS

Surveys are renowned for their versatility and as a systematic way of collecting information in different disciplines ranging from health, education, psychology and law to name but a few (Meadows, 2003a). Historically surveys were carried out using postal questionnaires. The era of telephones then introduced telephone interviews (often used in market research) and now online or web-based surveys are a common occurrence. Web surveys have an advantage over mail questionnaires because they cut out the need for printing and mailing questionnaires, and collating and manually transferring data into an electronic version.

Surveys are widely used – for example, the population census is a national survey of all households in the United Kingdom that provides vital information used by governments for service planning. Patients can be surveyed to find out their views on the standard of care they receive from their healthcare providers. Some surveys take a descriptive approach, looking at the population's health or health behaviour in relation to lifestyle choices or the emergence or prevalence of diseases. Studies of association can also be classified as a survey (Green and Browne, 2005). Association studies can look at, for example, sex education and the incidence of teenage pregnancies or poverty and unemployment. Figure 12.2 illustrates the three main categories of surveys, summarising their main uses.

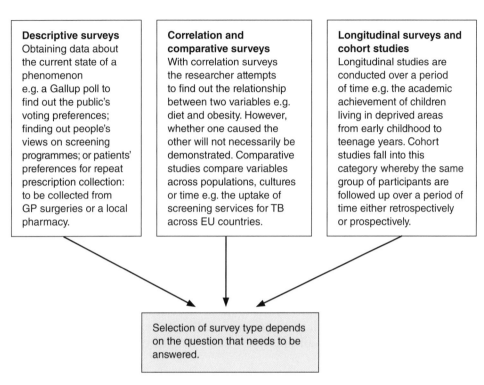

Descriptive surveys
Obtaining data about the current state of a phenomenon e.g. a Gallup poll to find out the public's voting preferences; finding out people's views on screening programmes; or patients' preferences for repeat prescription collection: to be collected from GP surgeries or a local pharmacy.

Correlation and comparative surveys
With correlation surveys the researcher attempts to find out the relationship between two variables e.g. diet and obesity. However, whether one caused the other will not necessarily be demonstrated. Comparative studies compare variables across populations, cultures or time e.g. the uptake of screening services for TB across EU countries.

Longitudinal surveys and cohort studies
Longitudinal studies are conducted over a period of time e.g. the academic achievement of children living in deprived areas from early childhood to teenage years. Cohort studies fall into this category whereby the same group of participants are followed up over a period of time either retrospectively or prospectively.

Selection of survey type depends on the question that needs to be answered.

Figure 12.2   Types of survey

Key features of survey method

Each survey, irrespective of the size and scope, should meet the following criteria (adapted from Meadows, 2003a):

- Clear measurable objectives.
- Robust design.
- The sample or population to be studied must be appropriate and clear criteria have to be used for their selection.
- The questionnaire or scales used to collect data must be reliable and valid.
- Data should be analysed to meet the objectives.
- The findings must be reported in the correct way.

Sampling

There are two types of sampling used in surveys – probability and non-probability sampling. Probability or random sampling has already been discussed when we looked at experimental design. When non-probability sampling is utilised, the same generalisation of findings to the target population cannot be made (Campbell and Swinscow, 2009). Non-probability sampling includes convenience, snowball and quota sampling. Snowball sampling is used when the researcher does not have access to the sampling frame or when it is difficult to contact the entire population – for example, the homeless or traveller communities due to the lack of a fixed address. Convenience samples are groups who are available and easily accessible. Quota sampling is equivalent to stratified sampling in experimental design where the researcher imposes greater control on the process by determining the most important variables which need to be captured in a proportional way when the sample size is known. These approaches to sampling are also utilised in qualitative research (and discussed in more depth in Chapter 11).

Deciding on the size of the sample

When deciding the size of the sample within survey research, consideration should be given to the sampling frame. This should be in relation to the sampling technique, whether it is probability or non-probability (for example, a random or a convenience sample), and if all calculations are study specific.

Data collection methods in surveys

One of the most commonly used methods of data collection in social health and epidemiological research studies is questionnaire surveys which can be administered by post, in person, by telephone, or via email or other virtual means. Bowling (2005) identified web-based questionnaire surveys that used varied formats such as computer assisted face-to-face interviewing, computer-assisted telephone interviews, self-administered computer methods and audio computer-assisted self-administered interviewing. With increasing and improving technology the methods for administrating questionnaires will diversify, but researchers need to ensure that the chosen approach fits with the research objectives and can accommodate the target population.

Questionnaires

Survey questionnaires can be used to measure knowledge, attitudes and beliefs, and quality of life (QOL), amongst other things. Standardised questionnaires are now available for researchers to measure phenomena such as patients' coping styles/strategies when living with chronic long-term illnesses, using for example the SF-36 (Doll et al., 2000). This tool has been widely used in various areas of healthcare and found to consistently provide accurate measures – it is therefore considered to be valid and reliable. (The need for validity and reliability is discussed more extensively in Chapter 8.)

Likert scales provide ordinal data (the natural ordering of information) and measure levels of agreement with a series of statements (Gerrish and Lacey, 2010). Likert scales in questionnaire surveys can be effective in eliciting respondents' attitudes and can also be sensitive to extreme views, and can identify attitudes and beliefs that respondents had not fully appreciated existed. Likert scales can be used across the age continuum (Laerhoven et al., 2004), and across different cultures, with varying degrees of success (Lee et al., 2002). An example of a study where a Likert scale was used is shown in Figure 12.3, which looked at student nurses' attitudes to research: as the figure shows, a series of statements were provided and respondents were asked to indicate their answer by stating how much they agreed or disagreed with each statement. With Likert scales there is no right or wrong answer to each statement. However, on analysing the responses there is a need to provide a rationale as to how the responses were interpreted.

The type of questions asked within a survey can range from 'open' to 'closed' depending on the nature of the survey being undertaken. Closed questions are often

Statements	Strongly agree	Agree	Neither agree nor disagree	Disagree	Strongly disagree
1. Research is not relevant to every day nursing practice					
2. Research expertise is taken into account in promotion to senior posts					
3. Nursing should become a research based profession					
4. Nurses are too busy delivering care to spend time reading research					
5. Research often leads to real practical advances in nursing care					
6. Research expertise is of value to the nurse in clinical practice.					
7. In practice very few nurses use research findings					
8. Research experience should not be taken into account in promotion to senior posts.					

Figure 12.3 An example of a Likert scale

used to obtain attitudinal or factual information where there are pre-determined answers or choices making up an integral part of the questionnaire. Open-ended questions by contrast do not have any fixed answers, thereby giving respondents greater freedom to answer the question asked in their own words. This type of question requires more effort on the part of respondents and therefore it should be limited to a few questions in self-administered questionnaires (Meadows, 2003b). Questionnaires with mainly open-ended questions are more suited to face-to-face interview-type surveys as they are more time consuming as regards administration and analysis. However, these limitations can be offset by the quality of answers given because the researcher is available to clarify the questions (Gerrish and Lacey, 2010). Questionnaires presenting both closed and open-ended questions give respondents the opportunity to expand on their answers (Gerrish and Lacey, 2010). The way the open-ended questions are analysed depends on whether the data generated are coded and entered into a statistical analysis package or treated as qualitative data and analysed qualitatively (see Chapter 11 for qualitative data analysis).

Data analysis

The thinking behind how survey data are analysed starts during the design phase of the study. Data analysis links with the research question, objectives and design of the questionnaire. With all research data, there is a need to make sense of those data – a process that involves descriptive statistics, as discussed in Chapter 4 (mean, median, mode range). Descriptive statistics provide basic information about the frequency of an occurrence (or how often something happened). This is a crucial step before more advanced statistical analysis is carried out on the data. Due to the sheer quantity of data generated from surveys, statistical packages such as SPSS or Minitab are used to manage the data and facilitate analysis. As discussed in Chapter 8, with descriptive statistics it is important to find out the frequency of an occurrence, the middle or average point in the data sets, and how wide a spread the data are from the average to decide the significance of the findings.

There may also be a need to make comparisons between and within populations to identify similarities and differences between gender, age, or ethnic group. Such tests may involve carrying out correlations between variables, such as the relationship between genetic inheritance of cardiovascular disease and lifestyle (Munro, 2004). Determining the most appropriate statistical analysis for any data set is dependent on the study's aims and objectives and will vary from study to study. It is, however, extremely important that data analysis is considered from the planning phase of the study, as discussed earlier, and especially in the questionnaire design, otherwise there is a risk that the questions posed cannot be analysed or the answers obtained are not valid and not fit for purpose. It is vital that all questionnaires are tested for validity and reliability following the same principles as discussed under quality of methods. To summarise, Table 12.1 provides an overview of the strengths and limitations of survey methodology.

Table 12.1 Strengths and limitations of survey methodology

Type of survey	Strengths	Limitations
Postal	Reach large numbers of respondents relatively cheaply	Poor response rate
	Covers a wide demography	Non-response bias in relation to incomplete questions
	Anonymised	Respondents unable to seek clarity of questions
Telephone	Reach large numbers of respondents relatively cheaply	Poor response rate
		Not anonymised
	Covers a wide demography	Response bias in relation to the type of people who would participate
Web-based	Reach large numbers of respondents relatively cheaply	Response bias in relation to the type of people who would participate – IT literacy and perhaps generational bias
	Anonymised	

QUALITY OF METHODS

Although the quality issues relating to quantitative methods have already been mentioned in Chapter 8, it is an area that should be revisited at all stages of the research planning and process. Therefore it would be remiss not to discuss quality issues relating to the specific quantitative methods mentioned above.

Validity

Validity refers to the accuracy of how the research methods chosen for the study are able to perform and ultimately answer the hypothesis and research question. All stages of the research process will contain areas where validity will be important. The sample should ideally be randomly selected from the population of interest or the reasons for another type of sample (e.g. a stratified sample) should have a justified rationale. If this is not the case, it will limit the researchers' ability to make general assumptions from their results to the wider population. This is known as 'external validity' (Parahoo, 2006). External validity should also be considered during the randomisation of the sample into intervention and control groups within experimental research.

Validity should also be considered at the data collection stage of the study. Flaws within the data collection methods (e.g. equipment which is not calibrated, or incorrect test measurements or questionnaires that have not been piloted and amended prior to use in the main study) may bias the results of the study. In the design of the data collection method not every factor may have been considered and this could interfere with the results. This is known as 'internal validity' (Parahoo, 2006). For instance, within the working example discussed in the RCT section, it may be that not all the data relating to 'confounding variables' (pets in the home, family history of asthma) have been included.

Within the data collection phase of the study, the validity of the questionnaire used is vitally important. There are three specific areas of validity:

1   *Content validity* – This refers to the need for questions within a questionnaire to be interpreted by the respondent in the way intended. It is often termed as 'face validity' – namely, 'it does what it says on the packet!'
2   *Criterion-related validity* – This is concerned with how well the data from one data collection tool relate to another form of data collection measuring the same outcome.
3   *Construct validity* – This is the hardest form of validity to assess as it is concerned with how well the questionnaire measures the particular outcome.

The use of a previously validated questionnaire where possible, as discussed in the survey section, is good practice within research where the questionnaire has undergone rigorous statistical testing and has been used in other studies to ensure its validity within the population of interest (Meadows, 2003b).

Validity is also key when analysing the results of a study. The data should all be checked for accuracy prior to the statistical analysis to ensure that all errors have been identified and corrected. There should also be a system for incorporating missing or incomplete data into the analysis – it is also important to identify the number of non-respondents as in the case of surveys and, where possible, the reasons for this. The researchers should be sure that they are using the correct statistical test for the outcome of interest and within this have a systematic method of preparing the data set and including additional data, to ensure the most valid results possible, which will ultimately eliminate bias. Finally, the researchers should ensure that they are able to interpret their results with confidence.

Reliability

Reliability refers to the consistency of methods used within a study and is most important within the data collection phase of the study (Moule and Goodman, 2009). The tool, apparatus or scale that is being used to measure and collect the data for the study should consistently provide the required results each time it is used. The reliability of a questionnaire can be assessed using a test-retest procedure where a participant can complete the questionnaire on two or more occasions and the comparison of responses from these occasions should be the same. As with the validity testing of a questionnaire, there are statistical tests (such as the Kappa statistic) which will assess how reliable the data collection tool is – thus ultimately adding to the quality and rigour of the research study.

PILOT STUDIES

Pilot studies are required in quantitative research to test the questionnaire or to act as a trial run for the methods designed for a larger study (van Teijlingen and Hundley, 2001). Within pilot studies the questionnaire is tested for validity and reliability, but in addition to this the questions used can be tried to ensure that they answer the main aims and objectives of the study. No matter how readable and interesting a questionnaire is, if the answers generated cannot be coded and analysed to answer the questions set by the aims and objectives of the study, then they should not be included. Pilot studies are also conducted to ensure that they are financially viable due to the large sums of money invested by funding bodies, as well as to make certain the findings are worthy of informing evidence-based practice.

ETHICS

All research projects require ethical scrutiny and permission from local and/or national ethics committees. Because of this it is vital to ensure that ethical issues and principles are addressed during the planning stage of a quantitative project. (This will be discussed in more depth in Chapter 13.)

You have now had a chance to look at the key aspects of quantitative research. The next two activities are designed to enable you to consolidate your learning. We know that at this stage in your career you are unlikely to be undertaking research, but we also know that you will be using research in your daily practice to ensure that it is evidence-based. The activities below should help you to really think about the issues raised within this chapter and allow you to feel more confident in your understanding of quantitative research.

Identify a quantitative research question from practice, then from the design and methods above decide on the most appropriate approach to undertake this research study. Identify:

- A question or hypothesis.
- A design (for example, you should include sample, data collection and analysis, reliability and validity, ethics).
- The reasons for your choices.

ACTIVITY 12.2

Case study

A recent academic review of students' views on the quality of assessment feedback identified dissatisfaction with the content of the feedback, primarily because students did not understand:

1 How to improve their next submission.
2 What they needed to do to achieve a higher grade.
3 What the markers meant by 'need to improve critical analysis'.

To that end the University of Wild Forrest has planned to undertake a university-wide study to find out students' views on what constitutes quality assessment feedback.

Questions

1 Between the two types of quantitative research methods discussed in this chapter, identify the most suitable method to undertake this study.
2 State the reason for your choice.
3 What would be the research question (hypothesis), aim and objectives?
4 Identify the main features of your methodology, including your sampling frame (if applicable) and technique, mode of data collection and analysis, ethical considerations, and the possible limitations of your proposed approach.

SUMMARY

This chapter has provided an overview of the two main designs used in quantitative research and when they should be used, and has detailed the processes for their adoption. The critical points for your learning so far are:

- The main purpose of quantitative research is to produce evidence that can be generalised to reach the larger population, however, as discussed within survey methods this may not always be the case due to the type of sampling used.
- Experimental designs normally assess cause and effect, and what possible impact the intervention would have on the population of interest, while surveys demonstrate versatility in a wide range of non-experimental-type studies by identifying their main scope and purpose.

FURTHER READING

There are numerous books and articles that can provide detailed information relating to quantitative research. Some of the most useful resources we have found are:

Berry, J. (2005) Quantitative methods in educational research. [online] Available at: www.edu. plymouth.ac.uk/resined/Quantitative/quanthme.htm Plymouth: University of Plymouth (last accessed 18 January 2013).
The material within this web resource was prepared by the University of Plymouth and is aimed at Master's level students, but there is a useful description of the terminology.

Coolidge, F.L. (2013) *Statistics: A gentle introduction* (3rd edition). London: Sage.
This is a useful text to explain statistics in a simplified form. The use of exemplar tables and graphs throughout help the reader to understand and interpret statistics relating to the given examples.

Moule, P. and Goodman, M. (2009) *Nursing research: An introduction*. London: Sage.
This is a useful text for some aspects of quantitative research, however, you will need to read further to access some of the specialised areas of quantitative research.

REFERENCES

Bowling, A. (2005) Mode of questionnaire administration can have serious effects on data quality, *Journal of Public Health*, 27 (3): 281–291.
Campbell, M.J. and Swinscow, T.D.V. (2009) *Statistics at square one*. Oxford: BMJ Books.
Doll, H.A., Petersen, S.E.K. and Stewart-Brown, S.L. (2000) Obesity and physical and emotional well-being: Associations between Body Mass Index, chronic illness, and the physical and mental components of the SF-36 Questionnaire, *Obesity Research*, 18 (2): 160–170.
Gerrish, K. and Lacey, A. (2010) *The research process in nursing*. Oxford: Wiley-Blackwell.
Green, J. and Browne, J. (2005) *Research design: Principles of social research*. Berkshire: Open University Press. p. 32.
Groves, R.M., Fowler, J.R., Couper, F.J., Lepkowski, M.P., Singer, J.M. and Tourangeau, R. (2009) *Survey methodology*. Hoboken, NJ: Wiley.
Herald, J.M. and Peavy, J.V. (2002) Surveys and sampling, *Field Epidemiology*: 196.
Holland, K. and Rees, C. (2010) *Nursing: Evidence-based practice skills*. Oxford: Open University Press.
Laerhoven, H., Zaag-Loonen, H.J. and Derkx, B. (2004) A comparison of Likert scale and visual analogue scales as response options in children's questionnaires, *Acta Paediatrica*, 93 (6): 830–835.
Lee, J.W., Jones, P.S., Mineyama, Y. and Zhang, X.E. (2002) Cultural differences in responses to a Likert scale, *Research in Nursing and Health*, 25 (4): 295–306.
Martin, D. (2000) Towards the geographies of the 2001 UK Census of Population, *Transactions of the Institute of British Geographers*, 25 (3): 321–332.
Martindale, S., McNeill, G., Devereux, G., Campbell, D., Russell, G. and Seaton, A. (2005) Antioxidant intake in pregnancy in relation to wheeze and eczema in the first two years of life, *American Journal of Respiratory and Critical Care Medicine*, 171: 121–128.
Meadows, K.A. (2003a) So you want to do research? An introduction to quantitative methods, *British Journal of Community Nursing*, 8 (11): 519–526.
Meadows, K.A. (2003b) So you want to do research? Questionnaire design, *British Journal of Community Nursing*, 8 (12): 562–570.
Moule, P. and Goodman, M. (2009) *Nursing research: An introduction*. London: Sage.
Munro, B.H. (2004) *Statistical methods for health care research*. Philadelphia, PA: Lippincott Williams and Wilkins.

Neale, J. (ed.) (2009) *Research methods for health and social care*. Houndsmills: Palgrave Macmillan.

Parahoo, K. (2006) *Nursing research: Principles, process and issues*. Houndsmills: Palgrave Macmillan.

Petticrew, M., Chalabi, Z. and Jones, D.R. (2012) To RCT or not to RCT: Deciding when more evidence is needed for public health policy and practice, *J Epidemiol Community Health*, 66: 91–396.

Turton, A.J., O'Leary, K.O., Gabb, J., Woodward, R. and Gilchrist, I.D. (2010) A single blinded randomised controlled pilot trial of prism adaptation for improving self-care in stroke patients with neglect, *Neuropsycological Rehabilitation*, 20 (2): 180–196.

Uijen, A.A., Bischoff, E.W.M.A., Schellevis, F.G., Bor, H.H.J., Van Den Bosch, W.J.H.M. and Schers, H.J. (2012) Continuity in different care modes and its relationship to quality of life: A randomised controlled trial in patients with COPD, *British Journal of General Practice*, 62 (599): e422–e428.

van Teijlingen, E. and Hundley, V. (2001) The importance of pilot studies, *Social Research Update*, (35): 1–4.

Watson, R., Atkinson, I. and Egerton, P.A. (2006) *Successful statistics for nursing and healthcare*. Basingstoke: Palgrave Macmillan.

13

ETHICS IN HEALTHCARE RESEARCH

ANDREW MCKIE

Chapter learning outcomes

On completion of Chapter 13 you will be able to:

1   Outline the scope of ethics for healthcare research.
2   Discuss the impact of ethical theories and principles on the research process.
3   Identify landmark events in the history of ethics in healthcare research.
4   Highlight key ethical issues pertinent to the research process.

Key concepts

Ethical theories, ethical principles, informed consent, ethical review.

INTRODUCTION

The purpose of this chapter is to help you explore ethical issues. These ethical issues may apply to research that you go on to undertake and will also apply to your understanding and critique of any research that you access. The significant place of ethics in professional healthcare itself was highlighted in Chapter 7, but you may have arrived at this conclusion yourself from your own studies and recent clinical experience. In this chapter various definitions of ethics are presented, several important philosophical and ethical theories are considered, a brief survey of the history of ethics in healthcare is conducted, and several ethical issues are reviewed and related to the research process. Finally, I shall take you on an 'ethical journey' with Joan, a professional healthcare researcher, featuring her ethical reflections upon conducting her own research. This journey aims to 'make real' the ethics in research from a researcher (student) perspective.

DEFINING ETHICS

The topic of ethics may, like philosophy itself, appear somewhat daunting to you. There are so many theories, perspectives and learned opinions! In addition, there appear to be so many complex ethical problems or dilemmas: for example, end-of-life issues, genetic screening, abortion, and organ transplantation, to name only a few. This is a common and quite understandable reaction.

Think back to Chapter 7 and recall the discussion on the place of purposes, or aims (ends – *telos*), in philosophical enquiry. If the practice of nursing possesses several particular ends (e.g. the relief of patients' suffering, promoting health), ethics may be considered an activity that is concerned with more generalised 'ends' of the 'good' or 'best'. Thompson et al. (2006: 2) assert that ethics is concerned with the 'conditions for human flourishing', whilst Vanier (2001: 13) centres more on the *means* towards achieving such an end: ethics 'helps us to clarify what is truly a human act'. The 'means/end' axis, or equation, is important in ethical reflection.

The practice of ethics, however, brings these larger concerns about human life (ends, purposes, values and aspirations) to everyday human activity itself, including research projects. The Greek philosopher Plato's most famous pupil, Socrates, stated that the focus of such an enquiry was on 'nothing less than how a man should live' (Plato, 1971: 106). Although ethics may resemble philosophy as a 'second-order activity', Socrates' view suggests that ethics has the potential to impact upon every aspect of the lives of men and women. From such a position emphasising an 'end' of human flourishing, researchers have the opportunity to view their practice in new, fresh, and critical ways. Now consolidate your initial thinking on ethics by completing Activity 13.1 below.

ACTIVITY 13.1

What do you understand by the term 'ethics'?
Outline the potential relevance of ethics for:

- Your own professional life as a nurse or healthcare practitioner.
- Your own personal life.

Try to raise some of the issues in conversation with your friends at the weekend. You may find it interesting to see the perspectives that others have.

An introduction to some new terminology should help you think some more about the ethical dimensions of research. You may know some of these terms already, but the discussion here will relate them to key aspects of the research process itself.

Ethical theories

Ethical theories are often neglected in discussions upon ethics in healthcare research. Nevertheless, addressing these can help you achieve a more critical understanding of the key features in research ethics. The first major theory to consider is *utilitarianism* or, as it is often called, *consequentialism*. According to this theory, any action should be evaluated in terms of its consequences or intended effects. The English philosopher John Stuart Mill (1806–1873) argued that people should act in ways which maximise human happiness or pleasure. The phrase 'the greatest happiness for the greatest number' became the central motivation of a nineteenth-century social ethic intent on improving the lives of men and women via social, health, and educational reforms. Its influence on British social policy since 1945 can be seen in the welfare state provision of universal healthcare, comprehensive education, and social benefits. Nurses can consider the ways in which utilitarian theory might contribute to their intention to provide good nursing care to all patients or to more specific groups – e.g. to a community nurse's caseload of older patients.

It is possible to ask some critical questions of utilitarian theory itself. Here are a few:

- What exactly is human happiness or pleasure?
- Who decides upon such an aim?
- Is it possible that the welfare of the majority of people might overlook the interests of the minority?

For the purposes of research, utilitarianism is given a sharper focus when its *consequentialist* dimensions are considered. By making the consequences, or effects, of human actions the main ethical focus, some pertinent ethical questions can be asked about the justification, or rationale, for carrying out any research project. In particular, these might include:

- What is the purpose of the intended research?
- What are the aims and objectives of the project?
- Who are the intended beneficiaries of the research?
- Could any *unintended* consequences result from the conduct of a particular research project?

Addressing such questions at the beginning of a research project permits the purposes (ends) of any activity to be kept firmly in view. By considering the consequences, the desire for knowledge can be located within the wider contexts of communities (public, private), potential respondents, and fellow researchers (colleagues, institutions). Reflect on the implications of this theory for research by completing Activity 13.2.

Using one of the research articles that you have looked at for a previous activity (or a new one if you wish), reflect on the impact of consequentialism upon:

- The justification or rationale for undertaking the research.
- The research aims and objectives.
- The suitability of the participants for the research.

The second ethical theory is known as *deontology* (*deon*: duty). In contrast to consequentialism, deontology centres attention upon the quality of an action itself and not on any intended (or unintended) consequences. Derived from the work of philosopher Immanuel Kant (1724–1804), deontology argues that the ethical evaluation of an action must be applied in *all* instances (the technical term is *universalising*). If truth-telling, for example, is considered to be a noble and proper action, then deontologists would argue that the truth should be always told in every situation without exception. People cannot simply choose to tell the truth on one occasion, but then do otherwise the next time.

Along with utilitarianism, deontology is open to criticism. To return to the example of truth-telling, this might be held up as a laudable and universal action. But you might also think of situations in nursing when truth-telling as an action needs to take account of contextual issues, for example when communicating 'bad news' to a patient in sensitive ways. In addition, viewing certain actions in 'duty' terms might lead to people neglecting to ask why such actions are being carried out in the first place.

Deontology's influence on research ethics centres upon the ethical quality of human actions (means). Actions should not compromise or threaten the dignity or humanity of others. Kant's famous Categorical Imperative (or Humanity Formula) interprets the interplay between means and ends: 'so act that you use humanity, whether in your own person or in the person of any other, always at the same time as an end, never merely as a means' (Kant, 1785). Accordingly, the research participant is given a pivotal place in terms of respect, dignity, and recognising individual rights. The ethical principle of autonomy derives from deontology and its outworking in research design seeks to ensure that the participant is provided with all the necessary information to allow them to decide whether, or not, to take part (informed consent). Now consolidate your thinking on deontology by completing Activity 13.3.

Consider deontology as an ethical theory. Try to think of examples of actions in nursing and healthcare practice that might be based on this category.

- Might there be exceptions to these actions?
- Try to justify these exceptions.

Consider Kant's Humanity Formula a little more. Discuss whether it might be permissible for human participants in research to be considered as means to an end as long as certain ethical safeguards are put in place.

The interaction between the ethical theories of consequentialism and deontology has a potential impact on ethics in research. Considered together, these two theories bring the collective perspective of consequentialism alongside deontology's focus on action and respect for human autonomy and rights. Researchers can perform an ethical 'cost-benefit' analysis of their design in terms of deontology (cost) and consequentialism (benefit) respectively.

The third ethical theory to consider is known as *virtue ethics*. In contrast to the features of results and actions in consequentialist and deontological theories respectively, virtue centres primarily – but not exclusively – upon the character of the person (ethical agent) carrying out a particular action. Virtue shares much in common with consequentialism and deontology in being a 'purposive disposition' (Aristotle, 1983: Book Two, p.101). Appropriate and contextualised actions are directed towards a goal or good. In emphasising such moral virtues as honesty, truthfulness, faithfulness, courage and modesty, virtue ethics has made a recent impact on healthcare ethics by reinstating the humanity of the professional and in recognising the importance of contextual factors at work in ethical deliberation.

In research ethics, virtue recognises the key role of the researcher throughout an entire project. Ethical issues cannot simply be addressed procedurally at the beginning of a project (for example, through participant recruitment or ethics panel approval). Highly complex and sensitive ethical decisions will often need to be made throughout a project. Virtue ethics reminds researchers to constantly review their position within the research project alongside its wider ends or purposes. Now summarise your learning about virtue ethics by completing Activity 13.4.

What virtues might a researcher need to practise at different stages of a research project?

ACTIVITY 13.4

ETHICAL FRAMEWORKS

Two particular frameworks may help you to further explore the place of ethics in research. Both frameworks draw upon strands of the three ethical theories discussed above. As you consider each framework, try to identify their potential impact upon research.

Principlism

The ethical principles, often gathered together under the title of 'principlism', were first discussed in Chapter 7. Viewed as general and universal guides for action, they build upon a 'common morality' applicable to, and across, different cultures and contexts (Beauchamp and Childress, 2009). These principles are extensively utilised in healthcare ethics, in particular in the field of bioethics – a term which often incorporates the interests of medical ethics, nursing ethics, and research ethics. These principles, usually outlined as four, are listed in Table 13.1 below.

Table 13.1   Ethical principles (source: Beauchamp and Childress, 2009)

Principle	Definition
Autonomy	Enhancing the decision making capacity of autonomous persons
Beneficence	Promoting good
Non-maleficence	Doing no harm
Justice	Distributing benefits fairly

In the specific area of research ethics, the four principles are often translated into what are known as the 'regulative principles' as follows:

- Free and informed consent.
- Privacy and confidentiality.
- Protection from harm.
- Avoiding a conflict of interest.
- Avoiding deception.
- The provision of information/debriefing.

It is possible to identify the influence of the ethical principles on the regulative principles. Securing participants' free and informed consent, maintaining their right to privacy, and handling all information received in confidential ways can be considered the distinguishing features of any promotion of the principle of autonomy in research. Similarly, the principle of beneficence can be mapped onto the need for researchers to provide participants with essential information about a study itself and debriefing as part of the dissemination of findings after that study is completed. The principle of non-maleficence can be seen in the requirement to protect participants from harm and deception, in addition to the responsibility of researchers to ensure that their own participation addresses any conflict of interest. Continue your reflection on these issues in Activity 13.5.

ACTIVITY 13.5

Consider the ethics within a research article of your choice. Outline the possible implications of the regulative principles for the study.

One notable feature of the use of principlism in research ethics centres around its rationalist and ordered approach (you will recall this feature in the critique of rationalism in Chapter 7). The principles shared in rationalist approaches to knowledge can be described as abstract and detached. The ethical principles, being *general* approaches to action, may lack essential details in helping persons to know how to act in particular situations. The ethical principle of autonomy is often operationalised by ensuring that researchers obtain freely given consent from participants based on the best information available. Think, however, about the issue of consent for a moment. Several questions may be asked here:

- What is meant by consent that is 'free'?
- How can it be ensured that potential participants will understand what it is that they are consenting to?
- In what ways might the consent of participants from certain client groups (e.g. older people, people with learning difficulties) require particular safeguarding and added attention?

The principle of autonomy is central to bioethics with its features of scientific measurement, rationality, and control. Its tendency, however, is to limit ethics in research to addressing certain well-recognised markers of a research project via an institutional ethical review: a robust research design, participant involvement and consent, sound data collection methods, and clearly stated outcomes. While important, such an approach may underplay the need for careful ethical reflection to be continued throughout a research project itself.

Hermeneutic ethics

A second approach suggests that research involves an 'ethical process' rather than merely being a study with a set list of projected outcomes. Hermeneutics (interpretation) is therefore a process in which the researcher actively engages with key participants and other salient factors of the research project. Clegg (2004: 186) notes that hermeneutic ethics 'preserves a bridge between philosophy and the human sciences, enlarging the limited horizon from which the problematic meaning arose'. In this ethic, the researcher's ethical participation involves reflexivity, taking responsibility, and practising the virtues described earlier in order to help address large (macro), as well as smaller (micro), issues about the research itself.

Clegg (2004) observes that the bioethical principle of autonomy may be of limited value in research involving persons with learning difficulties. Traditional notions of gaining consent may be limited with people for whom certain degrees of dependency on others in everyday living is simply a given. A hermeneutic ethic, on the other hand, seeks to involve the researcher, potential participants, and all relevant others in working together to ensure that research is relevant and remains sensitive to participants' needs.

In summary, both approaches (principlism and hermeneutics) are key in research ethics. Broad principles are required to frame (regulate) research, but so are interpretive approaches which will help researchers to be flexible and sensitive to the changing contexts of research itself. These approaches are summarised in Table 13.2.

Table 13.2 Ethical research methodology

Reflective research

➢ Listening and learning
➢ Interviewing
➢ Transcribing
➢ Interpretation
➢ Reading and writing
➢ Dissemination

Ethical review procedures

➢ Access to site
➢ Recruitment of samples
➢ Informed consent
➢ Maintaining confidentiality
➢ Research methods

A BRIEF HISTORY OF ETHICS IN HEALTHCARE RESEARCH

In part, the history of ethics in healthcare research represents the development and refinement of key ethical themes (e.g. autonomy, confidentiality, consent) and their incorporation into professional codes of conduct and protocols for practice. This history of practice has not always been positive. In this section, several key events are presented and certain issues will be considered arising from one famous research narrative: the Stanford Prison Experiment of 1971.

The events of the Second World War represented a watershed in the development of healthcare research ethics. At the Nuremberg Trials of 1946, 23 German Nazi physicians, medical scientists and administrators were found guilty of initiating and participating in 'experimental research' with prisoners, involving systematic torture, non-consensual surgical interventions, compulsory sterilisation, and killings. Two major documents addressing professional conduct in the practice of research in healthcare emerged from these events: the Nuremberg Code (1947) and the Declaration of Helsinki (1964). The Nuremberg Code (1947) addressed governance issues in the practice of healthcare research. Its main principle (one of ten) focused upon the requirement of obtaining the voluntary consent of participants in any research project. No guidance, however, was offered to address participants unable to give consent and confidentiality issues were not mentioned.

The Declaration of Helsinki (1964: latest revision 2008) was published by the World Medical Association (WMA) as a medical profession response to the Nuremberg Trials and Code (see www.wma.net/en/30publications/10policies/b3/17c.pdf). Therapeutic and non-therapeutic research was sharply differentiated and informed consent as the central ethical theme in research was emphasised. Surrogate consent was also included to address research participants deemed incapable of giving consent or when viewed as incompetent (e.g. a young child).

Several other events deserve noting. The Tuskegee Study began in 1932 but was only exposed in 1972. This study involved 399 black men in Alabama, in the USA, being 'treated' for syphilis and promised various inducements. In reality, however, these men were simply being observed and denied access to antibiotic treatment in the 1950s. Tuskegee's main outcome was the requirement for an institutional ethical review and the approval of all research projects.

The Thalidomide tragedy involved the birth of deformed babies in Europe and North America during the 1950s. Thalidomide was an approved sedative drug taken by pregnant women for morning sickness, the taking of which resulted in birth defects in their babies. The main outcome from this tragedy was stricter scrutiny of product marketing by drug companies and the requirement once again for informed consent to be obtained from all participants using experimental drugs.

Finally, the continuing relevance of ethics in healthcare research needs to acknowledge the controversies around the Bristol Heart Hospital and Alder Hey Hospital in Liverpool in 1999, when it was revealed that hearts and organs of deceased babies had been retained for further use by medical researchers without the knowledge and consent of parents.

Research narrative

In this selective look at the history of ethics in healthcare research, several ethical features of the Stanford Prison Experiment (SPE) are examined. The study was carried out by Professor Philip Zimbardo and colleagues of Stanford University in California in 1971. It involved the setting up of a mock prison and the recruitment of ten psychology students who were randomly selected into two groups of prisoners and guards. The main purpose of the research was to study the 'prisoner experience' over a two-week period, but the study had to be stopped after five days following complaints from one member of the research team. The participants had begun to take on 'real' behavioural attributes of prison guard control, involving acts of aggression, violence and intimidation towards the prisoners. In turn, the latter began to display disturbing behaviours of passivity, trauma, depersonalisation and deindividuation as a result of the treatment they received at the hands of their prison guards (Zimbardo, 2009). Certain key ethical aspects of the Stanford Experiment are significant for your consideration, and while this is an extreme example of experimental research, the issues highlighted are relevant to healthcare research. Consider these in Activities 13.6 and 13.7.

In the SPE, the student volunteers could have elected to quit at any time. No guns or legal statutes bound them to their imprisonment, only a subject selection form on which they promised to do their best to last the two full weeks. However ... the prisoners came to believe that it was a prison being run by psychologists and not by the State. They persuaded themselves ... that no-one could leave of their own volition. (Zimbardo, 2009: 222)

Discuss this excerpt in the light of participants' free and informed consent in research and their right to withdraw from a study at any time.

It should also have been apparent to me that we were losing the scientific detachment essential for conducting any research with unbiased objectivity. I was well on the way to becoming a prison superintendant rather than a principal investigator. However, even psychologists are people, subject to the same dynamic processes at a personal level that they study at a professional level. (Zimbardo, 2009: 99)

Discuss the conflict of interests that Zimbardo experienced during this experiment.

ADDRESSING KEY ETHICAL ISSUES IN RESEARCH

Several ethical issues will now be considered which need to be addressed at different stages in any research project. These combine the principlist and hermeneutic approaches outlined earlier, as well as insights from the ethical theories of consequentialism, deontology, and virtue.

Ethical issues in research design

Ethics should be central to the early thinking about any intended research. You will have seen from working through this chapter that it is not possible to compartmentalise ethics into certain stages of a research project and then to simply forget about this. Although researchers are required to address certain formal stages of ethics (e.g. submitting a proposal to an ethical review panel for approval and obtaining consent from participants), the insights gained from hermeneutic ethics and virtue ethics will indicate that ethical issues require attention to be paid *throughout* the entire research project, up to – and even beyond – the dissemination of results.

Ethical review

Submitting a research proposal for ethical review, whether via an NHS local ethics committee or a university faculty ethics panel, can be a daunting prospect. Completion of the necessary paperwork is often complex and challenging. However, this ethical review is not only a legal requirement, but it also provides the researcher with an invaluable quality review of the research project at the early design stage. In submitting a proposal, the researcher should try to make the application process as smooth as possible by complying with all the panel's requirements, including the submission date, online application, supply of 'hard' copies, and other relevant documents (e.g. copies of access letters to gatekeepers, invitation letters to potential participants, consent forms, information sheets, and questionnaires). Some panels will ask a researcher to appear in person whilst the application is being considered. Some typical responses from ethics review panels are listed in Activity 13.8.

Consider what ethical issues might be involved in the following ethical review comments:

'The information sheet for potential participants does not explain why the study is needed'.

'The consent form is minimal and lacks detail'.

'Please consider whether harm may be a possibility due to participants' exposure to a different set of circumstances from their usual practice'.

ACTIVITY 13.8

Sample recruitment

Recruiting a sample, in terms of appropriateness and size, is rarely straightforward. Ethical issues will often centre upon ensuring that the participants have fully consented to taking part in a research study. However, consideration may also have to be given to the ways in which the field of research is accessed – for example, by seeking the permission of 'gatekeepers' such as medical consultants, nurse managers, and care managers. In addition, the desire to undertake research in the researcher's own area of nursing practice may raise a conflict of interest between the role as practitioner and that of researcher. It is important to consider this issue when evaluating a particular research study for use in your own practice.

Informed consent

The significance of obtaining informed consent from research participants as a feature of promoting autonomy has previously been noted. Key issues for consideration by the researcher may include: the amount/level/extent of information given to potential participants to enable their choice to be properly informed; the mode of information used (a card, single sheet, booklet, online); and consideration of the type of participants within the sample (e.g. older people, ethnic groups, people with learning difficulties or mental health problems). Consider these issues by completing Activity 13.9.

You want to conduct some research into mental health users' perspectives on medication information given by community mental health nurses in your own practice setting. You consider, however, that the active recruitment of participants by yourself as a researcher might compromise the therapeutic relationship which you have established with clients. In what ways might you address this sensitive ethical issue?

As a nurse interested in researching the psychological impact of chronic conditions in young adolescents, you add as a 'reward' a gift token at the end of your publicity poster as a means of boosting recruitment to a focus group. Consider the ethical issues involved in adding such an inducement. Try to reach a decision and then justify your answer.

Ethical issues during the research process

It has already been noted that the consideration of ethical issues in research cannot be confined to the research design stage and the formal aspects of submission to an ethics review panel. Most research projects will undergo changes as they progress and researchers need to be aware of any ensuing ethical implications. A number of ethical issues pertinent to carrying out research itself shall now be considered.

The position of the researcher within the research project itself has important ethical dimensions. This is no less so when a nurse researcher is engaged in quantitative research with its features of objectivity and detachment. (Recall the significance of 'personal' knowledge and its impact on the selection of the research topic and the stance of the researcher from Chapter 7.) Many researchers in nursing and healthcare are actively *involved* in the research process itself. Such involvement may have significant ethical implications. Consider the ethical issues raised by Clancy (2011: 117; see also Box 13.1 below) in her narrative account as an observer in research being undertaken within a nurse-led family planning centre.

Box 13.1   Research in a nurse-led family planning centre (source: Clancy, 2011: 115)

'The nurse and teenage girl are chatting away about a new prescription for the contraceptive pill. Again I have problems observing. The situation is not intimate or sacred; "matter of fact" is a better description. The girl comes with a requirement, and the nurse complies and executes the order. The proximity of the nurse and girl disturbs me. I have been brought up to observe rules of common courtesy; it is not polite to stare'.

The ethical tension in research between pursuing a perceived benefit (increased knowledge) and upholding participants' rights is often demonstrated in one-to-one and group interviews. Talking to people during a semi-structured interview, or with others in a focus group about their health or experiences of nursing care, may yield many different results. The participant has the right to withdraw from the study at any time without it having any bearing on their present (or future) status. Researchers also need to be aware of the possibility that the research methods may cause harm to the participants and take steps to prevent this. Consider this issue further in Activity 13.10.

As a researcher in mental health nursing, you have carefully recruited eight participants for a focus group exploring the experiences of young adult suicide 'survivors'. Outline and justify what actions you might put in place to address potentially difficult outcomes in this situation.

ACTIVITY 13.10

An additional ethical issue centres around the storage of data. Researchers will gather data from a variety of different sources (e.g. demographic information about participants, survey information, transcribed interview data, policy documents, and key stakeholder views on practice issues). Data, even if anonymised, may be highly sensitive in respect of participants' personal details, attitudes, values, and beliefs. Like all information obtained in the public domain, the researcher's responsibility lies in protecting the participants by ensuring that access to data is restricted by utilising storage in locked cupboards and password protected files, and by using means in reporting to enhance anonymity and confidentiality. An institutional audit of funded research projects also seeks to ensure that these principles are being followed.

Finally, the ethical implications of revisions made to a research project must be noted. This may mean returning amendments to appropriate ethics review panels for further scrutiny and approval. Often, however, researcher reflexivity may simply allow a response to smaller-scale changes in sensitive and nuanced ways. The concept of 'continuing consent' is one way of ensuring that the participants are kept informed of, and give their approval to, changes made to a research design.

Addressing ethical issues on completion of the research process

There are several key ethical issues to consider on completion of a research project. One of them is the ethical imperative, via the principle of beneficence, to disseminate the research findings to a wider audience. This is, of course, ethically qualified by *which* findings the researcher chooses to publish and *how* they go about doing so. Nevertheless, the researcher has a responsibility – to the participants, sponsoring institution/funding body, profession, research community, ethical review panel, and society – to ensure that the research findings are made widely accessible for their implementation, discussion, critique, and further development.

Alongside dissemination of the research, important ethical issues surround the implementation of research findings: this is an area that you will become more familiar with as you use research in your own practice. Within contemporary care settings the emphasis is on practice being *evidence-based* and this raises issues around the types of evidence used and how implementation takes place. Note that the issue of ends (*telos*) discussed earlier is relevant here: namely, how does a particular piece of research evidence contribute to an end of patients' welfare/wellbeing or staff's enhancement of their skills?

THE 'ETHICAL JOURNEY' OF A PROFESSIONAL HEALTHCARE RESEARCHER: AN INTERVIEW WITH JOAN

In this section, key issues involved in research ethics are explored in an interview with Joan, a professional healthcare researcher. Joan has given her ethical permission to include this interview and anonymity has been addressed by using a different name.

Joan: I'll talk about my PhD project. My project was about bereavement care for older people. It was about how healthcare staff interact with relatives: before the death, at the time of the death, and after the death of somebody's relative. The participant groups included were hospital staff, nursing home and care home staff, general practice and community nursing staff. I also included a small sample of older people who had had bereavements. It was a qualitative interview study and people took part in an interview. From the data collected, I developed a guideline for bereavement care which staff could use and inform the care they provide for bereaved relatives.

Andrew: In your early thinking about your PhD, what part did ethics have to play?

Joan: The relatives were the key concern really. I had access to staff areas through people I had known previously. I wasn't very happy to 'cold call' relatives. I couldn't get access to who they were because of the Data Protection Act. You can't go to a General Practice and ask for a list of people bereaved during the last year. I actually ended up accessing them through the staff that had taken part in interviews.

Andrew: Were there specific ethical issues in gaining your sample?

Joan: The thing about bereaved relatives is when you would contact them. I was very concerned about causing distress. I wanted the healthcare staff to talk about their experiences professionally, rather than personally.

Andrew: Were there instances in carrying out the research when you had to stop someone being interviewed or refer them to other services?

Joan: That was all written in the planning. If someone did get distressed you would stop recording. The other thing I proposed initially was having a focus group with relatives around the guidelines. I planned to have two researchers (one of them my supervisor) because if somebody did get distressed in a group, you have somebody to take them away to a quiet area.

Andrew: Can you outline your experience of submitting your proposal to an ethics review panel?

Joan: My research involved NHS staff and people who had access to the NHS services so I had to go the NHS REC [*NHS Research Ethics Committee*] for approval. It's a bit of a long protracted process. Actually, it helped me to develop the study properly. Earlier on it was a proposal, but I hadn't thought through step-by-step how I was going to approach the project. Filling in the ethics form developed that.

Andrew: Were there specific issues to address following the ethics review?

Joan: I actually went to the ethics review panel meeting. The only person who had a question was one of the lay members. This was about when I would approach the relatives. His opinion was that it wasn't long enough. He had recently lost his wife himself and at three months he wouldn't have been ready to talk to a researcher. So I said that I wouldn't approach any relatives until they had been bereaved for six months or more. That was the only thing that changed after the ethical review. But I felt they were quite supportive.

Andrew: Some people view ethics panels as a bit like the police, rather controlling. Is that a correct view?

Joan: Not in my experience, no. The paperwork is large and cumbersome. But I was reassured because my research was in such a sensitive area. I think it needs more than your supervisors or your research team to say that it's fine because the ethics committee come from a wider perspective. They are not so engaged in your area of work and I just find it reassuring that somebody from another perspective gives permission for your work to go ahead.

Andrew: Were there any other ethical issues which emerged when carrying out your research?

Joan: There were a few actually. One lady I went to see, this is around informed consent. She knew why I was coming so immediately she opened the door she started talking about her loss, her husband, and when he died. Talking in quite good depth, but I hadn't switched on the recorder, I hadn't completed the consent form. I was just basically in the door, and she started. I had to stop her. The other thing was she prepared us tea and cakes, she was chatting all the way through tea and I had to stop her and go through all this stuff about recording and filling in the informed consent. She read all this information. She just really wasn't interested. After I did set the recorder going, but she wasn't talking. I did feel that it interfered in that particular interview.

Andrew: Did you use this rich data not formalised in the interview?

Joan: I did try to make some notes afterwards. The other thing that ethically I found difficult was that she was obviously lonely and looked on me as a friend. She stayed in sheltered housing and I was invited back to visit. I found that really hard. I never went back really because she didn't live in town, quite a distance away. But at the same time, you have that researcher participative relationship.

Andrew: In research, is there sometimes a clash of interests between your roles as a nurse and as a researcher?

Joan: I have previous experience of this. I went to collect data from a lady at home and her husband was in the end-stages and was in a bed in the living room. I ended up helping her to turn him before I left. Another thing I find difficult is that you go in to do an interview and I feel that it's sometimes a 'smash-and-grab' thing. I always send a thank-you note afterwards. You've opened up a lot of issues with someone, then you never have any contact with that person again. I struggle with that.

Andrew: One of the key issues in research ethics is about the autonomy and the dignity of the person. We have to see the person as an end, and not as a means. Clearly it has been an important issue for you.

Joan: It is and I will continue to struggle with it. One of the nurses I interviewed started crying as well and I am all right with folk crying. When you open up issues of bereavement people will cry, but she started bringing personal issues into the questions I was asking. I wanted to keep it on a professional basis.

Andrew: For all researchers, we need to be open to the unintended or the unexpected. That means that our ethical sensitivity must be very high.

Joan: Then there's myself as well, interviewing all these folk about bereavement. We did in the initial proposal have somebody identified to provide support to me. But this wasn't someone that I knew. I knew when I wrote it down in the proposal that I wasn't going to do it. Because I am not good at opening up to other people. I know more people around the university now.

Andrew: On completion of your research, were there ethical issues to address with regard to the publication and dissemination of results?

Joan: I think confidentiality and anonymity are quite important. I didn't want anything presented to be identified. I told them (the participants) that it would be confidential. Initially I gave them study numbers so that only I could work it. When I presented them on PowerPoint, I said: 'Female, sixties'. I didn't give them pseudonyms.

Andrew: Are novice researchers always aware of the central role of ethics?

Joan: I think they are aware of ethics, but until you actually do it proper ... As you engage in research, you do come across a range of issues that you maybe hadn't anticipated. It makes you aware of the difficulties around some of the things we try to do. I think it is important to get advice from people who have been there: a good supervisor and ethical committees. They are all there to support and I don't think we should hold back to ask for advice.

Andrew: Thank you very much.

SUMMARY

This chapter has provided you with learning related to addressing key ethical issues within the research process. An 'ethical checklist' is provided for your use at the end of the chapter (see Box 13.2). It is hoped that it will act as a reminder and will be of use when you are critiquing others' research. The critical points to reflect upon are:

- The scope of ethics in all healthcare research.
- The place and impact of ethical theories and frameworks upon the research process.
- An appreciation of the history of research in healthcare which accords a prominent place to ethical reflection.
- Recognising that an ethical journey should characterise the whole of a research project.

Box 13.2   Ethical checklist

This ethical checklist is not intended to be an exhaustive list of all the ethical issues which you might expect to address in a research paper. It may, however, help you to identify key ethical issues within the research process itself.

☐ Is the purpose of the intended research clearly stated in the paper?
☐ Are the aims and objectives of the research clearly outlined?
☐ Do the authors make the intended benefits/beneficiaries of the research obvious?
☐ Is there evidence of the research undergoing institutional ethical review?
☐ Are the informed consent procedures clearly mentioned?
☐ Does the research narrative demonstrate the attention paid to, and necessary action arising from, the 'regulative principles' (e.g. privacy and confidentiality, protection from harm, avoidance of conflict of interest, avoidance of deception, debriefing arrangements for participants)?
☐ Does the presentation and discussion of the research findings in the paper demonstrate appropriateness and ethical sensitivity?
☐ Does the paper itself indicate researcher reflexivity to the changing context of the research actually carried out?

FURTHER READING

Chadwick, R., Have, H.T. and Meslin, E.M. (eds) (2011) *The SAGE handbook of health care ethics: Core and emerging issues*. London: Sage. A detailed, but readable, handbook addressing current issues in healthcare ethics.

Oliver, P. (2003) *The student's guide to research ethics*. Berkshire: OUP. A comprehensive text to guide the student through ethics in research.

Thomson, I.E., Melia, K.M., Boyd, K.M. and Horsburgh, D. (eds) (2006) *Nursing ethics* (5th edition). Edinburgh: Churchill-Livingstone Elsevier. A readable account of key ethical issues pertinent to nursing practice.

Zimbardo, P. (2009) *The Lucifer Effect: How good people turn evil.* London: Rider. A detailed account of how 'experimental research' can go badly astray.

REFERENCES

Aristotle (1983) *The ethics of Aristotle: The Nicomachean ethics.* Harmondsworth: Penguin Classics.

Beauchamp, T.L. and Childress, J.F. (2009) *Principles of biomedical ethics* (6th edition). Oxford: Oxford University Press.

Clancy, A. (2011) An embodied response: ethics and the nurse researcher, *Nursing Ethics*, 18 (1): 112–121.

Clegg, J. (2004) Practice in focus: a hermeneutic approach to research ethics, *British Journal of Learning Disabilities*, 32: 186–190.

Declaration of Helsinki (1964) *Declaration of Helsinki: Ethical principles for medical research involving human subjects.* New York: World Medical Association.

Kant, I. (1785) Groundwork of the metaphysics of morals. Reprinted in W. Weischedel, *Werke in Zwolf Banden,* Vol. 7. Frankfurt: Suhrkamp.

Nuremberg Code (1947) Reprinted from *Trials of war criminals before the Nuremberg military tribunals under control of council law* (1949), No. 10, Vol. 2. Washington, DC: United States Government Printing Office.

Plato (1971) *Gorgias.* Harmondsworth: Penguin Books.

Thompson, I.E., Melia, K.M., Boyd, K.M. and Horsburgh, D. (eds) (2006) *Nursing ethics.* Edinburgh: Churchill-Livingstone/Elsevier.

Vanier, J. (2001) *Made for happiness: Discovering the meaning of life with Aristotle.* Toronto: Anasi Press.

Zimbardo, P. (2009) *The Lucifer Effect: How good people turn evil.* London: Rider.

14

PREPARATION FOR YOUR DISSERTATION

COLIN MACDUFF

Chapter learning outcomes

On completion of Chapter 14, you will be able to:

1 Appreciate what your undergraduate dissertation involves and why you are being asked to write one.
2 Reflect on your characteristic approach to learning and consider how this might work or need to be adapted for the dissertation.
3 Reflect on what you want from the dissertation personally and professionally.
4 Identify the main sources of knowledge and help that you can use on this journey.
5 Identify three common dissertation pitfalls and a five-point strategic plan for success.

Key concepts

Dissertation, preparation, self-knowledge and motivation, academic writing, supervisory relationship and expectations, achieving focus, time management, other sources of knowledge and help, planning for success.

INTRODUCTION

'Dissertation' is a word that can have an aura about it: on a good day it is surrounded by light – the fruit of your academic work budding near the top of the learning tree – but on a bad day it can seem dark and heavy – like the sound a big casebound book makes if it's dropped on the floor.

The aim of this chapter is to help bring more light to the dissertation process and final product through successful planning. In this way you can actually enjoy the dissertation experience and further both your learning and, hopefully, your career. To do this I want to help you to think proactively in a number of different ways, and so the chapter is divided into five distinct sections in order to achieve this.

Firstly, we will look at what a typical dissertation involves and why nursing education programmes may require that you write one. One of the ways of thinking about the dissertation that will recur throughout this chapter is to see it as a journey. Then in the second and third sections of the chapter you will be encouraged to prepare for that journey by first looking backwards to reflect on your characteristic learning style (in Section 2), and then forwards to imagine where you will go and what you will achieve (Section 3). As you begin to do this it is essential to be aware of the main sources of knowledge and help you can use to travel towards your destination (Section 4). Finally, a map of the terrain will prove invaluable and Section 5 provides this by helping you to chart the best route using six strategies for success and avoiding the most common pitfalls. At various points in the text the voices of past students and present supervisors are used to give this guidance and cause for reflection.

THE DISSERTATION: WHAT IS IT AND WHY DO I HAVE TO DO ONE?

The word 'dissertation' can mean different things in different countries. In the USA it is typically used to describe the final large piece of the self-directed study and writing that PhD students have to produce. In the UK, however, it usually refers to the final substantial piece of study and writing required at Honours or Master's level. In the context of most undergraduate nursing courses, the following definition is useful:

> ### Box 14.1   Definition
>
> A dissertation is a substantial, structured piece of writing that develops a reasoned line of thought, going into depth and detail where relevant to explain and justify.

Typically it will build from your undergraduate work to date and involve you in:

- Sourcing and critically reading relevant literature on a specific topic or question.
- Thinking critically about the issues this raises and considering their relative strengths and weaknesses.
- Writing an extended piece of work (usually around 10,000 words) that explains what sense you have now made of the topic or question, and which methods you used to collect and evaluate your evidence.

As the above definition suggests, a dissertation is often seen as the culmination of your academic study as an undergraduate. In this piece of work your university are challenging you to demonstrate that you can reason in a sustained and systematic way and that this is based on sound evidence. This will be one of your main attributes as a graduate embarking on a career in nursing, so it is important that you can show this.

However, it may not always be obvious to you as a student, to some clinical staff, and maybe your family and friends, why a nurse or any other health professional might need to carry out such an extended piece of work. Surely there will be no time or need in clinical practice for this sort of scholarship? And shouldn't nurses just be getting on with it rather than trying to be scientists or artists?

If you can, get together with some peers/colleagues in a group.

To begin with, thinking of the dissertation activities listed in the previous 'Definition' box and the necessary attributes mentioned above, try to list how these could be useful in future situations as a nurse.

Then share your lists as a group, discussing how these skills might inform nursing or healthcare work in clinical, management, educational, or research settings.

Finally, consider as a group some of the possible patient, public, professional, and personal benefits.

ACTIVITY 14.1

Hopefully the above exercise will highlight that the skills you will develop and demonstrate through doing your dissertation are some, though not all, of the very skills that patients, your colleagues and the public will not only value but also positively require. In the modern healthcare context these parties need healthcare professionals who can find the evidence by consulting widely and appropriately, who can think critically and logically about what is needed, who can advocate in a sustained and reasonable way on this basis, evaluate the impact of their actions, and reflect on what this means for others and themselves.

So even if you never need to produce such an extended demonstration of your thinking in this format again in your career, these skills of analysis and synthesis will stand you in good stead. Indeed, it is interesting that many experienced nurses who qualified years ago come into higher education today in order to try to deepen their knowledge and make sense of particular clinically relevant topics through study that involves a dissertation.

Having taken an initial look at what a dissertation is and why you are being asked to write one, let's now look in more depth at undergraduate dissertations.

It is now rare for undergraduate nursing students to be required to carry out original research for their dissertation. The challenges of obtaining the ethical approval for numerous students to gather useful data from people in healthcare, educational or public settings make this impractical in the 6–12 months that are usually available. Rather, your project will usually be based around a review of the existing research and related literature (Hannigan and Burnard, 2001).

In some universities, the whole dissertation will focus on an in-depth literature review as a means of addressing a specific question about a specific topic. In this case you need to demonstrate a systematic approach to literature review and interpretation, but you will usually have some choice over the topic and the question. For example, your experiences of nursing people who are receiving chemotherapy for breast cancer (general topic) may lead you to ask the specific question of whether scalp cooling is effective in preventing hair loss for these people. The remit here is to use the literature search and appraisal skills detailed in Chapter 4 so that you can bring together the best quality research evidence in a way that addresses the question. This will quickly give you the challenge of defining exactly what you mean by terms like 'scalp cooling', 'effective', 'preventing', 'hair loss', and even 'people' (see Macduff et al., 2003). However your concern for these people, and your curiosity to find the most helpful answer, will help to sustain you on this learning journey.

In some universities there may also be a choice to develop a research proposal for your dissertation. Although you will not usually be required to carry out the proposal that you create, the process has been designed to help you to demonstrate insight into realistic planning of necessary research. This is useful not only if you do go on to carry out research, but also if you are involved as a user of research findings. In this type of dissertation there is also a need for a substantial literature review as a basis for justifying your proposed approach to the topic and question. However, the literature review here is more of a means to the end of developing your proposal rather than being the study research method in itself.

In outlining these two main types of nursing dissertation one thing becomes very clear: the need to closely read and consider the guidelines that you will be given for the project. These should set out the learning outcomes that you are expected to achieve, the nature and scope of the dissertation itself, the format for presentation, and mutual expectations for student and supervisory staff. Typically the length of the dissertation will be anything from 10,000–15,000 words and there will be a need to cover key areas using a suggested structure with headings.

One of the best ways to start to understand what your nursing dissertation could look like is to examine a few recent examples from your particular programme. Many course leaders will make sure that a variety of good exemplar dissertations from previous years are accessible either directly from the department or via the university library. In some ways creating a dissertation or thesis is like building a house

(Macduff, 2008). Having a vision of the finished whole can help us understand how all the main parts need to fit together.

Having envisaged the nursing dissertation in its main forms, it is vital at this point to pause. Rather than rushing towards (or away from!) the prospect, it makes sense to first take stock of how you have reached this point, why you want to proceed, what you should take with you, and what help will be needed on the way. These aspects are now considered in the next three sections of this chapter.

WHAT WORKS FOR ME AND WHAT ELSE DO I NEED TO SUCCEED?

Take some time to reflect on the way you have approached essay writing up to now. How have you tackled these assignments? Do you:

- Make a work plan and work to it in a steady, progressive way?
- Rush in and try to get it over with?
- Put it off and cram the work into the last week or two?

Make a list of the strengths and weaknesses of your academic writing, drawing on any feedback previously received.

Now focus especially on your best piece of written work. How did you manage to achieve this? What strengths can you bring and build on for this more sustained piece of writing? (Don't be shy!)

So, looking ahead, how might you best plan for this dissertation journey?

ACTIVITY 14.2

Hopefully Activity 14.2 has got you thinking about a number of aspects that will be important for your success. Firstly, we will all bring to the task our individual histories of learning and characteristic behaviours so a knowledge of self is therefore important as a starting-point. Educational and psychological research provides a number of models that can help us understand how we characteristically approach learning across different contexts. For example, drawing on the theories of David Kolb, Honey and Mumford (1986) suggest four main learning styles that we will variously bring with us.

The *activist* approach engages openly and readily with a learning challenge such as the dissertation, getting going on the work, consulting others and not dwelling long on the planning. By contrast the *reflector* approach involves standing back to ponder the challenge and cautiously consider different angles and implications before starting out. Meanwhile the *theorist* approach also involves a lot of thinking, more specifically about underpinning assumptions and what theories could be brought to explain and structure the topic. Finally, the *pragmatist* approach involves focusing on what works so that a practical plan can be taken forward without ruminating too long on the possibilities.

From this way of looking at learning, it is clear that you will need parts of all of these approaches to succeed with the dissertation. While at this stage I am suggesting that the reflective and theorising approaches are most appropriate, there will soon come the time when a pragmatic plan and action are necessary. Honey and Mumford's work suggests that we all tend to be stronger in some of these four styles than others, so is useful to ask yourself *which of these are my characteristic strengths?* and *which will I have to work on most to make a success of the experience?*

The latter two questions are not only useful when thinking ahead to the overall dissertation journey, they can also be applied to specific aspects of it. Considering your strengths and weaknesses in academic writing in Activity 14.2 may have highlighted various aspects, such as a proven ability to think through and execute a clear essay structure using sub-headings, or a tendency to use description rather than critical analysis. We will return to academic writing later in the chapter when considering the sources of knowledge that can help along the way. In the meantime it is useful, as in many situations in nursing, to take a solution-focused approach. By this I mean that you should celebrate the strengths you developed and demonstrated in your best essays so far, and use these as the building blocks for further success.

Part of any solution-focused approach is knowing where you want to go and why you want to get there. In the next section of this chapter I want to challenge you to think more on these aspects.

WHAT DO YOU WANT FROM THE DISSERTATION PERSONALLY AND PROFESSIONALLY?

At first the answer to both parts of the above question might seem simple and obvious. Did I hear you say 'to pass'?! Certainly that would be a good bottom-line definition of success. However you could, and should, get much more out of the experience than this.

ACTIVITY 14.3

Thinking of your personal development, both now and in the future, how could the dissertation process and product be of help?

Thinking of your professional development as a nurse, both now and in the future, how could the dissertation process and product be of help?

Finally, are there any other potential beneficiaries for your work?

Hopefully Activity 14.3 has helped you identify a few more goals that the dissertation can help you towards. Aiming to publish a journal article after the dissertation is a real possibility. By that time, through your hard work, you will have almost all of the raw material for an article to hand. Although it may seem unlikely at the start of a dissertation, it may also motivate you onwards to undertaking more study!

> **Box 14.2   Student voice**
>
> ... I was excited to work towards this final piece of work and show everyone what I am about. Once I got started it was more a case of 'how am I going to get this down to the upper limit of 15,000 words?!' Ultimately I really enjoyed the experience and it has led me to undertake a Master's in Nursing degree. (Jennifer)

Being given the freedom to choose a topic area and research questions can be a very good motivator for many students. Not only does this give them the opportunity to focus on something that may have fascinated/puzzled/frustrated them in practice thus far, it also gives them a chance to become something of an expert in a particular area of nursing knowledge. With some foresight a good choice of topic could help you realise an ambition to work in a particular field of practice.

Nevertheless, this freedom may be a contrast to previous assignment experiences and bring its own challenges. We asked some recent graduates to recall how they felt at the start of the dissertation process. Their written comments are given in Box 14.3.

> **Box 14.3   Student voices**
>
> *Tracy:* Before my dissertation I felt:
>
> - Nervous I wasn't going to find a topic fast enough.
> - Anxious that other classmates had found a topic before me.
> - Concerned about what to write but not the length of the dissertation.
> - Worried that my references were not of a decent quality.
> - Concerned that I would fail.
> - Anxious as it would make up such a large part of my degree.
>
> *Fiona:*
>
> - I've never done any essay this HUGE before.
> - What will I talk about?
> - How do I decide on a topic?
> - How do I narrow it down?
> - In that timeframe?!
> - If it's an independent piece of work, how much support will I receive?
> - What have other people looked at in the past? How will I ensure that I am not replicating something that has already been done?
>
> *(Continued)*

(Continued)

Sushila:

- I felt anxious about choosing a topic as quickly as possible so I could get started, but that meant that I struggled to narrow down my area of interest which affected my literature searching as I wasn't sure what I wanted to do.
- I would recommend taking a little time to think about what you want to do because I ended up wasting time researching broad ideas, and when I went back to look at my notes they were so vague they were basically useless, and I had to re-read the articles I had found to see if I could actually use them or not.

Listening to these student voices it is clear that choosing a topic can initially be daunting. As a previous student, and as a supervisor, one of the key lessons I have learned is that focusing on a topic that is really of interest to you is one of the best ways of sustaining your curiosity and motivation over many months. Ideally if you can generate more than one potential topic of interest you can then evaluate which of these is the most viable. Box 14.4 exemplifies the subsequent process of moving from a broad topic/area of interest to a more focused study title.

Box 14.4   Vignette: From topic to working title

You might have developed a particular interest in the situation where someone with an acute mental health problem is hospitalised in a distant setting. Your interest may stem from personal knowledge (e.g. your neighbours on the remote island where you live have experienced this) or from professional experiences (e.g. working in a big city hospital with a remote catchment area).

In order to move from this general topic to a specific study title, and research question(s), you will need a more specific angle of enquiry.

A first step here would be to explore the nature and scope of the topic in the research and policy literature. What has been done before? How was it done, and how well? What was found? Is it helpful and relevant to your practice area and interests?

Sharing your initial findings with your supervisor, it becomes clear that perspectives from healthcare staff in Australia and Canada have been researched. However, there seems almost no relevant research on patients' or families' experiences of this situation.

After more reading and discussion over the next two weeks, you provisionally entitle your dissertation proposal:

'Families' experiences when a close relative is hospitalised in a distant setting due to a mental health problem: a Scottish study'.

It is a long title and it is likely to bring challenges, but it captures your interests. You have identified an important knowledge gap needing research and you now have a particular angle! Moreover, it may be an angle that can help others and yourself in your future career.

Hopefully the above vignette gives a sense of how you can move forward when preparing for the dissertation and then beginning it. Sometimes the use of a visual concept map can help you to focus on the particular area you want to research, and start to operationally define your main concepts. Applying this approach to the vignette above might result in something like the following (see Figure 14.1).

The concept map clarifies the areas of central focus for your study. Can you identify what should be entered in each of the blank sections where intersections occur in the above diagram? This helps clarify what is related to your core interest but is not of central/focal importance. This is very helpful for mapping the literature that you review. For example, the empty intersection in the upper right area of the diagram would locate literature that was about urban hospitals' provision of care

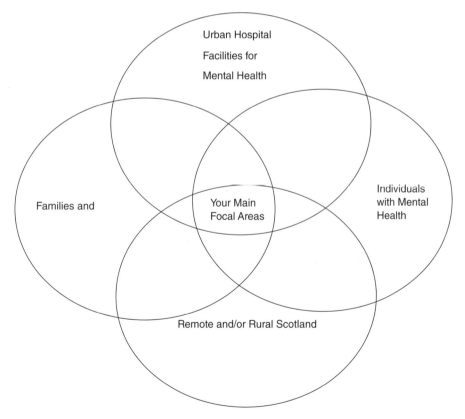

Figure 14.1 A visual concept map

for individuals with mental health problems, but had no substantive coverage of the experiences of families living in remote and rural Scotland.

Before leaving the example given above, what do you think some of the challenges would be in creating a realistic research proposal in this topic area?

As can be seen, one of the main lessons in all of this is that discussion and advice are important to help you best develop your research idea. Colleagues or your mentor on a practice placement may be helpful in suggesting a particular angle, and your academic supervisor should be a sustaining source of guidance.

In the next section of the chapter we will take a look in more detail at the sources of knowledge and help that should be integral to your dissertation experience.

WHAT ARE THE MAIN SOURCES OF KNOWLEDGE AND HELP THAT YOU CAN USE ON THIS JOURNEY?

As mentioned earlier in the chapter, if you read only one document at the very start of the journey, make it the dissertation guidelines. In addition to explaining the required content and format, they should also lay out the assessment criteria and weighting. This gives you a crucial steer as to where depth of coverage will be most important and valued. Again, if recent exemplar dissertations are made accessible to you, take the chance to explore how different students have structured their work in response to the criteria. A key aspect here is to compare, contrast and discuss the effectiveness, or otherwise, of approaches taken previously.

In many universities dissertation guidelines will also give detailed guidance on the structures, processes and intended outcomes of academic supervision over this 6–12 month period. As such, these would normally cover what you can expect from your supervisor and what s/he will expect from you. Box 14.5 provides some indicative examples of material from such a document.

Box 14.5   Examples from guidance document on student–supervisor expectations

Principles:

- Clarity of responsibilities for both the supervisor and the student.
- Co-ordination of the supervisory process in a consistent way.

Role in practice – the supervisor:

- The primary function of the supervisor is to maintain overall, general guidance of the project and to provide a critical and rational sounding board for student ideas.

> Role in practice – the student:
>
> - The prime responsibility for the management of the project lies with the student who must maintain a dialogue between him/her self and the supervisor. The responsibility for the work submitted lies entirely with the student.

Given that the dissertation usually accounts for a substantial proportion of the degree award, and given the relatively prolonged duration of the assignment, this is a relationship that works best when both parties enter into it with good will and energy. A classic text on PhD supervision (Phillips and Pugh, 2010) talks of 'managing your supervisor', and in some ways the need for this is also true for undergraduate students doing a dissertation. From a student point of view it is vital to remember that your supervisor is only human. Thinking back to our earlier consideration of Honey and Mumford's Learning Styles, it seems likely that your supervisor will also have their own characteristic strengths and preferences in terms of their approach to working together. Thus it is worth investing some time to negotiate the best mutual working approach. How often should you meet? Is it expected that some new work should be shared beforehand as a basis for discussion at the meeting? If your supervisor has a strong preference for reflective learning, s/he will most likely want the latter!

We asked some supervisors to comment on their experiences of supervising, and some of the highs and lows are presented in Box 14.6 below.

Box 14.6   Supervisor voices

Highs

Charlie: The opportunity to engage with students on a one-to-one basis and challenge them intellectually is very rewarding. It's great to watch over a period of time a small concept become a rigorous (hopefully) piece of work with strong practice implications.

Helen: Working with the students on a longer piece of work. Getting to know them and their abilities better and seeing them develop personally and professionally.

Denise: Use of learning contracts/log of meetings was helpful to both supervisor and student in setting deadlines and keeping a transparent track of discussions.

Lows

Terry: Students leaving things till the last minute rather than following the recommended timelines for their work can be frustrating.

(Continued)

(Continued)

Femi: Students waiting until February to start their dissertation despite me emailing them meeting requests three times from September, then expecting me to prioritise their draftwork to meet their deadlines.

From the comments above it can be seen that some clear themes emerge for supervisors in terms of motivations and frustrations. There is no doubt about the prizewinner in

Table 14.1   Time plan and log for a dissertation

1st Meeting (Month 1)	General discussion of dissertation. Decision making for proposal or review and consideration of question/objectives.	Agreed date
Key points of meeting Objectives/goals/ intentions for meeting 2		Date and initials
2nd Meeting (Month 2)	Review of literature for topic area and a consideration of the methodology (proposal or systematic review).	Agreed date
Notes from meeting Objectives/goals/ intentions for meeting 3		Date and initials
3rd Meeting (Month 3)	Specific development of methodology/method either for the proposal or a systematic review.	Agreed date
Notes from meeting Objectives/goals/ intentions for meeting 4		Date and initials
4th Meeting (Month 4)	Evaluation of findings/results and conclusion sections.	Agreed date
Notes from meeting Objectives/goals/ intentions for meeting 5		Date and initials
5th Meeting (Month 5)	Writing up the final dissertation – a consideration of all areas of the dissertation and presentation.	Agreed date
Notes from meeting Objectives/goals/ intentions for meeting 6		Date and initials
6th Meeting (Month 6)	Review and discussion of the final draft and submission.	Agreed date
Notes from meeting Objectives/goals/ intentions for completion		Date and initials

the latter category, so early engagement with your supervisor is likely to pay dividends in the longer term.

In the comments above, Denise highlights the potential value of a learning contract and keeping a log of meetings. Some universities will require that a specific learning contract is formally signed by both student and supervisor. Irrespective of whether a formal contract is required or not, the formulation of a mutually agreed plan for the dissertation work is of vital importance. One way of thinking about structuring this is to start from the final hand-in date and work backwards. An example of a highly structured time plan and log for a six-month dissertation campaign is given below. Note the central headings indicating key content as milestones for the different months.

While not every student and supervisor pairing will work best with such a prescriptive structured approach, a regular review and preview of work will be necessary for all. Moreover, keeping a record of meetings will be a vital help in this regard.

One of the areas of working together that is worth exploring at an early stage is the expectations around reviewing draft work. Generally speaking, a supervisor review of student draft work during the dissertation can be a very useful process. The student receives feedback on their developing work and the supervisor gains detailed knowledge of the student's academic writing and progress. However a balance needs to be struck in terms of how often such review can take place: for example, it would be unreasonable to expect a supervisor to undertake multiple reviews of each chapter in a six-month dissertation, and similarly, it would be unreasonable to expect the supervisor to feedback in detail on the spelling and punctuation in every piece of writing. Instead, you should expect to be directed to any strengths and weaknesses in these aspects, perhaps in relation to one or two specific examples. Conversely, however, if a supervisor refuses to ever review your ongoing work and give feedback, or is never available for consultation, s/he is not doing their job properly.

Clearly your supervisor is a key source of advice and help for the dissertation journey. However s/he is not the only source. Given that literature searching, review, analysis and synthesis are at the heart of any good nursing undergraduate dissertation, it is important that you further develop the range of skills detailed in Chapter 4. To make this work well you should engage at an early stage with the guidance provided by your university library. This will mean reading the key content and advice documents that are available on their web pages and may also involve seeking guidance directly from information-resources staff. In my experience these members of staff are typically very dedicated and derive their job satisfaction in being able to help students access and use resources optimally.

While all the material in Chapter 4 is relevant to the dissertation challenge, one of the most crucial habits to develop is managing the many articles and references that your literature review will generate. If you can establish a clear system early in your journey (e.g. by using REFWorks or a similar reference management system), this will pay dividends later on when you are synthesising your material and writing it up. One of the classic dissertation pitfalls is to seize on some key quotes from a text that you discover, but omit to fully record the source. This then leads to major frustration when you come to the later stages of writing up and can't locate the specific references. Again, a student voice (see Box 14.7) is helpful here.

> **Box 14.7   Student voice**
>
> I found having a sectioned project notebook helped as I could keep information for the different sections separated. Both this and colour-coding my notes with highlighters and Post-its helped me be more organised and keep on top of things instead of losing notes and panicking. (Dan)

A good referencing and recording system will also build a strong foundation for your academic writing. Although there is not the scope here for a full discussion of academic writing, there are some key points that are handy to know when preparing for your dissertation.

One of the most vital aspects in producing a long piece of writing such as a dissertation is being able to keep a clear thread of logical development running through the work. This helps to orientate the reader and make them feel that you are well in charge of your material and arguments. One of the most common problems that supervisors report finding in student dissertations is a failure to develop focus in the content matter (Hannigan and Burnard, 2001). Lengthy descriptions of the content of the literature you have covered will be of very limited value. Rather, your assessors will reward you for your critical appraisal of the material, i.e. the sense that you make of it in terms of its strengths, weaknesses and resultant value for developing understandings and building answers to your research questions. Thus good reference and recording systems are necessary – but not sufficient – foundations for success.

Finally, in thinking of sources of knowledge and help, it is easy to neglect those that exist outside the university buildings as well as those closest to home. As has already been mentioned, colleagues from clinical practice placements can be an invaluable source of expert advice on nursing topics. For example, a student who was interested in the experiences families had of end-of-life care in nursing homes used their initiative to consult with a range of experts in practice and education. This took in both the NHS and the private sector. Again, those with particular subject expertise were very happy to share this as it was being recognised, used and valued.

Given that the dissertation will usually involve over at least six months' work, it is vital to think of how this can best fit with commitments in your home life. Time management skills come to the fore here. Again, it is useful to reflect on your characteristic approach to assignments so far and to consider whether anything will need to change so that this more sustained piece of work can be developed. This may involve anticipating any periods where you may not be able to do much work because of a family commitment or something similar. Remember that there is scope to plan around these if flagged up in advance.

Moreover, you may be able to derive very useful support from your friends, peers and family if they understand the challenge you are embarking upon. A number of relevant studies (e.g. Lawton, 1996) have recognised the key supportive role that family and friends can play in supporting nurse education. Self knowledge will help and this can develop further as your journey progresses.

Box 14.8   Student voice

I was working a lot during my dissertation writing (and I should have put my foot down and said no to extra shifts) and I found that when I felt overwhelmed or I didn't feel I was getting anywhere with whatever section I was working on, I would save what I'd done, shut my laptop down and do something else for 15–30 minutes (went for a walk, phoned a friend, watched an episode of a TV programme, made lunch) and I then could get back to work with a clearer head. (Fiona)

As the example in Box 14.8 suggests, taking your dissertation work home with you is inevitable for most students and clearly this is not always a pleasure. At times the knowledge that you have to do more work on it may intrude on your enjoyment of other activities. However, there can be benefits when your dissertation starts following you around. Many students report that their best ideas come not when sitting at a desk formally trying to address issues head-on, rather they will encounter something in their other activities that then provides a spark or idea that can be transferred across to inform their dissertation work. Sometimes this can be a model or metaphor from another context or discipline. (The research pyramid in Chapter 10 may have arisen in a similar way!)

Indeed we can exemplify this now by using the idea of a pyramid to reflect in a different way on the journey taken in the first four sections of this chapter. In the first section we looked at the broad foundations for our preparation, considering what a nursing dissertation is and why it may be necessary to produce one. Gaining this initial elevation, we then looked back and around in Section 2 in order to think about previous journeys and how we had managed to successfully complete them. Section 3 took us a little further forward, considering why we wanted to reach the apex and how that might be beneficial. Finally, in Section 4 we looked upwards and around to think about what we would need, besides our own efforts, for the long haul ahead to reach the top.

In the concluding section of the chapter we will complete the map of the journey as if looking down and around from the summit. Looking back, what summary advice can be given to help plan such a journey, avoid the pitfalls, and build on success?

SUMMARY

A dissertation is a substantive part of your whole degree, involving an in-depth critical engagement with the research literature and sustained academic writing. It presents a real opportunity to focus on something that is important to you and others, and in doing so to further your potential as a nurse. Many of the skills that you develop further by doing the dissertation should be of value to yourself and others in the future – and therefore it makes sense to prepare as thoroughly as you can for this major piece of work.

Based on the content of this chapter, what you should avoid and what you should aim for can be summarised as follows:

In order to enjoy your dissertation and succeed, *remember not to:*

1 Procrastinate: putting off preparations and avoiding thinking about it is usually a recipe for future difficulty and frustration.
2 Plan to travel completely solo: if you set off in the wrong direction and are out of contact with your supervisor, it will be very hard to finish the journey on time and in good shape.
3 Underestimate the potential help that is out there: in terms of subject experts, knowledge resources, previous exemplars, and personal support from family and friends.

Finishing on the positive strategies ...
In order to enjoy your dissertation and succeed, *remember to:*

1 Engage early with the challenge in terms of the project guidelines, your topic interests, your supervisor, and your other sources of support.
2 Reflect on, and build from, the strengths that have brought you thus far, especially in terms of academic writing.
3 Pay attention to your motivation for the journey ahead and beyond – this can then sustain and reward you.
4 Plan your journey, set up systems, record your progress, and consult regularly with your supervisor along the way.
5 Strive for a topic focus using the ideas in this chapter.
6 Explain your challenge to family and friends – they may often be able to help in some way.
7 Put your whole self into the dissertation if you can – as is often the case, you will get more out of it if you do.

REFERENCES

Hannigan, B. and Burnard, P. (2001) Preparing and writing an undergraduate dissertation, *Nurse Education in Practice*, 1 (4): 175–180.

Honey, P. and Mumford, A. (1986) *Using your learning styles*. Maidenhead: Honey.

Lawton, S. (1996) *The effectiveness of educating community nurses by distance learning.* PhD thesis. Robert Gordon University, Aberdeen. Available at: https://openair.rgu.ac.uk/handle/10059/534 (last accessed 21 December 2012).

Macduff, C. (2008) Editorial: The PhD thesis as a virtual guest house, *Journal of Clinical Nursing*, 17 (18): 2381–2383.

Macduff, C., Mackenzie, T., Hutcheon, A., Melville, L. and Archibald, H. (2003) The effectiveness of scalp cooling in preventing alopecia for patients receiving epirubicin and docetaxel, *European Journal of Cancer Care*, 12 (2): 154–161.

Phillips, E. and Pugh, D. (2010) *How to get a PhD: A handbook for students and their supervisors* (5th edition). Berkshire: Open University Press.

PART 5

LET'S IMPLEMENT RESEARCH AND EVIDENCE IN PRACTICE

15

USING RESEARCH AND EVIDENCE IN PRACTICE

NEIL JOHNSON AND RUTH TAYLOR

Chapter learning outcomes

On completion of Chapter 15, you will be able to:

1 Define the terms 'research' and 'evidence dissemination and implementation'.

2 Identify the ways in which research and evidence informs national clinical guidelines, standards, and protocols in practice.

3 Understand the term 'research or evidence appraisal' and identify the tools used in this process.

4 Describe the models for research and evidence implementation.

5 Discuss the factors influencing the implementation of research and evidence in practice.

6 Discuss the importance of leadership and change management in the implementation of research and evidence in practice.

7 Identify methods of dissemination related to research, evidence, and other forms of scholarly activity.

Key concepts

Appraisal tools and skills, models of implementation, barriers and facilitators of research and evidence use, leadership and management of change, methods of dissemination.

INTRODUCTION

Up until this point in the book, the focus has been placed upon developing core skills and understanding related to research and evidence-based practice. With considerable volumes of research and other forms of evidence published annually, a key consideration now turns to getting research and evidence into practice. After all, the primary aim of all nursing research is to contribute to nursing knowledge and/or to serve to shape and improve the services that nurses provide to patients and the public group – namely, the final stage in the research process.

This chapter identifies the ways in which research and evidence can translate into standards and guidelines for practice at national levels e.g. via the National Institute for Clinical Excellence in Healthcare (NICE), the Scottish Intercollegiate Guidelines Network (SIGN), at a local level in the form of standards and protocols for practice, and globally via the work of organisations undertaking systematic reviews, for example the Cochrane Collaboration, the Joanna Briggs Institute (JBI).

The chapter primarily focuses upon the ways in which research and evidence translate into practice. Along the way, important considerations such as appraisal (judging the value of research and evidence) are discussed as well as conceptual models outlining the factors influencing implementation and that therefore ultimately have an impact and practice change. Furthermore, the significance of leadership and change management is explored and relevant links to the implementation of research and evidence are made. You may be wondering why a research textbook has included a chapter which aims to enhance your understanding of the implementation of research and evidence – after all, it is often assumed that this is someone else's business and as nurses we are the passive recipients of evidence. The standards of conduct, performance and ethics for nurses and midwives expressed within the NMC Code (NMC, 2008: 6) make reference to the need for nurses and midwives to 'provide a high standard of practice and care at all times', thereby ensuring they 'use the best available evidence' and that, as accountable practitioners, they keep their 'skills and knowledge up to date'. In introducing learners to research and evidence-based practice my message has always been to treat individuals with the highest standard of care that you can possibly provide and continually strive to enhance your nursing care by engaging and reading up to date sources of professional knowledge and evidence. This textbook has, until now, equipped you with the knowledge and understanding that will enable you to read and understand research and other forms of evidence. It will now enhance your understanding as to how to appraise or make a judgment on the value of research and evidence, as well as provide insights into the ways in which research can be implemented into practice and the factors facilitating and challenging this process.

A further consideration regarding implementation and basing clinical decision making on an evidence-informed basis is outlined in the NMC *Standards for pre-registration nurse education* (NMC, 2010), which emphasise the need for nurses to meet future challenges in healthcare, driving up standards of care and quality by adopting a range of roles such as practitioner, educator, leader and researcher. Although the NMC make explicit the fact that newly qualified nurses are not seen as having expertise in practice, leadership, education or research, preparation in regard to these roles as well as continued preceptorship and life-long professional development are central to ensuring that the public will be assured that new nurses will strive to (NMC, 2010: 5):

- Act to safeguard the public and be responsible and accountable for safe, person-centred, evidence-based nursing.
- Use leadership skills to supervise and manage others and contribute to planning, designing, delivering and improving future services.

It is therefore vital to consider (even if you read this as a nursing student, a newly qualified nurse, or even a nurse with some experience) your professional responsibility and accountability to contribute to continuous healthcare improvement through an understanding of research, evidence-informed decision making, and an awareness of the notion of implementation and the concepts relating to this latter subject. This statement is, of course, true for any healthcare professional.

CLARIFYING THE TERMINOLOGY

Before exploring the ways in which research and evidence are used in practice it is necessary to take some time to clarify the terms related to this notion (i.e. dissemination and implementation).

Dissemination refers to the communication or sharing of research. There are many ways in which this can occur (e.g. in a conference presentation, conference poster presentation, journal article publication). In addition, many organisations such as healthcare providers and educational institutions will facilitate ongoing seminar programmes, whereby professionals from a variety of disciplines can come together to learn about new research studies relating to their field of practice and gain an opportunity to discuss the study with the researcher(s). However, dissemination strategies such as those cited here will probably have little impact in terms of research being translated *directly* into practice (i.e. a single conference presentation or journal article publication is likely to have scant impact by itself). This is confirmed by the extensive work undertaken by the Centre for Reviews and Dissemination (CRD) at the University of York (www.york.ac.uk). The CRD have published guidance in relation to the dissemination of systematic reviews which is underpinned by both theoretical and empirical perspectives. (Further details regarding this approach can be found at the CRD website by accessing the publication 'Systematic Reviews: CRDs guidance for undertaking reviews in health care'.) It is generally accepted that passive methods of dissemination are generally ineffective in terms of translating into practice change/development, and therefore in recent years a considerable body of research has looked at approaches to translate research and evidence into practice change. Key to the success of translating research into healthcare practice is the sharing of findings with key stakeholders via appropriate methods, forums and publications (e.g. through policy makers, leaders and key professionals) and this is a key consideration for researchers if awareness of their findings is to be raised. It is therefore crucial for researchers to target specific publications and conferences where it is more likely that the audience will have a vested interest in the research itself.

ACTIVITY 15.1

Via your own library, or by reviewing your library electronic databases related to healthcare, identify:

- Which journals publish or communicate original nursing research studies?
- Which journals specialise in specific fields of professional practice (e.g. mental health, community nursing, specific elements of nursing, for example, wound care)?
- Choose one article from one of these journals, ensuring that it is an original research study.
- Reflecting back on your knowledge and understanding of research and evidence-based practice at the start of this text, how has your understanding and ability to interpret the structure and terminology used within this article improved? And has your ability to read research been enhanced?

Implementation, in the context of this chapter, is defined not simply as the translation of research and evidence into practice involving passive dissemination approaches and the direct application of research to practice, but as a process rather than a single entity. Wilkinson et al. (2010) view this process as a series of events by which the evidence, key stakeholders (e.g. nurses and other members of the interprofessional team), and the work environment (to include patients) are prepared to perform a change of practice. The process is seen as continuous, reflective of change management, in that the implementation is followed by an evaluation and the adjustment of practice. The process of implementation is complex and a number of models have been developed based upon empirical research to assist healthcare providers in planning this process (these are discussed later in the chapter).

SOURCES OF EVIDENCE IN HEALTHCARE

Reflecting back on my time as a student nurse in the late 1980s, as a learner sourcing and reviewing evidence in the form of research and other sources of professional literature, the experience of finding information pertinent to my questions was fraught with major challenges: limited electronic databases, limited internet availability, and rather basic library search resources all made this an arduous task! As has already been cited here and within other chapters, there is now an array of ways and means by which individual learners and professional nurses can access research and evidence that are related to their field of practice – often via the click of a mouse and in the comfort of one's own home. At an individual level this has assisted greatly in the dissemination of sources of research and evidence to enhance knowledge and understanding. For the learner there is an expansive array of sources that can help in understanding approaches to care within specific fields of practice or with particular service user groups. Access to individual research studies on a given topic can facilitate understanding and shape and influence attitudes, beliefs and values at the same time. On a higher level, a number of organisations have developed in response to the drivers for evidence-based clinically effective care and the minimisation of health inequalities and variations in care across various areas of clinical practice: the National Institute of Clinical Excellence (NICE), Scottish Intercollegiate Guidelines Network (SIGN), the Cochrane Collaboration and Joanna Briggs Institute (JBI) are good examples.

NICE was established in 1998 as a Special Health Authority in the UK with a remit to produce national, evidence-based guidelines for the National Health Service, local authorities and charities. NICE publishes clinical guidelines, clinical pathways and standards that are based upon the best evidence currently available. These publications provide guidance as to the most effective ways of preventing, diagnosing and treating disease as well as ill health. NICE not only develops and disseminates such guidelines, it also provides support and toolkits for the implementation of those guidelines in practice – ultimately the action on implementation is the responsibility of healthcare providers. The topics considered by NICE come from a range of sources including health professionals, patient groups, carer groups and the general public. More information about NICE Guidelines, Pathways and Standards, as well as information related to the implementation of NICE publications, can be found at www.nice.org.uk. This resource is extremely helpful not only for busy healthcare professional teams in identifying the best available evidence, but also for learners in key areas of learning.

Formed in 1993, SIGN (like NICE) has as its central objective the improvement of healthcare and the reduction in variations in practice through the publication of national clinical guidelines. SIGN's guidelines are directed toward the improvement of care for patients in Scotland and these usually relate to key health priority areas such as cancer, heart disease and mental health. Additionally, guidelines are developed, published and disseminated in relation to areas where variations in care are known to occur. SIGN (as well as NICE) develop guidelines that are based upon a rigorous and systematic review of scientific best available research evidence (and therefore less prone to bias). The topics suggested for SIGN guideline development will come from a variety of sources, however for consideration there must be evidence of:

- Current variations in practice.
- An extensive evidence base of research relating to effective practice.

The recommendations within the guidelines are graded and therefore these provide healthcare providers with a means of selecting and identifying the priorities for implementation. As with NICE, SIGN does not actively participate in the empirical implementation of guidelines, however the organisation does support NHS Health Boards in Scotland by disseminating recommendations, networking with relevant managed clinical networks, and providing tools that will assist in the implementation process. It would be worthwhile visiting the SIGN website at www.sign.ac.uk. By clicking on the guidelines tab on the SIGN home page you will be able to see the extensive range of guidelines that have been published to date – review this list and click on a guideline that interests you.

The Cochrane Collaboration is an international, non-profit making organisation which assists in the translation of evidence into practice by publishing systematic reviews in the Cochrane Library. The library helps healthcare providers to access and identify the most effective approaches to care and treatment, assists in decision making related to practice (e.g. issues of cost *vs.* clinical effectiveness), and informs patients and carers about the risks and benefits related to specific courses of care/treatment. Further information and explanation regarding Cochrane as well as access to a variety of resources can be found at www.cochrane.org. Again it would be worth your while to take some time to visit this website and explore the information and resources offered.

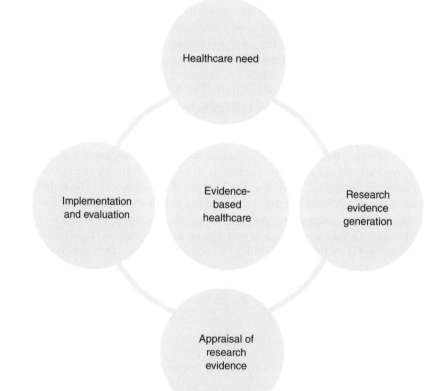

Figure 15.1   An evidence-based healthcare cycle (adapted from the JBI)

Based in Adeleide, Australia, but with collaborating centres globally, the Joanna Briggs Institute (JBI) is a non-profit making organisation which assists in the systematic review, synthesis and implementation of evidence into practice with the aim of improved healthcare outcomes. For more information visit www.joannabriggs.edu.au (please note, a subscription is required to access specific resources. However the website will provide you with an overview of the work of the JBI). The JBI provides a suite of resources to assist collaborating centres in the implementation of evidence and does so by adopting a cyclical process (see Figure 15.1). This cycle is similar to other approaches to evidence-based healthcare such as that of Dawes et al. (2005: 3), where the process is seen as:

1 The translation of uncertainty into an answerable clinical question.
2 A systematic retrieval of the best evidence available.
3 A critical appraisal of the evidence for validity, clinical relevance and applicability.
4 An application of the results in practice.
5 An evaluation of performance.

The JBI therefore provides the evidence generation, evidence appraisal, and evidence transfer (e.g. best practice guidelines/protocols and tools) to assist in the implementation of evidence, as well as an evaluation of the impact in terms of healthcare outcomes. Within the JBI approach to evidence-based healthcare, consideration is given not only to the strength of the evidence but also to the preferences of individuals, professional decision making, and the context in which healthcare is being provided (see Figure 15.2).

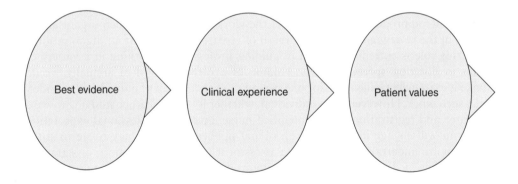

Best evidence

Clinical experience

Patient values

Figure 15.2 The essential elements in clinical decision making (adapted from Melynk and Fineout-Overholt, 2005)

Evidence-based healthcare is not simply a prescription to care – a set of rules or guidelines that must be followed in a systematic and detailed manner for all patient and clients regardless of their individual health needs, values and preferences. The translation or implementation of evidence into healthcare *must* consider the individual in clinical decision making and care planning must take note of this fact.

There are therefore a number of organisations that will assist healthcare providers in ensuring their services are the most effective or appropriate and in doing so promote the desired healthcare outcomes.

ACTIVITY 15.2

Identifying and using clinical guidelines in practice

Perhaps even without realising it, it is likely that you are working or learning in a clinical environment that has implemented or is planning to implement clinical guidelines published by organisations such as NICE or SIGN:

- Which clinical guidelines have been implemented in the clinical environment?
- When were these guidelines published?
- Using an appropriate internet search engine, find the guideline that has been implemented and review its content.
- Finally, can you determine how this guideline has improved care and how this is being evaluated in terms of clinical outcomes?

CRITICAL APPRAISAL

Thus far the chapter has focused upon the role of national and global organisations that provide guidance to healthcare providers in relation to the most effective or appropriate approaches to care. Part of the work undertaken by such organisations is that of the review and critical appraisal of research evidence. At an organisational level this role is extremely helpful in guiding professionals working in a variety of areas in differing specialities. The volume of evidence published annually would make it extremely challenging for one person or even a group of individuals to undertake such work. However as an individual, whether it be as a learner studying toward a degree and registration or as a qualified nurse, there is a professional expectation that you will engage in reading professional publications: this may relate to study that you are undertaking for a course assessment (e.g. an essay, report, dissertation, or a project), or that you are working upon with others with a view to improving practice. As such, reading and understanding research evidence is one thing. But being able to read it with a critical eye in terms of the strengths and weaknesses of a study is another. To do so, a basic understanding of the research design and method is required and earlier chapters of this text will help you in this respect.

So how are you, as a practitioner, able to know which evidence is good or bad or good/bad? The risks of just trusting in a 'hunch' may mean at worst that the feedback on your essay states that you have not been critical in your discussion of the research evidence. However, the consequences of going with this 'hunch' in practice could have far-reaching outcomes for individual patients and clients. But what is the difference between simply reading a research paper or guideline and critically appraising it? The difference consists of the application of a set of consistent and structured questions that will enable you to judge the strengths and weaknesses of the paper or guideline you are reading (or will enable you to judge the applicability of the evidence or guideline as regards your own specific patients or clients). A critical appraisal of evidence such as research papers or guidelines can be distinguished from simply reading in the following ways:

- A critical appraisal focuses on the quality of the evidence in terms of its relevance and the audience the evidence is directed towards;
- A critical appraisal focuses on the internal quality of the evidence e.g. in primary research papers, the study design and method;
- A critical appraisal sets aside any bias or subjectivity in terms of viewing the worth of the evidence.

We would therefore appraise evidence for its:

- Strength.
- Quality.
- Applicability.
- Validity or trustworthiness.
- Reliability.

A critical appraisal enables you to evaluate evidence which is of a high *quality* and *relevance* to your respective fields of practice. It also enables you to exclude poorly designed studies or evidence of a low quality, as well as limit the amount of evidence reviewed, and therefore it focuses your time and energy on systematically reviewing the evidence that matters most. It is useful to think about this in relation to what the Joanna Briggs Institute terms 'Healthcare Practice Interests'. A useful acronym (FAME) is used to categorise these interests which may relate to the areas of:

- Feasibility.
- Appropriateness.
- Meaningfulness.
- Effectiveness.

These interests are usefully related to research approaches and will be helpful in guiding your own critical review of evidence in relation to your clinical questions (i.e. depending on your question being one of feasibility, appropriateness meaningfulness, or effectiveness):

- Feasibility (e.g. critical inquiry, policy analysis).
- Appropriateness (e.g. ethical inquiry, philosophical inquiry).
- Meaningfulness (e.g. interpretive inquiry, phenomenology).
- Effectiveness (e.g. cause and effect inquiry, RCTs, cohort studies).

To ensure that the critical appraisal of research evidence consistently asks the right questions, there are a number of tools or checklists that have been developed to assist in this process. These checklists have been devised in order to appraise differing types of study – tools and checklists for randomised controlled trial (RCT) studies, tools for cohort studies, tools for qualitative studies, to name but a few examples. SIGN provides a range of checklists that should be carefully selected so as to ensure that the correct checklist is being applied to the correct type of study. The SIGN methodology checklists can be accessed at the following URL link: www.sign.ac.uk/methodology/checklists. html. These can be downloaded and saved, thereby enabling the reviewer to actively enter their responses directly onto the downloaded file: this then assists in the storing and tracking of any papers reviewed. Alternatively, other checklists are provided by Solutions for Public Health (NHS) via their Critical Appraisal Skills Programme (CASP). For CASP you will need to access the following URL link: www.casp-uk.net/ find-appraise-act/appraising-the-evidence.

Finally, in relation to a guideline appraisal the AGREE II (Appraisal of Guidelines Research and Evaluation) tool can be used, and this can be accessed at http://agree. machealth.ca/players/open/index.html.

At this stage it would be useful to familiarise yourself with these tools as they will assist you greatly in the appraisal of research evidence which will in turn help to develop your critical reading, thinking and writing skills, as well as avoid the risks of simply accepting the evidence and going with the aforementioned 'hunch'.

ACTIVITY 15.3

Applying critical appraisal skills in reading research evidence

Utilising the skills you acquired through reading and engaging in activities in earlier chapters of this book, you should now attempt to source, read – and crucially here – appraise an original research article. Remember that this should be an article that provides an abstract, the study aims/objectives, and background, methodology and discussion. This could be a quantitative study (e.g. RCT) or a qualitative study (e.g. phenomenology). Once you have selected a research article you must also choose an appropriate appraisal tool (e.g. a SIGN methodology checklist for RCT, or a CASP checklist for qualitative studies).

- Read the article.
- Look at the article again, but on this second reading try to answer the questions posed by the chosen relevant appraisal tool.
- What are your main conclusions following this process: what are the strengths and/or weaknesses of the article?
- What do you think your views or opinions of the paper would have been without your use of the appraisal tool?

Critically appraising research is a skill that all graduate and undergraduate nurses will develop at some point in their studies. You can probably see how the appraisal of one article in Activity 15.3 has perhaps enabled you to read research in a different light. If you think about an educational or practice-based project, there will likely be multiple sources of research evidence to source, read, and critically appraise. A common mistake made by many learners is that of ineffectively managing their reading/review, and although there are software packages to assist in this respect, my advice to many is to consider some form of evidence or appraisal table so that your growing body of research evidence can be managed, handled and utilised in a more effective way (see Chapter 6 which looks at practical approaches). A simple study skills tip is to construct a table whereby you will identify the source or reference, the study design, and the main findings and recommendations, as well as the strengths and weaknesses of the study (based on your appraisal of course). An example of what this table may look like is presented in Table 15.1. Obviously with three sources (hypothetical studies) this is not presented as a final version, but hopefully it provides an idea of how such an approach may look in the early steps of development. It needs to supply a good overview of your emerging evidence base.

Table 15.1 The evidence or appraisal table

Author/title	Study design	Main findings and recommendations	Study strengths and weaknesses
Eboh, W. and Mowatt, E. (2006) *The lived experience of students' learning research design*	Qualitative. Phenomenology. Two focus groups: each comprising ten students in their final year of study. Semi-structured interviews. Thematic analysis.	Students perceive research as an important subject for their future professional roles. Students felt that learning in small groups made the subject more interesting. Students initially found the subject challenging, but once they understood the key terms their learning was enhanced. Teachers as role models – seeing teachers as research active was important.	Structured, open-ended interviews allowed the researcher to clarify questions if respondents were unsure and also clarify the answers given. Data were validated by two researchers independently analysing those data. A recognised tool was used to analyse the narrative data. A convenience sample resulted in no male participants – not reflecting the total population.

(Continued)

Table 15.1   (Continued)

Author/title	Study design	Main findings and recommendations	Study strengths and weaknesses
Johnson, N. and Adams, D. (2009) *Teachers of research – challenges, barriers and facilitators*	Quantitative. Questionnaire survey. A questionnaire was sent to all education institutions which provided undergraduate nurse education programmes. Likert scale. Descriptive statistics.	Teachers' attitudes toward research varied – 50% felt it was relevant and 50% felt it was not. Teachers preferred to teach the subject face to face as online learning did not help students. Being a research-active teacher enabled the subject to be delivered in a more appropriate and meaningful way. Students had difficulties in sourcing research-based articles.	A pilot study was undertaken. The study only gathered data from three institutions and therefore the findings cannot be generalised. The response rate to the questionnaire was only 29%. The questionnaire was sent to teachers who did not have responsibility for teaching research, therefore some of the responses lacked validity.
Mayo, J. and Miles, K. (2009) *Student nurses' attitudes toward research.*	Qualitative. Phenomenology. Ten undergraduate student nurses in year 1 of their programme. Individual unstructured interviews. Thematic analysis.	Questioning relevance – students could not see the relevance of the topic to their course at first. Teacher influence – the students learned more from teachers who made the subject come to life and made it more interesting. Learning styles – students benefited from a range of teaching approaches, both face to face and online. Seeing real world research – students' attitudes were influenced by them seeing research in action in practice.	Pilot interviews were conducted. The small sample means that the findings cannot be generalised. The study took place outwith the UK in a differing educational system, therefore the findings may not be contextualised to the UK because of this factor. There is no indication as to which data analysis tool was used or how the validity of the data analysis was addressed. Some of the findings do however corroborate with other studies of this type.

Up until this point in the chapter I have discussed the notion of implementation, identifying some examples of organisations which provide evidence-based guidelines and recommendations as well as looking at your own individual skills of critical appraisal. Let's now turn our attention in the final sections of the chapter to the process of implementation and dissemination, stopping along the way to explore the relevance of key concepts such as leadership and change management. We will start by exploring models and frameworks of implementation.

MODELS AND FRAMEWORKS OF IMPLEMENTATION

The implementation and evaluation of evidence-informed practice are a considerable challenge to nurses and organisations responsible for healthcare provision. Key issues relate to the consideration of what facilitates implementation as well as which outcomes from that implementation should be measured. In an earlier chapter you considered the notion of the impact of research evidence at different levels (i.e. conceptual and instrumental: see Nutley et al., 2007):

- Conceptual impact is seen as the ways in which research evidence can shape and influence not only knowledge but also attitudes and values.
- Instrumental impact is seen as the ways in which research evidence can actually demonstrably change practice.

With these concepts in mind it is more useful to consider implementation as a process. In doing so we can plan and implement evidence-informed practice in a more effective manner. To this end, models of implementation can serve to guide this process in practice as well as trace this process as a learning model. So models are useful as practical as well as educational tools. Whilst it is not the scope of this chapter to explore *all* the models that inform the process of implementation, it is acknowledged that many others exist (e.g. the IOWA Model, the Stetler Model, the Ottawa Model, and Diffusion of Innovations). For a further discussion of such models we would recommend that you read Chapter 3 of Wilkinson et al. (2010).

Within this chapter two models/frameworks have been chosen as examples and both provide useful insights into the implementation process as well as the factors facilitating and acting as barriers. The two models discussed here are the Modified Pipeline Model (Wimpenny et al., 2007) and the Promoting Action of Research in Healthcare Services (PARiHS) Framework.

Glasziou (2005) proposes that this implementation pathway is likened to a 'leaky' pipeline along which evidence flows. He identifies specific stages along the pipeline and suggests that there are points at which leakage occurs, resulting in a limited impact on clinical outcomes. These stages have been expanded from work by Pathman et al. (1996), who define four stages from evidence to action: aware, agree, adopt and adhere. Further stages were added based on a systematic review of barriers to using evidence (Cabana et al., 1999) with the result that seven stages were included in Glasziou's model (see the bulleted list below).

- Awareness of relevant, valid evidence by the practitioner.
- Acceptance of the evidence by the practitioner.
- Applicability to practice for that group of patients.
- Availability of resources and ability to carry out the intervention in that context.
- Acted on by the practitioner.
- Agreed to by patients in the light of available decision aids.
- Adhered to by patients who follow the appropriate regime.

Thinking about implementation as a *process* rather than an *outcome* will encourage you to identify the key stages, barriers and facilitators, and trace and explore each stage as it presents itself in your own projects or learning. Questions around the seven stages of this model assist in being both proactive in planning for change and tracing and evaluating impact at different points in the process.

The model can further assist in an assessment of the impact of evidence at both conceptual and instrumental levels. Further exploration of this concept by Wimpenny et al. (2007) led to the development of a Modified Pipeline Model, whereby Nutley's conceptual and instrumental impact continuum is incorporated into this process. They argued that the earlier steps in the process could have an impact at a conceptual level (i.e. changing and shaping knowledge and beliefs), whilst later stages (e.g. agreement and adherence) may represent an instrumental impact. This is deemed important as it re-emphasises the point that research evidence and its implementation can influence professional attitudes and beliefs.

Glasziou's seven stages are depicted within the context of process in Figure 15.3, and following this representation, Figure 15.4 illustrates how Wimpenny et al. incorporated the conceptual/instrumental impact continuum.

ACTIVITY 15.4

Reflecting upon the research impact

Firstly, consider the ways in which your readings from research have impacted upon you personally. In what ways have these readings shaped and changed your attitudes, beliefs and values? For example, how have these readings changed your attitudes toward certain groups in society, how have your readings enabled you to gain insights into the lived experiences of others, and how have these readings enhanced your self-awareness as a developing professional?

The model as proposed by Glasziou demonstrates a potential loss of transfer at specific points in the pipeline which results in low levels of adherence at the point of implementation. The model as modified by Wimpenny et al. (2007) has the potential for tracing evidence implementation and loss, as well as exploring the impact beyond implementation in terms of not only patient outcomes but also in examining changes in the attitudes, beliefs and behaviours of healthcare providers – something that other models do not address within their conceptual framework. These conceptual impacts

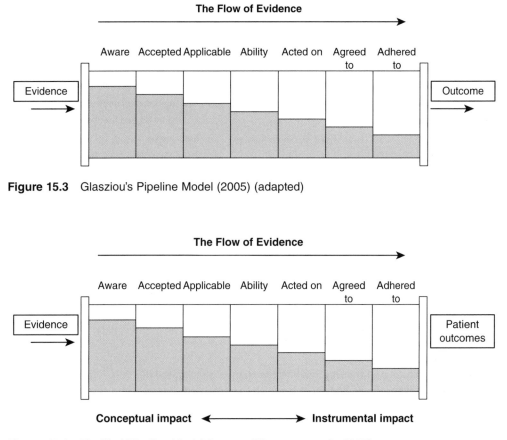

Figure 15.3   Glasziou's Pipeline Model (2005) (adapted)

Figure 15.4   Modified Pipeline Model (source: Wimpenny et al., 2007)

are seen as being worthy of evaluation as they are often the determinants of sustained change in the healthcare setting.

The model therefore serves a number of useful purposes but primarily it is seen as assisting in tracing and evaluating the impact of implementation at a number of levels. Whilst the facilitation of implementation is promoted it must be acknowledged that a number of facilitators and barrier factors will also influence this process. In their study of the 'Determinants of the sustained use of research evidence in nursing', Davies et al. (2006) help you to consider the barriers and facilitators. These are listed in Figure 15.5. This is by no means an exhaustive list and I am sure, particularly if reading this as a registered nurse, that you can also consider factors that are perhaps specific and unique to your own practice setting.

One framework which provides a means of identifying and analysing these factors is the PARiHS Framework (Promoting Action on Research Implementation in Health Services: see Kitson et al., 1998). Further developed by Rycroft-Malone

Facilitators	Barriers
Leadership;	Changes in staffing and structure;
Management support;	Lack of sustained leadership;
Ongoing staff education;	Heavy workload and limited time;
Guidelines integrated in policies and procedures;	Limited ongoing staff education;
Staff buy-in and ownership;	Lack of follow-up and feedback;
Synergy with partners and external influences;	Staff resistance;
Guideline characteristics;	Limited management commitment;
Multi-disciplinary involvement.	Guidelines not integrated into policy, procedures and documentation.

Figure 15.5   Barriers and facilitators to research evidence implementation (Davies et al., 2006)

(2004), the framework considers three elements which have a dynamic relationship with one another in terms of the levels of success relating to implementation.

This framework sees successful implementation (SI) as a function of three elements:

- The evidence (E).
- The facilitator and the way in which the change is facilitated (F).
- The context or the environment in which the proposed change is implemented (C).

Therefore, $SI = f (E, C, F)$.

Within this model the evidence is seen as a combination of research, clinical experience, patient experience and information pertaining to the local context (remember that evidence is not a straightforward prescribed transfer of protocols or rules). The context relates to the organisational culture, leadership, and the appropriateness of evaluation and feedback systems, whilst facilitation relates to the need for skilled facilitators with a specific focus upon the facilitation of change. Each of the three elements work dynamically and each can score high to low on a continuum where successful implementation is a function of each scoring highly. For example, Rycroft-Malone states that successful implementation is more likely to occur when:

- Research evidence is derived from a number of sources and is of a high quality.
- There is critical reflection, and consensus following debate and discussion has taken place.
- Patient preferences (e.g. narratives) are adopted in the decision making.
- There is the use of local information or evaluation data which has been systematically gathered and analysed then reviewed.
- An organisational culture exists where the culture is conducive to change.

- Transformational leadership exists with clear roles and effective teamwork occurs.
- There are environments with robust and broad systems of evaluation.

It can be seen from this type of framework as well as other theories of change that a key central element is that of leadership, and it is worth now turning our attention to this as Ruth provides the following discussion.

LEADERSHIP AND CHANGE MANAGEMENT IN THE IMPLEMENTATION OF RESEARCH AND EVIDENCE IN PRACTICE

The models of implementation that are cited within this chapter have, as a central recurring theme, the importance of considering the roles of those key stakeholders involved in the change and in particular the role of leadership and change management.

As a student nurse, and as you move into qualified professional practice, you will have a key role in implementing evidence in clinical practice. One of the aims of this book is to equip you with some of the knowledge and skills required for implementing evidence in practice. For example, you have developed your skills relating to the ability to critique evidence – both qualitative and quantitative research – so that you can make informed judgments about the value of particular research findings for your own practice. Being able to critique evidence is key to your professional practice. What you then need to do is to implement that evidence where appropriate. You may feel that this should be fairly straightforward, but it is likely that there have been times where you have encountered a resistance to change – perhaps you have observed a qualified nurse working with colleagues to implement a new guideline or policy where this has not been immediately welcomed. But did you see this member of staff using skills to encourage those colleagues to embrace the required change in practice? What we are talking about here is clinical leadership in action.

Clinical leadership can be defined as 'the leadership that takes place within any clinical setting and which aims to enhance care and lead to positive patient outcomes' (Taylor and Martindale, 2013). One of the key aspects of clinical leadership is that anyone who works in clinical practice can be a clinical leader. If you think about the activities that you undertake on a typical shift on placement, you can probably think of lots of times where you or a less senior member of staff have led the care of particular patients. You can also probably think of clinical staff who have been assigned the responsibility for leading specific areas of practice (for example, the development of a policy in practice). The clear message here is that you as a student nurse, and when you are newly qualified, have a role in clinical leadership. Healthcare professionals are committed to delivering safe, effective, person-centred care – to achieve these aims clinical leadership is crucial.

This section does not aim to provide a detailed discussion of clinical leadership. However, a brief overview of the key attributes is provided below with a more detailed discussion of change management (within the context of implementing evidence in practice). Box 15.1 provides a synopsis of the attributes of clinical leadership – within a framework of quality (Taylor and Martindale, 2013). While all of these attributes are important for you as a healthcare professional, we have highlighted some that will have a particular bearing on the role of the clinical leader in implementing evidence into practice. You will see that these focus on a knowledge of evidence and quality processes, and personal attributes that lead to effectiveness when working with colleagues in the process of change.

Box 15.1   Attributes of clinical leadership within a framework of quality

Safe

- Recognition of clinical excellence in practice.
- Expert clinical skills.
- Ability to create an environment conducive to safety – a vibrant, research-based, evidence-based practice culture.
- Authority to act as a manager, co-ordinator, case manager, project leader, team leader, etc.
- Knowledgeable about the quality processes.

Effective

- Ability to adjust to service demands through flexibility and imagination.
- Ability to adapt and seize opportunities within the healthcare system.
- Ability to demonstrate the influence that nursing care has upon patient outcomes and organisational efficiencies.
- A continuous quality improvement focus.
- Direction and modification of policy and patient care.
- Strategic thinking – able to link the current work to goals and prospective outcomes.
- Decision making skills.
- Change management and liaison skills.
- Influence and political skills.

Person-centred

- Mentorship, supervision, feedback, support of colleagues.
- A positive orientation and inspiration to others.
- Excellent interpersonal skills which ensure team engagement and participation.
- Authenticity – being true to self and values.
- A patient focus with patients as participants in care (co-production).
- Vision, stamina, dynamism, confidence, selflessness, assertiveness.
- Collaboration, innovation.

Having reviewed Box 15.1, you may wish to take the opportunity to reflect on your own skills and attributes – remember that these are ever-evolving as a healthcare professional, and you will find senior colleagues striving to continually improve their skills in these areas throughout their careers. You will have a chance to think more about how you achieve your potential as a student and then a qualified nurse or healthcare professional in the final chapter in this book.

Change management

Having considered clinical leadership and its focus on practice development and enhancement, it is worth your while to spend a bit of time considering the types of skills and knowledge that you will need when you wish to make a change in practice through the implementation of evidence. Again, this is a brief summary of the key issues as you will have an opportunity to explore the theory and practice of change in other aspects of your learning.

Change is, rather obviously, when something happens to make the current situation different, and this can relate to anything from a change in the way a placement area is organised to a change in a particular approach to care. It can therefore impact on the entire clinical team, which means that the person or people making that change need to plan it effectively so as to ensure that the impact of the proposed change is fully assessed. One of the key problems associated with change has already been alluded to – that of the human reactions to a change in practice. Inevitably, some people will be cautious of change whether that is a particular change or change generally. This is understandable as change pushes people out of their comfort zones and unavoidably means that they themselves will need to operate somewhat differently. Added to this, some people will have had bad experiences of change where the impact was not fully reviewed and unforeseen consequences led to further challenges in practice rather than improving the situation. So as you can see, the clinical leader (or the change agent) has to have the following:

- Knowledge of the context and the evidence relating to the proposed change.
- Skills and attributes to work with people in the change management process (i.e. the planning, implementation, and evaluation of change in practice).

You have already explored the first point in detail as you worked your way through the other chapters in this book – knowledge of policy and practice drivers that lead to the need for change in practice, and the ability to critique evidence which relates to service development. You have also briefly reviewed some of the skills associated with change management in other sections of this chapter, and these as well as others are listed again for you here:

- An ability to share the vision for change across a diverse team and within potentially challenging clinical situations.
- Interpersonal skills for team engagement, participation, collaboration and conflict management.

- Liaison and networking skills to bring into play relevant people, teams and organisations for the benefit of the change.
- Political and influencing skills to assist in others recognising the need for change, and in gaining the required resources to implement the change.
- A positive orientation and influence towards others to facilitate the ownership of change and persuade people of the need for change.
- Innovation and creativity to enhance the nature of the change and to engage the enthusiasm and motivation of others within the change process.
- Analytical and decision making skills to establish the potential outcomes of the change, alongside an ability to communicate this analysis to a wide range of staff: 'bringing choices into awareness' (Iles, 2011: 22).
- Authenticity and the demonstration of a caring approach to help with developing relationships and trust across the team.
- Mentorship skills to work with team members so that they have the skills and knowledge to take forward the change.
- 'Sitckability' – a determination and self-motivation to continue to take forward the change so that it is implemented.

DISSEMINATION

We will end this chapter by considering in a little more depth the notion of the dissemination of research findings. This is a crucial step in the research process as there is little point in undertaking research and then not share and communicate the findings to a wider audience. Indeed many bodies commissioning research would require that the findings are disseminated in appropriate ways. However the manner of such ways differ:

- Research can be published in professional journals as standalone studies where readers can review the research and decide how best to use the findings.
- Research studies can be presented at conferences and other seminars in:
  - a poster format;
  - workshops;
  - seminars;
  - presentations.
- Research can be shared at journal clubs based in educational institutions, clinical settings, or as collaborations between both.

As a student you may be unsure as to why this may be relevant to you, but it would be anticipated that many students will at some point in the future work toward publication or a conference presentation either on their own or as part of bigger team. Alternatively you may be a nurse working in practice who is engaged in both a clinical and research-based career.

CONFERENCE PRESENTATION

To the relative novice, presenting at a conference can at first seem a daunting prospect. Standing up in front of an anticipatory audience, sometimes containing experts in the subject field, is naturally going to convey some feelings of anxiety. What must be remembered here is the original contribution that you and your team's hard work has to offer to the specific subject discipline, and, as well as this, many will want to hear what your study findings are as your sharing of knowledge will benefit others either conceptually or in terms of them considering the ways in which your work contributes to the bigger picture of knowledge and understanding. Furthermore, you will gauge the audience feedback toward your work and this combination of disclosure (sharing research) and feedback is vital in your personal professional development. A little anxiety can also help to focus the mind! Considering which conference you wish to present at is important as you will want to reach out to those individuals who are most closely aligned with your area of research. This will then facilitate your engagement with the audience and the audience's with you. There are various conference events organised annually, both locally and globally. These can range from educational conferences to conferences related to specific fields of practice. Conference calls, as they are known, will usually publish requests for abstracts where the conference organising committee will consider whether or not to accept your paper. It is vital to read the conference call carefully as it will provide details as to the nature of the conference, any theme groups that are to be provided within the conference, and crucially, the format of the abstract. This usually follows a standard convention:

- The title of the study.
- Background/context/rationale.
- Method.
- Key findings.
- Recommendations.

If accepted, guidance will be provided regarding the length of the presentation, the medium (e.g. PowerPoint), and the length of time allocated to questions and the discussion. You should read the guidance carefully and plan your presentation accordingly. Good presentation skills are necessary in terms of clarity, your awareness of non-verbal communication, and capturing your audience's attention. You may wish to reflect on these skills at this point.

Poster presentations differ in that the poster is usually the medium by which information is conveyed, and again guidance is likely to be provided related to the size, format and space. You may also be required to talk briefly about your research and field questions from conference participants. Some artistic ability helps here – you want to capture the audience's attention and most educational institutes and healthcare providers will have an IT team who can help you in this respect. Allow some time in the planning phase for consultation, development, proofing and printing.

WRITING FOR PUBLICATION

While this is perhaps a little less anxiety provoking, writing for publication is nonetheless challenging and time consuming. The length, style and format are conventions that will be guided by the publisher so don't drift away from the guidance! A report that is well written and published in a professional journal has the potential to be read and accessed by a larger population either in hard copy or an electronic format. If you are new to writing for publication, it may be useful to identify collaborative projects where you will benefit from the guidance and experience of more experienced writers. Within my own institution there are many good examples of academic/clinical/student collaborations in relation to written papers. These serve as a good example of how scholarship can be demonstrated in a collaborative manner with outcomes often being reinvested in the curricula. The general convention in terms of structure of a research article is:

- A written abstract or summary of the entire study.
- The research aims and objectives.
- A background literature review section providing the context and rationale for the study – this should present all of the literary sources and reports that are relevant to the research question.
- Research design and method – this will include the discussion around the methodology selected and present subsections related to the ethical considerations, sample framework, data collection, data analysis, and findings.
- Discussion – the findings should be discussed fully, and depending upon the chosen method, these may vary in the way in which findings are discussed in light of what is known about the research topic to date.
- Limitations – the article should acknowledge any weaknesses as reported by the researchers.
- What the study contributes – more and more, articles are challenged to discuss and highlight how the study contributes to the professional discipline or subject area.

Written publications undergo a rigorous review process once submitted and prior to this most editors will decide whether your paper should be sent to reviewers who will undergo a blinded review process (i.e. they will not know the identity of the author(s)). This blind review process may lead to a number of possible outcomes including acceptance, acceptance based upon the comments and recommendations of the reviewers, or rejection. Even when rejected, an editor may provide guidance as to where else the paper could be sent for further consideration.

SUMMARY

Whilst there are a number of organisations that have become nationally and globally responsible for the synthesis of research evidence, careful consideration must be given to how this is implemented in practice. Implementation is not simply a translation of evidence in the form of guidelines and protocols into practice, but must instead take into consideration the evidence, the patient or individual client preferences, the context, and the clinical experience of healthcare providers. Models can help us to understand this process, however we are all as healthcare professionals accountable for the care that we provide and responsible for our own professional development. As a healthcare professional, you owe it to yourself, your colleagues, and most importantly patients, that you engage in research evidence as a reader and/or contributor.

- A number of key organisations generate, appraise, synthesise and collate research evidence to assist healthcare professionals in clinical decision making.
- Implementation is a complex process, one which is dependant upon a number of factors that will work dynamically with one another. One key factor here is leadership and change management.
- Critical appraisal skills enable individual nurses to read and review research evidence and promote an active engagement with the literature rather than passive reception.
- There are a number of ways in which dissemination can take place.

FURTHER READING

Listed below are a number of useful links, some of which were cited within this chapter, that will assist in your understanding of the generation of evidence, implementation and appraisal:

Access to the Cochrane Collaboration: www.cochrane.org/about-us
Access to NICE: www.nice.org.uk/
Access to SIGN: www.sign.ac.uk/
Access to JBI: www.joannabriggs.edu.au/

REFERENCES

Cabana, M.D., Rand, C.S., Powe, N.R., Wu, A.W., Wilson, M.H., Abboud, P.A. and Rubin H.R. (1999) Why don't physicians follow clinical practice guidelines? A framework for improvement, *JAMA*, 282 (15): 1458–1465.

Davies, B., Edwards, N. Ploeg, J., Virani, T., Skelly, J. and Dobbins, M. (2006) *Determinants of sustained use of evidence in nursing. Final Report. Canadian Health Services Research.* Ottawa: Foundation and Canadian Institutes for Health Research.

Dawes, M., Summerskill, W., Glasziou, P., Cartabellotta, A., Martin, J., Hopayian, K., Porzsoly, F., Burls, A. and Osbourne, J. (2005) Sicly statement on evidence-based practice, *BMC Medical Education*, 5 (1): 1.

Glasziou, P. (2005) The paths from research to improved health outcomes (Editorial), *ACP Journal Club*, 142 (2): A8–A10.

Iles, V. (2011) Leading and managing change. In T. Swanwick and J. McKimm (eds), *ABC of clinical leadership*. Chichester: Blackwell. Chapter 5.

Kitson, A., Harvey, G. and McCormack, B. (1998) Enabling the implementation of evidence based practice: A conceptual framework, *Quality in Health Care*, 7: 149–158.

Melynk, B. and Fineout-Overholt, E. (2005) Transforming health care from the inside out: Advancing evidence-based practice for the 21st century, *Journal of Professional Nursing*, 21: 335–344.

Nursing and Midwifery Council (NMC) (2008) *The Code: Standards of conduct, performance and ethics for nurses and midwives*. London: NMC.

Nursing and Midwifery Council (NMC) (2010) *Standards for pre-registration nurse education*. London: NMC.

Nutley, S., Walter, I. and Davies, H. (2007) *Using evidence: How research can inform public services*. Bristol: Policy Press.

Pathman, D.E., Konrad, T.R., Freed, G.I., Freeman, V.A. and Koch, C.G. (1996) The awareness to-adherence model of the steps to clinical guideline compliance: The case of paediatric vaccine recommendations, *Med Care*, 34: 873–879.

Rycroft-Malone, J. (2004) The PARiHS framework: A framework for guiding the implementation of evidence-based practice, *Journal of Nursing Care Quality*, 19 (4): 297–304.

Taylor, R. and Martindale, S. (2013) Clinical leadership in primary health care, *Primary Health Care*, 23(5): 37–7.

Wilkinson, J., Johnson, N. and Wimpenny, P. (2010) Models and approaches to inform the impacts of implementation of evidence-based practice. In D. Bick and I.D. Graham (eds), *Evaluating the impact of implementing evidence-based practice*. Chichester: Wiley-Blackwell. pp. 38–67.

Wimpenny, P., Johnson, N., Walter, I. and Wilkinson, J. (2007) Tracing and identifying the impact of evidence in practice: The use of a Pipeline Model, *Worldviews on Evidence Based Nursing*, First Quarter 2008: 3–12.

PART 6

ACHIEVING YOUR POTENTIAL

PART 6

16

ACHIEVING YOUR POTENTIAL

RUTH TAYLOR

Chapter learning outcomes

On completion of Chapter 16, you will be able to:

1 Identify ways that will enable you to achieve your personal and professional potential so that you 'stand out' from the crowd.
2 Implement leadership skills from and for research that will enable you to make a positive impact on clinical practice.
3 Plan the next steps for your learning and development.

Key concepts

Personal and professional development, leadership, potential.

INTRODUCTION

This chapter is somewhat different in focus from all the previous chapters. It is written from a personal perspective and (as I hope you will be able to tell) comes from a passion that I hope will speak to you as an individual. The approach that I take here may not be for you (and if this is the case I think you will recognise this fairly quickly), but if you are interested in engaging in this chapter's activities, you will need to consistently think about how they relate to your role as a health professional and as a user/implementer of research in clinical practice. The chapter aims to encourage you to think about the ways in which you can work towards achieving your potential – both personally and professionally. It is a very personal chapter, one that comes from a lifetime of striving always to be better than I am and from the recognition that there is absolutely always more to be done to achieve this desire! If I come across as a little evangelical, it is because I have had the privilege of seeing many students who have sometimes not believed in themselves go on to achieve extraordinary things. I believe that with the right focus and a number of tools, people can make changes that will impact positively on them, their important others, and the people that they come into contact with professionally.

So, in this chapter I will be putting forward a number of points relating to the benefits of striving to achieve your potential and identifying what your potential is (although this will change and grow as you change and grow), and ending by relating this back to research and evidence for practice – your leadership role. Please don't think that I am suggesting you are not focused on being the best you can be: I am sure that this is the case, and what a fantastic starting-point that is. All I want to do here is shine a light on what you are doing so that you can perhaps think differently about what you could achieve in life, and offer you some thoughts on how you might go about this. In my case it is a lifelong commitment and one which brings with it numerous rewards – for example, feelings of energy, enthusiasm and motivation that are sustaining for the self and nurturing for others.

A STARTING-POINT

Before I begin putting down some of my thoughts, complete Activity 16.1. This aims to set out clearly where you are now, where you want to be, and some early ideas about how you plan to do that. As you work through the subsequent activities, you will have an opportunity to come back to this activity and build on these thoughts.

ACTIVITY 16.1

Write down what you would like to be doing – personally and professionally – five years from now. I challenge you to be brave and to come up with things that might take you out of your comfort zone!

What kinds of qualities and skills will you need to develop to enable you to achieve these ambitions?

How many of these skills and qualities do you have now, and which do you feel that you need to develop further?

If you had asked me those kinds of questions when I was a student nurse, I am not sure that I could have answered them properly. Certainly my responses would have changed over the years, and they will continue to evolve as I make my way through life. I have asked these questions of my students and Box 16.1 is a vignette that offers a changing perspective on the ambitions that one student I know set out over the four years that she was a student. The 'quotes' are synthesised from the various conversations that I had, but they aim to convey the sentiments that she expressed to me.

Box 16.1   Vignette: Student voice (Rosie)

Year 1, week 2 of the nursing course:

> I want to try and understand what I need to know so that I can go into practice and do things properly. I guess that in five years' time I want to have a job as a nurse – it seems so far away that I can't imagine it.

Year 2:

> I want to be working where I can make a difference to the care of older people. I want to make sure that I provide the best care that I can, and that it makes a difference to the patients' experiences.

Year 3:

> In five years' time I want to be a charge nurse so that I can lead changes in practice that will make a difference to older people. I am really understanding the need for evidence-based practice and I want the clinical area that I am working in to be offering the best evidence-based care.

Year 4 (just about to start a newly qualified role in a setting for older people):

> In five years' time I want to be a charge nurse in a similar area to the one I am about to start working in. I want to lead evidence-based practice as a caring and compassionate professional. I also want to have completed a Master's degree and undertaken some research into the experience of older people so that I can really make a difference to the experiences of the people I care for. Hopefully my research could make a difference more widely.

Can you see how this student's views on her potential changed incrementally over time? I would suggest that part of the reason that her views changed relates to the transformation that can take place through educational experiences (both in the university and in practice), as well as the innate motivation for the profession that she clearly demonstrates. Can you relate to any of what Rosie told me over the years? Feel free to go back to Activity 16.1 and make any amendments that you wish as you continue through this chapter – being bold in your ambitions for personal and professional development will enable you to achieve your true potential.

WHAT ARE THE BENEFITS?

There are a number of points that can be made in relation to the benefits of achieving your potential. Some of them will appear to be so obvious that they hardly seem worth mentioning – but I am going to anyway! Seeing the whole picture and building your own view of the benefits will act as a motivator for you. Some of these motivators are intrinsic (the things that make a difference to how you *feel* about yourself and your work). Others are extrinsic and relate to the kinds of tangible outcomes that come from achieving your potential.

- Your CV will stand out from other people's.

If you are able to demonstrate a progressive engagement with the evidence base and with making an impact on clinical practice (e.g. through your portfolio), you will be able to tell a powerful story within your CV. You will be able to highlight some of the necessary skills and attributes of a healthcare professional – for example, the ability to critique policy and research, the capability to make effective changes in practice, and the talent to evaluate the impact that you make in any practice situation. Let's also remember that future employers will also be interested to know about the additional aspects of your character that can be demonstrated through engaging with 'extracurricular' activities and interests – as part of your drive to achieve your potential you may decide to become involved in the work of a charity or voluntary organisation. Translating the skills that you can gain through these kinds of experiences onto your CV shows any future employer that you are committed to making a difference.

- Employability and the opportunity for promotion or progression.
- The development of transferable skills – useful for the various roles that you will undertake in your career.

Similar to the last point, but taking it a little further, the ways in which you continually develop (both personally and professionally) are likely to be recognised if they are expressed to the right people and in the right way. This book is not about CV writing, but the key point here is that you can make yourself more desirable to any future employer (and to a current employer who is looking to promote a member of staff) by taking on opportunities that will prepare you for the next step. In the context of research and evidence-based practice, you could think about how you use your reflective portfolio to demonstrate learning and development in particular aspects of your practice. You can then use this learning to put forward an evidence-based proposal for a practice development. Chapter 15 explored some of the ways that you can go about this.

- Personal satisfaction.
- Increased motivation, energy and enthusiasm.

I often think to myself that I am extremely privileged to have had the career that I have had so far. I am lucky to wake up in the morning and feel enthusiastic about going to work. I am sure that I feel this way because I get a lot of satisfaction out of what I do. You need to think about what it is that provides you with personal satisfaction. One of my students eloquently told me about what gave her personal satisfaction:

> 'I am so glad that I decided to do nursing. The best thing for me is when I can see that I have really helped someone. They don't have to say anything – I can just tell. It makes me always want to do my best when I am on placement.' (Lynne)

Where you feel great satisfaction from what you do on a daily basis and through your ongoing development, it is almost inevitable that you will also feel more motivated and enthused. Your energy levels will feel higher and you won't be able to help but convey this to the people that you work with – both patients and other professionals.

- Better relationships – both personal and professional.

It's rather obvious, but if you take a lifelong approach to achieving your potential it is very likely that you will develop certain skills that will enhance your relationships. There is plenty of evidence to support the need for the use of excellent interpersonal skills in care delivery (see, for example, Brunero et al., 2005; Benson et al., 2010). This aspect of your development will probably take prominence throughout your career and will only serve to enhance your own personal experience of being with people both personally and in a professional capacity.

- Ability to deliver and lead better care.
- Role model for others – both personal and professional.

The activities and information in this book have had a particular focus – to equip you with some of the skills and knowledge that you will need to deliver care to a high standard. One of the important messages that runs through the book is that a critical, open and questioning mind is crucial for evidence-based practice. With these skills, and with a commitment to continued development, you will be in an excellent place to deliver the best care that you can. What this also means is that you are likely to be a role model for those around you. Being the best you can be, delivering the best care that you can, and operating in a way that is true to your values will mean that inevitably you will become a role model.

- Recognition from others – feeling valued.

Working out the kinds of things that motivate you as an individual is crucial in all of this. Again, your motivators can change over time. For example, as a student you may currently be highly motivated by the thought of being newly qualified and gaining employment, in part so that you are better-off financially. Later in your career your motivations may relate to being offered the opportunity to take on new things within a role so that you learn new skills, make new networks, and impact positively on the patient experience. Have a think about the things that motivate you currently and consider how you can use these to influence your approach to developing your potential.

So have these points convinced you that a clear and focused approach to personal and professional development is worthwhile? Building your responses to Activity 16.1, take some time to make a few notes for Activity 16.2.

ACTIVITY 16.2

Thinking about the areas that you have identified for your own personal and professional development, make a list of the motivating factors (the benefits) for you as you continue to build on your potential. Be as specific as you can – picture those benefits and make sure that they are meaningful to you.

IDENTIFYING YOUR POTENTIAL

You have now had a chance to think about where you see your potential – hopefully in a little more detail than you had done previously. Now it's time to move on to thinking about other aspects relating to your potential, namely how you can identify these and start to use them in a positive way, so that you can continually shift your view of your potential in ways that will repeatedly push you to strive ever further. I am very aware of the focus of this book and aim to keep bringing you back to its purpose and relating this discussion to research and evidence-based practice. One way that I can do this is to present some of the evidence that exists around the facilitators and barriers to you achieving your potential. Think back to the section that you read on change management in Chapter 15. You can apply some of that theory to the aim of this chapter – after all, any personal or professional development will change you inwardly and has the potential to make a difference to what you actually do. Box 16.2 provides an overview of the key facilitators and barriers to change based on Figure 15.5 in the previous chapter – you will recognise everything on the list and be able to relate to the evidence base for these change factors. Once you have read through these, complete Activity 16.3.

Box 16.2   Facilitators and barriers to change

Facilitators	Barriers
Leadership	Changes in staffing and structures creating uncertainty
Management support	
Ongoing staff education	Lack of sustained leadership
Guidelines and development to support the implementation of policies and procedures	Heavy workload and time commitment required for the change and relating to current commitments
Staff buy-in and ownership of the change	Limited ongoing staff development
	Lack of communication or ineffective communication
Synergy with other initiatives and directives that relate to the change	Staff resistance
Whole team (including the inter-professional team) involvement	Limited management commitment
	Lack of integration with other aspects of the service

The list in Box 16.2 is not an exhaustive list – you may have some other points that you wish to add. Now is your opportunity to do that. Make a list in each of the columns of the things that will help you achieve your personal and professional potential (facilitators), and those that may inhibit your development (barriers).

Facilitators	Barriers

ACTIVITY 16.3

You may have come up with a long list of things that might help – for example, a supportive family, a professional team that are enthusiastic and motivated, or a clear sense of what your goals are. You might also have noted that there are some things that may get in the way – such as a busy schedule that involves juggling your work, study and family life, or a lack of clarity about how to take your development forward. Whatever you have written down will be helpful as it will enable you to be clear about where your support lies and where you may perhaps need to address certain barriers. You can give this some thought just now if you like. Here are some suggestions that come from working with my students when they were feeling that things were rather challenging at particular points:

- Clarify your goals (these will change over time) and split them into bite-sized pieces so that you can see progress over the short term.
- Find ways (that suit you) of being as organised as you can be. We are all different and some of us like to complete things early while others are more last-minute. Whatever your preferences, you need to be able to work with them and yet still achieve what you set out to do.
- If there are issues with your workplace, discuss them with the relevant person (your mentor, your boss) in a way that will enable a critical discussion to take place with some solutions identified for going forward.
- You can't always change your personal circumstances, so find ways that let you have a few minutes to reflect on your goals and what you need to do to achieve them. This might literally be only five minutes before you go to sleep, or fifteen minutes as you eat breakfast. Again, everyone is different and you will need to find what works for you.
- Reward yourself when things go well, but don't worry too much if things aren't going to plan. Simply take another look at what has happened and refocus! You just knew that your reflection skills would come in handy here somewhere didn't you!

ACHIEVING YOUR POTENTIAL

There are a number of tools or approaches that you can use in this lifelong journey. I have listed some of them in Box 16.3 below and hope that they act as a catalyst for you to try one that you aren't already using.

Box 16.3   Reflection

A reflective diary can be useful as a tool for personal and professional development. You can write down:

- Your personal goals.
- The approaches that you plan to take to achieve these.
- A strategy for managing the barriers and using the facilitators.
- A record of your progress: the learning and the achievements.
- The changes to your goals as you progress.

Remember to mark your entries with a date so that when you look back you can see what you have achieved within the timescales. Sometimes I use my reflective diary to simply brainstorm new ideas or to get a few things off my chest when things aren't going to plan. It's surprising what these notes can reveal!

You might want to go back to Chapter 6 where you had the opportunity to explore reflection and consider some of the tools that can make the process both easier and more useful.

Coaching/mentoring/critical friend

First, definitions are provided (you will see that there are some similarities – and I would say that as long as you and your supporter understand the purpose of the relationship, it doesn't matter too much what you call him or her!):

Coach: A person who will work with you in a way that challenges your thinking, stimulates your ideas, and uses tools, that enables you to focus on your potential and guide you through this process.

Mentor: Variously defined as someone who teaches you, facilitates your learning, challenges you to move out of your comfort zone, and provides the environment for you to develop in specific areas.

Critical friend: A person who will help you to critically reflect on your practice (and your thinking) and challenge you in ways that are supportive.

It is important that you have your supporters with you as you work your way towards your goals. The benefits that these people will bring to you are:

- Someone who has your interests at heart and is committed to your development.
- Someone who can offer advice where needed, or guide you to find solutions to your own issues.
- Someone who can offer an alternative viewpoint and help you see things differently.
- Someone who gives you the permission to spend time thinking about your personal and professional development.

Other approaches

There are many approaches to thinking about your development. What you could do is look at some of the personal development literature and use the techniques that work best for you. Here are a few suggestions, but there are many more out there and it is vital that you find the approaches that suit you most.

- Goleman, D. (1996) *Emotional intelligence: Why it can matter more than IQ*. London: Bloomsbury. What I like about this book (and I know it has been around for a few years) is that it acknowledges that potential is achieved through a wide range of characteristics and attributes.
- Covey, S. (1999) *The 7 habits of highly effective people*. New York: Simon and Schuster. Covey's approach is still widely taught and used for personal and leadership development. The book offers an integrated approach to self-development.

- The King's Fund is an independent charity that aims to improve health and health-care in England. It has a strong leadership focus and if, in the future, you are considering how to develop your leadership potential, you might want to visit the website (www.kingsfund.org.uk/leadership).

You have had a short trip through personal and professional development here. What is important is not so much that you do all the things that are suggested in this chapter, but that you find your own way to continue to work towards the achievement of your potential. However you do this, you should make sure that it offers you sustenance and motivation, and ramps up your energy for the challenges that you will come across in all aspects of your life. Bringing it back, finally, to the focus on research and evidence-based practice: there will always be a need for healthcare professionals both to undertake research and to implement research findings in practice in ways that will lead to increased quality for the patient experience. You are in a position to be part of the leadership for practice development through what you know now, what you will know in the future, and through making decisions about the type of healthcare professional that you want to be. Exciting times!

SUMMARY

The key points in this section include:

- A lifelong commitment to the achievement of your evolving potential will ensure that you are in a position to continually drive up the standards of care.
- Leadership for research and evidence-based healthcare practice is crucial for its ongoing development – you can make the decision to be part of that leadership.

REFERENCES

Benson, G., Ploeg, J. and Brown, B. (2010) A cross-sectional study of emotional intelligence in Baccalaureate nursing students, *Nurse Education*, 30 (1): 49–53.

Brunero, S., Lamont, S. and Coates, M. (2005) A review of empathy in nursing, *Nursing Inquiry*, 17 (1): 65–74.

GLOSSARY

Action research research that aims to solve problems in practice situations through a process of planning, implementation, and an evaluation of change.

Aesthetics and ethics the particular values which we hold about the world and ourselves.

Algorithm has a specific meaning in mathematics and computing, but in general refers to an unambiguous, step-by-step process to solving a problem or making a decision. It is used in medicine as a series of questions asked of a patient, the answers to which can help achieve a diagnosis.

Anonymity the process by which participants' identities and views/information are hidden so that they cannot be recognised by readers of the research.

Applied research the outputs from research that are utilised in/applied to practice.

Athens widely used among universities and by the NHS in the UK to provide an identity management and authentication access solution to electronic journals and databases. It has an international customer user base that has made the phrase 'Athens password' very well known indeed. Named after Athena, the Greek goddess of knowledge and learning, the Athens service originated in 1996 at the University of Bath, and was provided free to UK Higher Education Institutions until 2010.

Audit professionally-led initiative which seeks to improve the quality and outcome of patient care through the examination of practice.

Authentication and identity management these are methods used by organisations to provide access to electronic journals and databases to their members, usually students and staff at universities, and health services employees, students and partners. Methods include Athens, Shibboleth, IP address, and Edugate in Ireland.

Authoritative in the context of information resources this means highly reliable and of high quality. It is synonymous with 'an excellent source of information'.

Autonomy promotion of the decision making capacity and independence of individuals.

Beneficence promotion of the good in every situation.

Blinding within an RCT (**randomised controlled trial**) blinding is considered to minimise bias within the study. This is the process by which either the participant or the researcher is unaware of which group the participant is assigned to. When both the participant and researcher are unaware, this is called 'double blinding'.

Case study research an in-depth exploration of a well-defined phenomenon (usually a specific group or situation) from multiple perspectives.

Clinical effectiveness the term 'clinical effectiveness' is considered as an overarching term to describe the activities, tools and skills used in the pursuit of quality improvement.

Clinical trial an ethically approved research study undertaken to determine the safety and effectiveness of a health intervention (drugs or therapy, etc.).

Complex intervention study an experimental study with one main outcome, but there are several factors to be considered within the intervention.

Confidentiality the way in which a researcher deals with data gained from participants in order that they are assured that these are used in only the way specified and are not given to anyone outside the research team.

Confirmability if a study demonstrates **credibility, dependability,** and **transferability,** it can be said to possess confirmabilty.

Confounding variable any variable(s) that may interfere with the hypothesis, but are not directly the variable under consideration.

Consequentialism an ethical theory focusing on the consequences, or outcomes, of an action.

Construct validity this is concerned with how well the data collection tool measures the specified outcome.

Content analysis the process of organising narrative qualitative information according to categories, themes and concepts.

Content validity this refers to how well the data collection tool is interpreted by the respondent in the way intended. Also known as 'face validity'.

Control group within an RCT the participants within the control group have no additional intervention given within their care or service. They continue with the normal care or treatment.

Convenience sample a sample based on the ease of accessibility with which the recruitment of participants can take place in a study.

Credibility allows the research user to have confidence in the truth of the data and research findings.

Criterion-related validity this is concerned with how the data from one data collection tool relate to another form of data collection measuring the same outcome.

Crossover RCT design an RCT study where the participants are assigned to one of two groups which will contain the intervention for part of the trial period and crossover to the control for the other part.

Delphi method a consensus approach that aims to come to a point of common agreement on a particular issue, usually through the use of surveys.

Deontology an ethical theory focusing on the quality of an action itself.

Dependability (or auditability) the audit trail that demonstrates the procedural routes to decisions made by the researcher at every stage in the research process.

Dependant variable the outcome variable in which a change can occur, for example disease present or absent.

Descriptive statistics describe simple summaries from the sample from which the data are taken.

Diary a written document that enables participants in a research study to record their thoughts, views or experiences in relation to the phenomenon under investigation.

Distribution the frequency of the occurrence of scores or values in a sample.

Documentaries the use of existing documents or records which are investigated, and analysed, in order to investigate a particular phenomenon.

Domain names the equivalents of internet addresses giving a strong indication of the ownership of a website. Their use has evolved as the internet has evolved. There were originally seven generic top-level domains .gov (Government) .edu (Education) .com (Commercial) .mil (Military) .org (Non profit organisation) .net (Internet service providers) and .int (Intergovernmental), along with the top-level country codes. In the UK, the domain name .ac.uk indicates the website belongs to an academic institute of Higher Education. The fact that the domain name signifies something about the website means this is a factor in terms of evaluating the information contents.

Empiricism a school of philosophical thought in which knowledge is derived from observation, experience and experiment.

Epistemology what we mean by our pursuit or attainment of knowledge.

Ethnography aims to study culture and cultural groups through the observation of behaviours, rituals, customs, and practices.

Evaluation research research that aims to determine the impact (or otherwise) of nursing and healthcare practice.

Evidence-based practice a process of making decisions about the care of patients based not only on the best available valid research, but also on a consideration of professional expertise, and the particular patient's needs, abilities, preferences, circumstances and beliefs.

Experiment a quantitative research design that enables the researcher to test hypotheses through the application of an intervention within a particular context (usually **randomised controlled trials**, and also **pre-/post-test experiments** and **quasi-experiments**).

Focus group discussions that take place within groups of people (usually of around four to nine participants) in which the phenomenon under investigation is explored.

Grounded theory aims to generate theory by concurrently gathering and analysing data.

Hermeneutics the science and interpretation of oral and written texts.

Hypothesis a statement that provides a focus for a research project, usually about the relationship between one variable and another.

Independent variable the variable that can initiate a change to the dependant variable.

Inferential statistics used to test a hypothesis by drawing conclusions from the data within an element of certainty, ensuring the results have not occurred by chance.

Informed consent the process by which research participants are provided with the required information that enables them to make a decision about whether or not to become involved in a research study.

Interpretivist paradigm locates the researcher within, rather than outside of, the research enterprise itself.

Interval scales numbers that have a specific order with measures that are equal between each occurring value.

Intervention group within a **randomised controlled trial** the intervention group is the one(s) in which participants test a new intervention.

Interview allows data to be gathered through structured, semi-structured or unstructured conversations with participants.

Justice promoting fairness or the just distribution of goods.

Likert scales scales that provide ordinal data (a natural ordering of information) and measure levels of agreement with a series of statements.

Literature review a process by which the researcher locates the most relevant sources to determine what is known about the topic under investigation; this can be used as part of the analytical process.

Logic and reasoning the ways in which we think and make sense of the world.

Mean commonly known as the arithmetic average. This is calculated by adding all the scores in a distribution and dividing the result by the total number of scores. The mean uses every score in the distribution, so is usually a good representative value. The mean is however sensitive to 'extreme' scores, and in this case may not be useful as a true reflection of the average.

Measure of central tendency a way of working out a typical value for a distribution which can then be used to provide a simple description of an entire population – usually employs a mean, median or mode.

Median the score that divides a distribution exactly in half: 50% of the scores in a distribution will be above it, and the other 50% below it. Often used an alternative to the mean when 'extreme' scores are present in a distribution.

Mixed methods research research in which a number of research methods are utilised to address the research questions or objectives within a single study.

Mode the most commonly occurring score in a distribution. Very easy to calculate – you just look for the most common score! It works well with any scale of measurement. Often given along with the mean.

Multi-arm RCT design a **randomised controlled trial** with more than one intervention group and one control group. More than one hypothesis is likely to be tested in this design.

Nominal or categorical data labels (or names) which have an intrinsic order as such (e.g. gender, religion).

Non-maleficence the ethical principle of doing no harm to others.

Non-probability sampling the process of sampling that does not use random selection.

Observation used to collect data through a reseacher's prolonged immersion in the participants' natural setting. Observation can be participant observation or non-participant observation.

Ontology what we understand by reality.

Ordinal scales data that have named categories and are ordered.

Phenomenology a term that covers a range of research approaches that aim to investigate the lived experiences of people within the particular content of that experience.

Pilot study a 'trial run' to test questionnaires, or to test the use of methods for a study.

Population this is the entire group of individuals that a researcher wishes to look at. By the entire group, we literally mean every single individual.

Positivist paradigm a concern with the 'positive application of knowledge to assist human progress' (Cruickshank, 2012: 71). Focuses on 'objective facts'.

Pre/post-test studies data are gathered prior to the intervention with the same approach to data collection being used following the intervention, thus allowing for comparisons to take place between the two.

Presuppositions frequently unexamined assumptions.

Probability sample the process of sampling that uses any form of random selection so that any one 'unit' within the overall **population** has an equal probability of being selected.

Purposive sample a sample based on the selection of participants who have experienced the phenomenon under investigation.

Qualitative research research approaches that do not use numerical data, and usually use textual data to uncover meaning or experiences.

Quantitative research research approaches that use numerical data which are then analysed using statistical methods.

Quasi-experiment an experiment in which the 'rules' of a randomised trial (a true experiment) are not always followed.

Questionnaire a tool for the collection of data that can be delivered verbally, in writing, and/or electronically, which asks a series of questions relating to the research study.

Quota sample a sample based on the selection of participants from specific sub-sections of the general population based on common characteristics.

Randomisation the process by which participants recruited into an RCT are assigned to either the intervention group(s) or the control group.

Randomised controlled trial (RCT) an experimental study which tests a given hypothesis in comparison with what is already known.

Range the range of a distribution is measured from the highest to the lowest score. Gives an indication of the spread of scores within the distribution.

Ratio scales considered the strongest scales as these have an absolute zero starting-point, thereby enabling the distance between the points to be compared.

Rationalism a school of philosophical thought in which it is asserted that a legitimate source of knowledge lies within human reason itself.

Reliability whether the data collection tool consistently measures what it has set out to measure.

Research and development (R and D) refers to the process by which organisations, policy makers, practitioners and decision makers utilise research outputs to address the need for improved services to patients (quality improvement).

Research process the steps that enable a research study to be carried out systematically and coherently.

Rigour the way in which a research study is carried out that ensures it is of good quality.

Sample a subset of the chosen **population** that the researcher uses to investigate the area of study.

Single blinding this is when either the researcher or the participant is unaware of whether the participant is in the intervention or the control group.

Snowball sample an approach to sampling that involves the researcher identifying an individual or individuals who are then able to suggest other relevant participants.

Stratified randomisation ensures that equal numbers of participants with similar characteristics that may affect the outcome are assigned to each group. See also **randomisation**.

Surveys a research design that enables the researcher to collect data from a sample of the population.

Synonyms words which are different in their sound and spelling but which mean the same thing.

Thematic analysis the process of identifying, analysing and reporting patterns (themes) within data.

Theoretical sample a sample based on the selection of participants because of their potential manifestation or representation of important theoretical constructs.

Thick description the use of analytical data and other sources to provide a detailed description of the context and findings from a research study.

Transferability the degree to which the findings of a study can be transferred to other contexts or settings.

Triangulation the process by which two or more research methods are used within one study.

Trustworthiness indicates the level of rigour with which a study has been undertaken in relation to its credibility, transferability, dependability and confirmability.

Utilitarianism an emphasis on promoting human happiness or pleasure (see **consequentialism**).

Validity whether the data collection tool measures what it set out to measure.

Virtues moral dispositions towards achieving certain ends (e.g. courage).

APPENDIX

REFLECTIVE LEARNING JOURNAL TEMPLATE FOR RESEARCH AND EVIDENCE-BASED PRACTICE

The purpose of the template is to enable you to think about an issue or topic critically, to record these thoughts and therefore reflect on them, and to learn from this process as part of your approach to learning throughout your course (and afterwards!). You will be spending time reflecting on practice experiences. While this is not the purpose of this template, it is likely that there will be considerable overlap in your reflective activities.

Describe the issue or topic of interest [you may have identified the topic through an experience in practice, or as part of your overall learning a module].
Review the theories and concepts [you will need to access reliable sources of evidence to enable you to identify the key theories and concepts].

Include a list of the references for the reading that you have completed in relation to the topic.

Describe the learning [for example, what do you now know from your reading?].

Evaluate the learning by relating it to a real-life experience [consider the ways in which the theoretical learning has had (or could have) an impact in practice].

Analyse the learning to make sense of the issue [for example, what aspects of the learning have been relevant to the experience, and how has the learning enabled you to make sense of the original issue you wanted to look at?].

Draw conclusions relating to the real-life experience [building on the last point, how has the learning enabled you to think differently about practice?].

Action plan for your future learning needs [for example, do you need to do a further literature search to uncover more evidence to support your practice?].

INDEX

Note: Page numbers in *italics* indicate figures and tables. Page numbers followed by a "g" indicate an entry in the glossary.